Using Narrative Writing to Enhance Healing

Jennifer Lynne Bird
Oxbridge Academy, USA

A volume in the Advances in
Medical Diagnosis, Treatment, and
Care (AMDTC) Book Series

IGI Global
DISSEMINATOR OF KNOWLEDGE

Published in the United States of America by
IGI Global
Medical Information Science Reference (an imprint of IGI Global)
701 E. Chocolate Avenue
Hershey PA, USA 17033
Tel: 717-533-8845
Fax: 717-533-8661
E-mail: cust@igi-global.com
Web site: http://www.igi-global.com

Library of Congress Cataloging-in-Publication Data

Names: Bird, Jennifer Lynne, author.
Title: Using narrative writing to enhance healing / Jennifer Lynne Bird.
Description: Hershey, PA : Medical Information Science Reference, [2020] | Includes bibliographical references and index. | Summary: “”This book approaches healing through the fields of education and medicine”--Provided by publisher”-- Provided by publisher.
Identifiers: LCCN 2019035915 (print) | LCCN 2019035916 (ebook) | ISBN 9781799819318 (hardcover) | ISBN 9781799819325 (ebook)
Subjects: MESH: Health Education | Writing | Narrative Medicine | Personal Narrative
Classification: LCC RC489.W75 (print) | LCC RC489.W75 (ebook) | NLM WA 590 | DDC 615.8/5163--dc23
LC record available at https://lccn.loc.gov/2019035915
LC ebook record available at https://lccn.loc.gov/20190359

This book is published in the IGI Global book series Advances in Medical Diagnosis, Treatment, and Care (AMDTC) (ISSN: 2475-6628; eISSN: 2475-6636)

British Cataloguing in Publication Data
A Cataloguing in Publication record for this book is available from the British Library.

Advances in Medical Diagnosis, Treatment, and Care (AMDTC) Book Series

ISSN:2475-6628
EISSN:2475-6636

MISSION

Advancements in medicine have prolonged the life expectancy of individuals all over the world. Once life-threatening conditions have become significantly easier to treat and even cure in many cases. Continued research in the medical field will further improve the quality of life, longevity, and wellbeing of individuals.

The **Advances in Medical Diagnosis, Treatment, and Care (AMDTC)** book series seeks to highlight publications on innovative treatment methodologies, diagnosis tools and techniques, and best practices for patient care. Comprised of comprehensive resources aimed to assist professionals in the medical field apply the latest innovations in the identification and management of medical conditions as well as patient care and interaction, the books within the AMDTC series are relevant to the research and practical needs of medical practitioners, researchers, students, and hospital administrators.

COVERAGE

- Emergency Medicine
- Experimental Medicine
- Disease Management
- Medical Testing
- Chronic Conditions
- Disease Prevention
- Alternative Medicine
- Internal Medicine
- Cancer Treatment
- Diagnostic Medicine

IGI Global is currently accepting manuscripts for publication within this series. To submit a proposal for a volume in this series, please contact our Acquisition Editors at Acquisitions@igi-global.com or visit: http://www.igi-global.com/publish/.

The Advances in Medical Diagnosis, Treatment, and Care (AMDTC) Book Series (ISSN 2475-6628) is published by IGI Global, 701 E. Chocolate Avenue, Hershey, PA 17033-1240, USA, www.igi-global.com. This series is composed of titles available for purchase individually; each title is edited to be contextually exclusive from any other title within the series. For pricing and ordering information please visit http://www.igi-global.com/book-series/advances-medical-diagnosis-treatment-care/129618. Postmaster: Send all address changes to above address.

Titles in this Series

For a list of additional titles in this series, please visit:
https://www.igi-global.com/book-series/advances-medical-diagnosis-treatment-care/129618

Strategies to Overcome Superbug Invasions Emerging Research and Opprtunities
Dimple Sethi Chopra (Punjabi University, India)
Medical Information Science Reference • ©2020 • 284pp • H/C (ISBN: 9781799803072) • US $225.00

Advanced Applications of Nanotechnology in Cancer Detection ad Therapy
Alireza Heidari (Faculty of Chemistry, California South University, USA)
Medical Information Science Reference • ©2020 • 280pp • H/C (ISBN: 9781799801399) • US $275.00

Developmental Challenges and Societal Issues for Individuals With Intellectual Disabilities
Rejani Thudalikunnil Gopalan (Mahatma Gandhi Medical College and Hospital, India)
Medical Information Science Reference • ©2020 • 416pp • H/C (ISBN: 9781799812234) • US $265.00

Global Applications of One Health Practice and Care
Sandul Yasobant (Center for Development Research (ZEF), Germany) and Deepak Saxena (Indian Institute of Public Health Gandhinagar, India)
Medical Information Science Reference • ©2019 • 306pp • H/C (ISBN: 9781522563044) • US $245.00

Pre-Screening Systems for Early Disease Prediction, Detection, and Prevention
Thierry Edoh (Technical University of Munich, Germany) Pravin Pawar (Philips Research, India) and Sagar Mohammad (Philips Research, India)
Medical Information Science Reference • ©2019 • 395pp • H/C (ISBN: 9781522571315) • US $245.00

For an entire list of titles in this series, please visit:
https://www.igi-global.com/book-series/advances-medical-diagnosis-treatment-care/129618

IGI Global
DISSEMINATOR OF KNOWLEDGE

701 East Chocolate Avenue, Hershey, PA 17033, USA
Tel: 717-533-8845 x100 • Fax: 717-533-8661
E-Mail: cust@igi-global.com • www.igi-global.com

Table of Contents

Foreword

I dwell in Possibility-

A fairer House than Prose-

More numerous of Windows-

Superior for doors-

Of Chambers as the Cedars-

Impregnable of Eye-

And for an Everlasting Roof-

The Gambrels of the Sky-

Of Visitors- the fairest-

For Occupation- This-

The spreading wide my narrow Hands-

To gather Paradise-

-Emily Dickinson

Never before has humanity been in such a need for holistic healing through the power of mindfulness and innovative practices such as, journaling and creative expression. A treasure of mankind evolves from our creativity as it taps into unlimited imagination. Recognizing and utilizing this inherent ability opens possibilities through numerous windows and doors. It has been my privilege to collaboratively work with Dr. Jennifer Bird integrating literacy and visual art for over fifteen years. Her research on the healing process of language arts through narratives and creative journaling link closely to my own work on artistic journaling and visual art production as beneficial to this process. The approach described in this text melds her research on narrative writing with other researchers in this field. Dr. Jennifer Bird captures this method to healing and inspires others to lead healthy lives that positively impact the sense of self and build meaningful relationships with others. Many readers who themselves or who have loved ones that struggle daily through a myriad of illnesses will find that the approach in this book enhances their perspectives, sets a new framework in motion, and develops new pathways for seeking peace and the potential for healing. Extraordinary accomplishment can become an everyday occurrence by creating a new framework around a set of circumstances as your journey unfolds. Healthful living involves management of diverse roles developing new and existing relationships along with other factors of daily life. Imagination and inspiration can help balance our creative self and daily responsibilities. Through this approach tension and stress can be released and a joy of discovery permeates daily life. Playful exploration of the world around you opens doors and windows to possibilities. Opportunities are endless much like the vast sky described by Dickinson. I encourage readers to be open as the pages of this book capture Dr. Bird's energy, passion, and caring dedication blended with insight, research, experiences, personal revelations, and of course stories into a holistic healing approach.

Susannah L. Brown
Florida Atlantic University, USA

Preface

Dear Reader,

I wanted to share stories again. Five years after the original publication of *Innovative Collaborative Practice and Reflection in Patient Education*, I decided to revisit my writing. The new title, *Using Narrative Writing to Enhance Healing*, reflects the concept of using narratives to supplement healing from physical or emotional illness. Writing cannot take the place of a visit to a medical professional and compliance with a treatment plan, but it can help both the patient and the clinician during the healing process.

DISCLAIMER

The strategies and treatments discussed in this book do not take the place of a visit with a medical professional such as a physician, physical therapist, psychiatrist, nutritionist, or other trained specialist. As the editor of this publication, I do not advocate attempting any treatment plan on your own. I encourage you to feel inspired by the stories, but please consult a medical professional if you are experiencing physical or emotional pain.

THIS BOOK'S PURPOSE

I consider this book more of a reimagining than a revision, although revising writing became necessary throughout the process of putting this publication together. This book has the overall objective of connecting the fields of education and medicine to present eclectic and innovative approaches to health education. It compiles chapters which appeared in other IGI publications into one comprehensive narrative. For this book, I took previous chapters, combined similar content, and added new references with examples. While editing the writing of others gives me joy and allows multiple voices to express themselves, this time I wanted to focus on my voice and celebrate the contributions my colleagues and I made to the field since we first started this work seven years ago. For me, using writing to help people does not seem like work, but a calling. It makes sense to begin a book about narratives with a few narratives of my own which introduce the influences for my writing.

HOW TO WRITE A NARRATIVE

1. Begin by removing all distractions. Turn the TV off, put your phone someplace where you won't be tempted to read text messages, and try to wait to do this until kids and pets are occupied or sleeping! Instrumental music is ok if you prefer not to write in silence. This is being in the present moment.
2. Choose a simple prompt like "I am," "I want," "I need," or "I believe." You can take this in any direction you choose, or more than one direction. For example, "I am a teacher" creates entirely different writing than "I am proud to be part of my family." The key is to keep writing by asking yourself open-ended questions. Writer Anne Lamott (1994) calls this an "SFD" (an acronym for "stormy first draft," although Lamott uses a stronger cuss word that starts with s when working with adults) (p. 22).
3. Keep writing and don't judge yourself. Writer Natalie Goldberg (1986) believes that your first thoughts are the truest ones before the self-censor starts critiquing (p. 9). If you can't think of what to write about, write "I can't think of what to write about" until you do think of something.
4. Read your writing and see what statements are reflecting back to you. Writer Julia Cameron (1998) believes that in open, honest writing we can sometimes answer life's questions, or at least gain a new perspective on something (p. 65).
5. Actively listen to what you need. Writer Georgia Heard (1995) calls this honoring what is in your heart map (p. 2). Heard (2016) designed the idea to draw a heart and fill it with things that would make you happy in the present moment (p. 1). Then, go do something that makes you happy as an act of self-care!

JOURNEY TO ENGLAND

In the summer of 2018, I received an invitation to participate in a prestigious creative writing program at the University of Cambridge in England. In addition to receiving my first passport stamp, I would have the opportunity to once again put my writing theories into practice. It felt wonderful to write for several hours a day and learn from experts in the field. I also received the honor of reading a description of my childhood adventures with my grandmother in front of an international audience. As you read my words, I want you to know who I am, but each time I write, I rediscover who I am.

WORDS FROM MARILYN KEPLER BIRD

When I went away to college, my mom wrote me old fashioned handwritten letters. Even after she discovered email, she still sent letters. I attended college only an hour away from my hometown of Kettering, Ohio, but I lived on campus and her words provided comfort as I began a new chapter in my life. Now, the letters she wrote me feel like a gift. Her life ended, but her words remain. I loved her observations of daily life.

I picture my mom, sitting in her favorite chair, the beige recliner in the corner of the living room, writing her letters. Evening is her writing time. She reaches for the mug of coffee on the table next to her and turns her notebook to a new page. One of the family cats sits next to her. She loves to stay informed, so occasionally glances up when the television news catches her attention. She puts pen to paper and provides inspiration to her only child.

MEDICAL DRAMAS

"I never thought you would like a medical drama," my mom told me as I described the latest plot of the television drama *ER*. I compared setting the tone of a hospital like the doctors discussed to setting the tone in a classroom. A lover of literature and writing, I frequently experienced anxiety during my high school biology class. To this day, when I walk through the hallways of the high school where I teach English, I check to see my colleagues in biology aren't dissecting anything before I walk into their classrooms. Yet,

I love walking the hallways of the local hospital and praying with people. My mom and grandmother both volunteered at a hospital, although I never thought I would continue the tradition.

ARTIFACTS

My mom kept her brown jewelry box with the gold handles in the middle of her dresser in her bedroom. Now, the jewelry box has a place in my closet. I debated using the jewelry box as my own, but instead chose to use the gold jewelry box my aunt bought me as mine and kept my mom's on the closet shelf. My mom would have liked this; keep something that she loved while also honoring my own style. I did keep something of mine in Mom's jewelry box. My pin when I received my integrative health coach certification is next to her hospital volunteer badge.

WRITE THROUGH THE PAIN

Carrying heavy bags too often + neck pain = trip to physical therapy.

My neck pain journal started halfway through my physical therapy journey. My physical therapist, Dr. Eric Wanner, loved showing his patients a model of the spine to explain injuries. His explanation of the problems with the facet joints in my neck made it easy for me to comprehend my diagnosis. I felt nervous when I first handed my notes to Eric. What would he think? He read my notes for a few minutes, looked up and said something like, "I like it," and promptly changed some of my exercises based on the new information. I kept sharing more notes and Eric adjusted the treatment plan to help me become pain free. I appreciate Eric's faith in my writing and feel grateful our research continues to help people.

BE PATIENT WHEN BEING A PATIENT

As I prepared to conclude this book, I became a patient again. This time, I didn't just have neck pain. My medical odyssey led me to a variety of specialists; in a quest for a diagnosis I felt both grateful for and frustrated with the medical system. I watched my savings account drain as I paid copays at the offices of various doctors while simultaneously feeling grateful for health insurance and a savings account. I felt grateful I had a lighter schedule during the summer months because going for medical treatment started to feel like a part time job. I felt like a frustrated medical football being passed around from one specialist to another while simultaneously feeling grateful I finally got a diagnosis and that over time and with treatment, I could get better. I needed to find the inner strength I taught others to find. I needed to use my writing as healing research to help myself.

DESCRIPTION OF BOOK CHAPTERS

Each chapter tells its own narrative, but read in order, the book tells a larger narrative. *Narratives of Spirituality* provides an overview of an interdisciplinary collaboration as Eric and I reflect on both spirituality and our research experiences. *Narratives of Research Design* describes the thought process when designing an original research story. *Narratives of Health Coaching* explains why I decided to pursue National Board Certification as a health coach so I could help patients use writing in a similar manner that I help my students use writing. *Narratives of Emotional Truth* shows the value of creative nonfiction to present a narrative. *Narratives of Curriculum Design* illustrates the similarities between the program design process in the fields of education and medicine while introducing the PAGES program. *Narratives of Patient Care* explains how narratives relate to the medical field and why patients can use narratives to share additional information with their medical practitioners. *Narratives of Anxiety* discusses a research study illustrating how writing helped college students cope with anxiety and provides strategies which help with anxiety. *Narratives of Teaching Methods* presents methods from my English classroom demonstrating how writing helps with stress management. *Narratives of Journal Writing* shares practical solutions for implementing writing in different moments of life. *Narratives of Writing and Healing* tells the story of when I became a patient and describes how I needed to use everything I learned to help myself heal. It became a powerful full circle moment and a fitting conclusion to the book that my research of using writing to help with emotional and physical healing helped me heal when I became a patient!

Some of the themes, such as narrative inquiry and multigenre writing, appear in multiple chapters. The theory of narrative inquiry and the practice of multigenre writing provide the foundation for presenting research in an innovative method, as well as honoring the first person voice during the sharing of narratives. Narrative writing gives writers the opportunity to share part of themselves with the reader. Sharing part of my life in narratives led to the honor of collaborating with an outstanding team of writers. Thanks to my cousin Robin Perry Newkirk and my friends Claudia Jayne Brahler, Susannah Brown, Valerie Bryan, Ann Musgrove, Jillian Powers, Ryan Urenda, and Eric Wanner for writing the original IGI publications with me which inspired ideas for this book. I appreciate Eric taking the time to collaborate again on our chapter revisions. Thanks to my cousin Melissa Bird Teixeira for creating medical artwork from an X-ray of my spine that appeared on the cover of the original publication and which the publisher chose again for the revision. Thanks to my physical therapy team of Eric Wanner, Dak Adamson, David Fielding, and Ryan Urenda for all the great medical advice. Thanks to my colleague Susannah Brown for writing a beautiful forward.

I hope my narratives inspire you as the reader to reflect on your own narratives and use them to help you heal.

REFERENCES

Cameron, J. (1998). *The right to write*. New York, NY: Tarcher/Putnam.

Chulack, C., Crichton, M., Wells, J., & Zabel, D. (1994-2009). *ER* [Television series]. Burbank, CA: Warner Brothers.

Goldberg, N. (1986). *Writing down the bones*. Boston, MA: Shambhala.

Heard, G. (1995). *Writing toward home*. Portsmouth, NH: Heinemann.

Heard, G. (2016). *Heart maps*. Portsmouth, NH: Heinemann.

Lamott, A. (1994). *Bird by bird*. New York: Anchor Books.

Acknowledgment

Whenever I write a thank you page, I always hope I don't forget anyone! Thanks to the entire team of people who made this project possible.

Thanks to my editor at IGI, Halle Frisco, marketing assistant Brittany Haynes, and the rest of the publishing team who helped with this book. I have edited previous publications with IGI and it was wonderful to return for this one.

Every day I feel blessed to belong to my amazing family who supports my dreams and makes me feel I can do anything. Much love to Dann Bird, Diane McLoughlin, Susie DeBeck, Bill DeBeck, Robin Perry Newkirk, Derrick Newkirk, David Bird, Patricia Bird, Melissa Bird Teixeira, Erik Teixeira, Derek Bird, Gabrielle Bird, Marsha Bird, Sandy Bridges, Joanna Claridge, Carl Claridge, Erica Younkvich, Margaret Earl, Tim Earl, Michael Schafer, Cher Schafer, Benjamin Schafer, Crystal Schafer, Arthur Bruggisser, Brian Bruggisser, Amanda Bruggisser, the O'Connor family, and all the new kids in the family! And to Marilyn Kepler Bird, my mom and guardian angel.

I am writing these words now because of the support from all my friends, colleagues, and students throughout the years. The names are too numerous to mention in this space, but please know that I thank you for being part of my life and appreciate the role each one of you played in my journey throughout the years.

Jennifer Lynne Bird
Oxbridge Academy, USA

Chapter 1
Narratives of Spirituality

Jennifer Lynne Bird
Oxbridge Academy, USA

Eric T. Wanner
Palm Beach Sports Medicine and Orthopaedic Center, USA

ABSTRACT

How does spirituality inform narratives? Some readers may view the experiences survived by the authors as a series of random coincidences, but because religion plays a large role in the lives of both authors, they believe that their experiences happened for a reason. They are not trying to convert you to a certain religion but simply want to show the power religion can have. It is recommended to take out all prejudgments on this issue and read the chapter as is. After that, take out of it what you wish. When the authors conducted a research study, they discovered potentially groundbreaking implications for the fields of patient education and health education. The official narrative of the research follows the research project from the initial idea to the final statistical analysis. The unofficial narrative of the research illustrates all the moments that cannot be captured in a statistical table as the authors answer questions, share stories, and provide information of what they learned.

DOI: 10.4018/978-1-7998-1931-8.ch001

STRENGTH FROM SPIRITUALITY

This chapter symbolizes the strength of spirituality and what it can do from the perspective of two people who had near death experiences and life changing events. People might refer to a situation like this as a "Godwink" since they happened to collaborate in this writing. These are each very unique situations and the authors prepare you to ride first class in their experiences.

Godwinks are coincidences that symbolize signposts from God showing people the right path. Rushnell (2012) defines a Godwink as, "your destiny will not arrive in a limo to pick you up. Determining where you want to go in life is your job. And once you do – once you pull yourself from the curb and head in whatever direction your inner compass is telling you to head – the signposts will unfold…godwinks, all along the way. That's a promise" (p. 73). Godwinks enable people to see patterns in their lives. Godwinks can also provide hope for people unsure where the path of life may lead next or why certain things happen. Hale (2014) believes, "call it synchronicity or fate or, as I call it, divine order; every moment of your life pushes you toward your greater calling" (p. 12). In a moment we may not know why something happens, but the reason why it happened becomes clear later.

Life can feel stressful and chaotic at times, and Godwinks bring order to the chaos. As Heard (1995) writes, "synchronicity draws recognizable patterns on a sometimes chaotic universe. Writers need to pay attention to these synchronistic moments and events" (p. 104). These Godwink moments provide faith that the puzzle pieces of life will eventually fit together, maybe not in the current moment, but someday soon. Zimmermann (2002) reminds us to trust the journey because "the stars have lined up, and we had nothing to do with it. Some call it grace; some call it synchronicity; some call it serendipity; some call it a connection with the divine; some call it coincidence; some call it luck. If we stay open to life, unexpected gifts begin to appear" (p. 160). Sometimes we don't know why things happen. We don't get something we want, or a prayer goes unanswered. But looking back and mapping the Godwinks of an experience can show that perhaps not getting the thing we originally wanted led to something better down the road. Or as Hale (2013) powerfully states, "on the journey of life, sometimes it takes losing our way to find ourselves" (p. 177).

And sometimes losing our way can help us find our greater purpose in life. As Warren (2012) believes, "you will be most effective when you use your spiritual gifts and abilities in the area of your heart's desire, and in a way that best expresses your personality and experiences. The better the fit, the more successful you will be" (p. 246). He elaborates, "this custom combination of capabilities is called your SHAPE:

Spiritual gifts
Heart
Abilities
Personality
Experience" (p. 234).

For both of us as the authors of this chapter, we have used the SHAPE theory to inform our practice of research and writing. We find strength in spirituality and possess a passion for research. Eric's abilities as a physical therapist and Jen's abilities as a college English professor enabled us to learn from each other as we designed unique interdisciplinary research. We have the common personality trait of compassion for people, as Eric has made a positive difference in the lives of his patients just as Jen has made a positive difference in the lives of her students. And our individual life experiences led us to see research as part of a greater life's purpose.

Because we as the authors advocate the sharing of stories, we each share a story of how following the advice we share in this chapter helped us. Both of us have strong religious beliefs, and by telling our stories from a spiritual perspective we do not tell anyone else what to believe. Because research and writing feels like a larger purpose instead of just work, it translates into appreciating the moments when the puzzle pieces of ideas click into place to form projects that will help people. As part of our research we asked physical therapy patients and college students to write their stories, so we need to feel willing to write ours. Both of us survived incredible ordeals and our paths crossed so we could share our knowledge and help others.

Eric

As a Christian myself, I see the beauty of believing in God and what He can do. I was actually in a near death situation the summer after I graduated from The Ohio State University in 2008. I will tell you a very quick overview of my experience as I could actually write an entire book about this. I mainly just want you to realize the impact and beauty religion (God) can have for you. I went on a mountain climbing trip to the Grand Tetons with my dad. I climbed with a guide while my dad recorded me. The first day I climbed several mountain faces without falling one time. The climbs I did were several hundred feet at a time. But the next day, that is when my "magical" experience happened.

Day two of the climb my guide and I decided to climb one of the most challenging mountain faces in the Grand Tetons called the Open Book. My dad, my guide, and I started hiking to this mountain face at 6am. It took around 3-4 hours to get to the bottom of where the climb began. The mountain face was 1500 feet and completely vertical. No gradual incline at all. Also, there wasn't really anything to hold onto but cracks. This was crack climbing at its finest. To be able to climb this face you must use different techniques, such as finger locks and hand locks to proceed up the mountain face. The rope was around 200 feet long, so about every 150 feet we would have to redo the belay device (the lifesaver which helps stabilize the rope with which one climbs) so that we could continue spotting each other. My guide would climb first while putting in the holds, put the rope through it, and I would take them off while climbing. Then he would reattach us to allow us to belay each other, and we would start over again.

Once we got to 1000 feet up the mountain face went backwards. This means that the slope was to the point where your back was facing the ground. My guide climbed up this without a problem. Now it was my turn. To get past this point I would have to use a diagonal crack, but when it stopped, swing my body around to reach the cleft that was six feet away (the next hold). There was no foot hold and the backwards incline went about 20 feet back. When my guide made it to the top of it he re-belayed and was ready for me to begin. I made it past the crack, but now was my turn to swing my body to the cleft. Keep in mind I don't have a great reach for this move. I went to do this and my feet slipped out from underneath me. I was swung around on the rope about 30-40 feet away from the mountain face and was facing the other mountain range. While I was swinging from the fall I looked down and could see several thousand feet below me and noticed the absolute vertical of nothing but rocks at the bottom of this mountain face. Once my momentum stopped from the fall I was still around 20 feet away from the mountain face. To get back to climbing I actually had to swing myself toward the starting point and grab onto the wall.

When I made it back to climbing position I was pretty shaken up. That was absolutely the scariest thing I have ever experienced. I tried to mentally block it out, but knew that I had to make it on the next attempt or my grip strength would be shot. Every time you try to do a big move it takes a lot out of your grip strength.

So, I started back up again. My hands were shaking a little bit, grip strength was becoming worse, but I was determined. I made it to the same spot as the previous time. I went for it again, but again my right foot slipped at the same spot and I missed the cleft. Immediately I was swung back 30-40 feet from the mountain face. When this happened I looked up and the rope was fraying. Yes, FRAYING!!!! The part that went backward that the rope had to go over was a very big and sharp rock. I realized that I had to get back to the climbing position as quick as possible or the rope might break. This immediately became a life or death situation. I swung myself back to the spot to start but was holding on to a rock to prevent myself from swinging back again. There was not enough slack in the rope and my body was completely horizontal with my legs unable to touch. After what seemed like a minute of screaming to my guide to get me more rope I finally got more and was able to put my feet down. I couldn't blame him since it was really hard to hear each other at all. Because of where we were in relation to each other, it was a cave effect which pretty much muted each other out.

At this point I looked at my hands which were covered in blood. Apparently my skin got cut from the rock on my last attempt. I wiped the blood off on the mountain face and started praying. This was the first time in my life I truly did not think I would make it out alive. I prayed to God that he would either help me out with this situation if I was meant to live, or if the alternative was my destiny then so be it. Keep in mind that where I was, it was not possible to save me. A helicopter wouldn't be able to fly close enough to me without running into the sharp rock above, and the rescuers would have to swing back and forth from a bungee several feet to even come close to me (which could have brought down the helicopter due to the instability and increased risk). There was also nobody else at all who was climbing the same mountain face that day. I didn't know what else to do so I just kept praying and waiting about half an hour. I had to build up some more strength to make my best attempt for what could be the last attempt ever.

Suddenly I heard voices. A man out of nowhere poked his head up making it to where I was. He asked me if I was having troubles and if I needed help. I told him that I was pretty much stuck and couldn't get past where I was. I never had to climb with a backpack before this trip since I was from Ohio. The man and his friend informed me on how to pull myself up on the rope if I fell on the next attempt since they saw the rope was fraying. He also grabbed my backpack and told me he was going to give it to me at the top. Suddenly I heard another voice. "Eric, I'm going to pull you up!" It was my climbing guide. He actually detached himself from where he originally was to help me up. He did this knowing something was wrong. Keep in mind I didn't really fall the entire trip until this point. I told my guide to wait as the men I just met were telling me how to pull myself up in case I couldn't make it past on my next attempt. We had to yell back and forth until we came to the agreement that I had one more shot, and if I didn't make it the guide would pull me up. He didn't realize the rope would actually completely break if he did since it was already fraying on the sharpest part of the rock. The man and his friend next to me grabbed my backpack and wished me luck.

On my last and final attempt I began climbing. I knew if I fell I was dead, but also knew I couldn't think that way to make it all the way. The weight off of my back helped a lot and I felt like I was climbing Ohio style again. As I was climbing my legs and arms were shaking more than they ever have. Even though I knew I had to stay calm, my body wouldn't listen. I made it to the spot I couldn't get past and all of my fingers but my index finger slipped out of the crack. I felt a sudden bolt of power through my body and somehow threw myself on top of the cleft with one finger. I made it! My guide was amazed by the move although I felt like I was going to have a heart attack, and we ended up making it to the top. We received my backpack at the top from the men I met at the mountain and then they just disappeared.

Call it dumb luck, call it adrenaline, call it being at the right place at the right time, call it anything else. I call it as I saw it. I believe that man and his friend were Angels sent from above to help me get past a deadly situation. I don't think it was just a coincidence. This is why I believe that if you choose religion, it can do wonders.

Meanwhile, my dad was at the bottom of the mountain face. He was told to go over on the other side of the river. Yes, it was a frozen river and not really cold on that side so luckily the ice didn't break through. He actually was unable to see us since the guide didn't tell him to go in the right spot since they never had anyone try to film from the bottom at that mountain face before. My dad didn't see us the entire time, so he went back to where we started. He left a note on the guide's car that said if he didn't hear from us he would have the troopers find us by 6pm since it got dark a little after that. Luckily we made it back in time and got ahold of him and he was okay.

Again, I am not saying you have to believe what I took out of my real life experience. I am not saying that you should believe in what I do or another type of religion. What I can tell you is that if you believe in something, it can really help calm your nerves and help you more than you ever dreamed.

Jen

I too could write a book about my experiences. Sometimes I wonder if the tone of that book would be too sad, or if I should make it happier. But I can't write book chapters telling people to own their stories and not follow my own advice. I experienced heartbreaking moments in my life, but I experienced more moments of joy, when I felt at peace with the world and grateful for all the wonderful gifts and people in my life. Through everything, both good and bad, I've felt God with me. Faith means letting go and knowing things will be okay even when the road map disappears or prayers go unanswered. Even if I can't always see the purpose of my life, I believe God does. Each semester in class I give my students a small candle and remind them they can be the light in the lives of others, and if they are going through a difficult time a little light is enough to light the way until things get better. I am a woman who survived the death of her mom and an autoimmune disease, but I am also a Christian, a teacher, a writer, a singer, a dancer, and a researcher. I belong to an incredibly supportive family who encourage me to fly fast and far because they will always catch me if I fall. I hope my stories light the way for others.

Sometimes people who are not medical professionals can diagnose your health issues. My hairstylist ordered me to go to the doctor when large amounts of my hair fell out into her hands as she styled it. I soon began a medical odyssey that resulted in a quest to heal as I climbed my own metaphorical mountain of survival.

Sjogren's Syndrome is an autoimmune disease where the body's white blood cells forget their purpose and attack a person's own cells and tissues. If Sjogren's sounds familiar to you, tennis star and athlete Venus Williams has it and made the public more aware of the condition when she discussed her own case. There is no cure, and symptoms vary from person to person. Some patients only suffer from dry eyes and a dry mouth, while others endure complications in various organs.

I remember sitting on my couch staring at the wall after a discouraging doctor's visit. I secretly suspected the lab technician was a vampire because of the large amount of blood she took from me. I discovered I was more likely than the general population to get cancer. My doctor wasn't sure if I could ever have children. I was seeing a specialist for every part of my body and taking more pills than my grandma took. I couldn't even cry because my eyes wouldn't produce tears. The doctors said nothing I did or didn't do caused this autoimmune condition; it just happened. But the fact that I experienced physical health issues a couple years after an emotional trauma did not shock me.

My mom died suddenly of a carotid artery aneurism a few days before Thanksgiving in 2003. Earlier that day I remember thinking how incredibly happy I felt. My graduate studies at Miami University challenged me but I loved my classes and research, and I looked forward to the holiday break and spending time with my family. In one horrific moment, my life changed. I couldn't stop thinking that if anything had been different about that day maybe my mom would still be alive even though such thoughts wouldn't bring her back.

I wrote extensively about losing my mom to cope with my feelings. Sometimes I wondered if I wrote too much about it. I started to put my life back together with the support of friends, family, and an emotional therapist. However, my immune system was compromised due to all the stress and no matter how many people I told I felt fine, my body told me otherwise.

I find beauty and grace in religion because when I hurt so much I couldn't even think, I knew I was not alone. So I had a nice long chat with God. Actually it was a screaming rant at God for letting my mom die and letting me get sick, but letting everything go made me feel better. A wise minister told me my behavior was healthy because I was being honest and still talking to God. I remember wanting to live and feeling that I still had something to accomplish with my life. So I turned the out of control things over to God to worry about and changed the parts of my life I could control. A dancer my entire life, I took a dance seminar with professional dancers and pushed my body through exercise. I reworked my diet and became a vegetarian. I tossed items from my endless "to do" list and spent the time stretched out on my bed listening to music that inspired me. I spent more time with my family. I prayed several times a day. And I wrote about my experiences as well as poetry, songs, and a novel when writing my thoughts hurt too much. And one day when watching a really sad movie, I started crying. My eyes were producing tears again!

Remission happens infrequently for autoimmune diseases. It happened to me. Being healthy again feels like someone waved a magic wand over me, made my symptoms disappear, and gave me my life back. I don't take it for granted. My treatment plan worked for me, but I'm not a medical doctor so I can't tell other people to follow it and have the same results. I know there are hundreds of people who try various treatments without success, and I'm grateful there are specialists to help anyone who suffers from an autoimmune disease. I always say a prayer each year before I get my blood test results, feel lucky the only inconvenience in my life is taking a couple pills a day, and know I proved I can deal with whatever life throws at me. I knew if I survived the death of my mom and my health issues I needed to do something meaningful with my life, and writing chapters like this one to help others is part of my life's purpose.

RESEARCH REFLECTIONS

Eric

When writing my story I thought about the angels that I encountered. I keep trying to remember exactly what they looked like but cannot. All I remember is that they were around six feet tall, close to 200 lbs, wearing a helmet, backpack, harness, all the climbing essentials. They both had on sunglasses and a climbing jacket. There was so much adrenaline in my body that I had a hard time remembering more about their features. All I remember is how I suddenly felt comfort when I saw them. I remember that not only did they have to climb up the hardest part of the mountain after meeting up with me but climbed with my backpack as well (along with their backpacks). Once they met up with me at the top they gave me my backpack and climbed away the other part of the mountain. My guide and I went down the opposite side of where we climbed up since it actually had an angle to it (along with snow). We had to hurry down the mountain since it was supposed to rain and the clouds were moving in. With rain it would make the climb down much harder. We didn't have time to see exactly where they went but I just remember them suddenly disappearing into the mountains.

I remember praying to God that if I survived then I will be certain that He has more planned for me in life and that I still had a purpose for him. I think that is why I care so much about what I do and helping others get better in life. Whether physical therapy, research, or writing, I want to help people achieve their goals and come up with ways to continually improve their quality of life. I continually remind myself that if I help as many people as possible perhaps that is one of my purposes in life. Jen and I shared the same perspective about the research and writing which makes this a unique situation. It brought two completely different fields together and has led to groundbreaking results in both of our fields.

Jen

Helping as many people as possible is one of my purposes in life too. I feel grateful every day that on my last day of physical therapy treatment Eric suggested we still work together and use writing to help other patients. I smile whenever I think of all the people we have helped and will continue to help in the future.

I fell in love with the topic of using writing as healing when I wrote my doctoral dissertation about writing leading to emotional healing, but it never occurred to me that writing could help people heal physically, and the idea intrigued me. I felt one of life's full circle moments; my research came together in my hometown when I returned to Ohio from Florida in order to work with one of Eric's former professors. Even though my dad's career as a city planner took him to Indiana, he and my stepmom met me in Dayton so Dad could check on some buildings and projects he implemented there. After a successful research day, I left the University of Dayton and went to the cemetery to tell my mom the good news. I know she's not really there and knows what is going on in my life anyway. As if to prove that point, when I got to the cemetery, it started raining. Mom never wanted me to dwell on sad things and was telling me to leave the cemetery and get on with my life. When I shared the news with Eric about our research discovery, without even knowing my cemetery story he said the quick thought that I had must have come from my mom. It wasn't the first time I thanked my parents for helping me achieve my dreams.

This research journey helped other people, but also helped me discover my purpose in life. I process my experiences through writing, so in my role as a teacher, writer and researcher, I realized I could help others through difficult experiences because I survived one myself. Beck (2012) believes that "all these people can help others back from hell because they've found their own way back from internal, infernal experiences" (p. 244). Instead of falling apart after my mom's death, I wanted to use the pain to make a difference in the lives of other patients. As Warren (2012) writes, "In fact, your greatest ministry will most likely come out of your greatest hurt" (p. 244). My research and writing became intertwined with my story.

When I remember my mom, I smile thinking of the time we once went to the Kettering, Ohio bookstore, Books & Company, three times in one day for "the thrill of the magazine hunt." I remember our close relationship and her goal of getting me to enjoy life; whenever she saw me spending too much time studying, she would bring out a yellow cat puppet named Buttons to make me laugh. I don't want to define my life by her death and before this writing becomes too poignant perhaps I should prop Buttons up against the computer screen to remind myself to lighten up a little bit. Mom would love that.

My grandpa, a kinematics professor, discussed physics principles in his book such as, "dynamics deals with motion and the effects of forces acting on rigid bodies in motion" (Kepler 1973, p. 1). The same philosophy applies to both physics and life: A force causes things or people to move. I want to become a force for change. Using the power of my words to help others through pain has become part of my life's purpose; by doing so I hope to share enough of myself for people to know who I am. And that means stepping out in faith even if the path is unconventional for an English professor. I am reminded of the novel *Shoeless Joe* (which later became the baseball movie *Field of Dreams*), where Ray Kinsella follows his dream of building a baseball field in the middle of his Iowa cornfield no matter what anyone else thinks because he knows he is doing the right thing. For a moment, I am a kid again sitting next to my grandma in the stands at a Cincinnati Reds baseball game as I think of Kinsella (1982) describe life as "Heaven on earth, indeed" (p. 211). I love to teach students about the power of dreams in the scene from *The Great Gatsby* where Fitzgerald (1925) has Nick the narrator watch his friend staring at a light in the distance and observe, "I thought of Gatsby's wonder when he first picked out the green light at the end of Daisy's dock" (p. 189). No matter where life takes me, I can't tell students to reach for their dreams if I'm not willing to reach for my dreams too.

It seemed every book or magazine article I found referenced the research of James Pennebaker. The most powerful example of this was when I reread a writing book by Susan Zimmermann that my cousin Robin found and my Aunt Susie bought for me on one of our beloved shopping trips years before I knew I would ever research writing as healing. When I began this research, I remembered that book. What I didn't remember was that it referenced the exact study by Pennebaker I was investigating. It became another full circle moment that made me feel God knew what I was supposed to do with my life years before I did.

As a result of my research experience, I enrolled in a seminar at Duke University that referenced Pennebaker's research and began the journey to become a health coach using writing therapy to help heal people. Brown (2007) describes the feelings many patients have and shares, "there is nothing more frustrating, and sometimes frightening, than feeling pain and not being able to describe it or explain it to someone. It doesn't matter if it's physical pain or emotional pain. When we can't find the right words to explain our painful experiences to others, we often feel alone and scared" (p. 155). I dream about helping patients find the right words. I envision a future research project where patients at Eric's physical therapy clinic will write answers to *The Wanner Bird Healing Survey for Pain Recovery*. Eric will use their answers to adjust their treatment plans and help them heal physically, while I read their answers and counsel them to heal emotionally so they have a holistic approach to healing that achieves elite results.

Some people may say everything happened as a series of coincidences, but I prefer to see them as Godwinks affirming that even if at the time I don't understand why things happen, I end up exactly where I am supposed to be.

GODWINKS IN RESEARCH

This next section on Godwinks in research represents the retelling and reliving of a research story. Writers live stories once, and relive the stories when writing about them. Or as Goldberg (1986) states, "writers live twice" (p. 48). Life is a series of stories. The qualitative research theory of narrative inquiry embodies the sharing of stories. Clandinin and Connelly (2000) explain when describing narrative inquiry, "what may have appeared to be insignificant nothingness at the time they were composed as field texts may take on a pattern as they are interwoven with other field texts in the construction of research texts" (p. 104). Hindsight allows for patterns to emerge and additional understanding about the journey that took place. Writing becomes a time for self-reflection and self-awareness. Looking back and learning from an experience leads to understanding of how the puzzle pieces of a journey fit together.

Writing helps us process life events that occur so we comprehend our learning needs and cope with inevitable changes in life. Sometimes, we must look back to move forward. Writing helps us do this by setting any locked up feelings free so that we don't have to constantly carry them. Cameron (1998) explains, "because writing is a practice of observation as much as invention, we can become curious as much as frightened in the face of change. Writing about the change, we can help it along, lean into it, cooperate. Writing allows us to rewrite our lives" (p. 31). Carrying upsetting feelings, just like carrying a heavy bag, can create tense muscles and lead to physical pain. Cameron continues, "our bodies are storytellers" (p. 58). She elaborates, "your body will speak to you. It will tell you your own needs. It will tell you the cost of your life as well as what is priceless to you. Images and memories will arise at the touch of a finger. Muscles will unlock to whisper your pains and your dreams" (p. 58-59). Writing, such as creating a pain journal of symptoms, can provide information about the story the body tells. Clandinin and Connelly (2000) discuss, "in writing narrative research texts, we must be mindful of balancing the tensions of writing within the three-dimensional narrative inquiry space, of writing in ways that narratively capture the field experiences, and of balancing these with audience" (p. 154). Since narrative inquiry encourages first person perspective, you will see the stories shared in our own voices.

NECK PAIN LEADS TO RESEARCH

Bringing multigenre writing to the field of medicine began with Jen's neck pain. When Jen needed physical therapy for neck pain, she kept a journal of her symptoms to show Eric, her physical therapist. Part of the journal is included as an appendix at the end of this chapter, in case you would like to use the model for any pain you might be experiencing and share it with your doctor. Jen's pain level seemed all over the place. Why was it better or worse at certain times? Between treatment sessions, she wrote notes so she would remember what to tell Eric about her pain and decided to reorganize everything into a chart. Eric looked at Jen's notes and instantly diagnosed a pattern. He used the insights from her writing to adjust her treatment plan.

Multigenre papers find patterns in the form of narrative threads. Putz (2006) explains, "whereas traditionally a researcher begins with a premise and looks for evidence to support it, the multigenre researcher begins with an interest and discovers a unifying element along the way. It is this emergent theme that often suggests a thread with which the writer may create cohesion among the separate pieces of writing" (p. 2). In the case of Jen's neck pain, she lacked the expertise to find the narrative thread that explained the pattern to her symptoms. She needed to rely on Eric's expertise to find the unifying element that would explain her pain. Romano (1995) writes, "admitting people into the process of our writing, however, is a greater act of faith and fearlessness than writing about what we feel strongly but cannot yet envision" (p. 174). When Jen took a leap of faith and found the fearlessness to share her writing, she was happy Eric read it. Eric's goal became to help Jen find strategies to relax more (she's still working on that) and celebrate slow and steady progress in a theory he called "thinking like a turtle." So Jen found artifacts that made her happy, such as a playlist of her favorite songs, pictures of the beach, and a flyer for an upcoming concert. Her medical chart began to look like a multigenre project. Allen (2001) writes, "the best way I can describe a multigenre paper is to say that each piece in the paper utilizes a different genre, reveals one facet of the topic, and makes its own point" (p. 2). Each piece of writing Jen showed Eric provided one facet of the topic of her pain, which incidentally was caused by the facet joints in her neck.

After Jen healed and collected a few turtle necklaces and statues along the way, we decided to use her neck pain journal to help other patients. As Goldberg (2000) explains, "I believe that this is a primary commitment a writer makes to her writing, an essential commitment she makes to her reader: a willingness to be open to encounter, to experience – and to the suffering this may bring" (p. 86). By sharing their stories, some patients fear they will suffer more if they do not have a supportive audience; however, there are supportive clinicians who will hear what they have to say and help them heal. We believe in integrative medicine that encourages patients to collaborate with clinicians and create their own multigenre healing journals. We encourage readers of this chapter who experience physical and emotional pain to share their stories with supportive medical professionals, and for clinicians to value patients' voices and listen to stories shared so that a multigenre approach to medicine can provide education, hope, and healing.

Jen

As Eric once said, I help patients learn to conquer fragile moments in life with writing. He helps patients regain the ability to do what they want to be able to do again, and this holistic approach of emotional and physical health intertwines for our unique approach to health education.

I almost didn't write the neck pain journal that started this research story. Patients are supposed to go to medical facilities and follow established protocols, not ask their clinicians to spend extra time reading writing. During each of my physical therapy sessions for neck pain, Eric, my physical therapist, asked me to assign a number to the pain I felt in my neck. I would tell him the number of how I felt that particular moment, but maybe an hour or two earlier I would have said a different number. How was I supposed to remember all those numbers? When faced with a dilemma, I turn to writing. So on a sheet of paper, I wrote not only the number of how I felt at any given time, but also the activity I did to cause me to feel that number. I didn't know Eric well, so I had no idea how he would react if I showed him my journal. I took a leap of faith and shared my writing, because maybe there was something in those notes that could help him solve the mystery of my neck pain. Not only did Eric read every word, he encouraged me to write more and used my writing to adjust my treatment. Murray (1996) believes, "we all need to tell our stories and our stories need to be heard" (p. 7). I never would have healed from physical pain if I hadn't told the story of what was causing my symptoms, and I appreciated that the person who could help me heal wanted to hear my story.

Eric and I discussed academic articles we read during my treatment sessions, and I enjoyed those conversations that made physical therapy actually fun. On my last day of physical therapy, Eric asked me if I wanted to write something about my experiences. Why hadn't I thought of that idea? I'm happy he did. We wrote about my neck pain journal and wondered if my experiences with writing as healing could help other patients.

My mom died young of a carotid artery aneurism. After her death my dad found a journal of possible symptoms she kept and never shared with anyone. I will never know if her story would have ended differently if she shared her writing with someone in the medical field, but maybe I could help other patients rewrite their stories.

My neck pain journal also brought me back to a topic I loved. During my first couple years teaching at Florida Atlantic University, I focused on entertaining my students with various ideas; discussing the connections between Katy Perry's songs and literary inferences became a smash sensation with college undergraduates. I missed research, however, so when I returned to researching writing I rediscovered my purpose in life.

During this process I enjoyed working with Eric, who shared my passion for the topic. Sometimes collaborating with others can be frustrating when people won't complete their share of the work, but working with Eric has been easy and fun because we have the same strong work ethic and dedication to the research. Eric and I brainstormed ideas for the survey we designed and sent emails back and forth. He always responded to my ideas with a combination of positive comments and questions that made me think about more ideas. He even read my long emails that had Roman Numeral subheadings for each topic! We designed a survey we named after ourselves, *The Wanner-Bird Healing Survey for Pain Recovery*. I looked forward to seeing how patients would respond to our combination of numeric and written subjective questions.

Eric

As Jen discussed earlier we had an idea to do research together to collaborate ideas from two different fields. Physical therapists usually look more toward what recent research shows with objective tests and measures, and are just now starting to look at patients' expectations in physical therapy with measures such as the SETS survey (Stanford Expectations of Treatment Scale). After performing our research, I realized that physical therapists do not use the writing concept as much as they should. With our research, it showed that patients who used more artistic writing scored higher objectively on pre-existing physical therapy measures depending on their body part that was injured. We used the DASH (Disabilities of the Arm, Shoulder and Hand), NDI (Neck Disability Index), Modified Oswestry (for back pain), and LEFS (Lower Extremity Functional Scale) as our objective measures to compare with our survey.

It seemed to be clear that as patients had higher artistic writing scores, they also seemed to be objectively improving at the same rate. Also, patients who set clearer goals for themselves improved the most objectively as well. People seem to perform better when striving to reach a goal. Schunk (1990) discusses research performed where subjects that set higher goals tended to have higher self-efficacy. According to the findings, "when students perceive satisfactory goal progress, they feel capable of improving their skills; goal attainment, coupled with high self-efficacy, leads students to set new challenging goals" (p. 71). Patients also seem to do better with writing by allowing them to truly express how they feel. Becoming more aware of what is helping or hurting their recovery process makes them more accountable to do their recommended home exercises and makes them work harder while in physical therapy.

When we came to this realization, we wrote about our findings and ideas to help others get better with a few publications and presentations along the way. Our goal is to share with as many people as possible our groundbreaking research findings to help them either recover from an injury using our tactics in addition to what the physician recommends, or even in life in general.

When talking about sharing your life with a medical professional it may seem like a crazy idea. Most people believe they don't have enough time to ask their physician or physical therapist questions about their life. Most people allow stress to eat away at them until nothing is left. Recent statistics from the American Institute of Stress (2013) show that most people (77%) regularly experience physical symptoms caused by stress and 73% of people experience psychological symptoms caused by stress. (http://www.statisticbrain.com/stress-statistics/). But what if you actually decided to take the risk like Jen did and discuss pertinent information about your life? When does your pain feel the best? When does your pain feel the worst? These questions are actually key elements for people in the medical field to be aware of in order to find contributing factors to the patient's symptoms. Writing will help bring awareness to your situation prior to your medical visit and is actually very beneficial. It might even remind you to ask certain questions since writing down ideas helps you remember. Perhaps you might not see a pattern for why you are feeling the way you do at certain times of the day and think that it doesn't relate. You might be listening to certain types of music or hanging out with friends who make you feel better, or you might feel stuck staying in a job you continue to dislike. These things could actually lead to more or less pain overall. It is beneficial to first make a list of internal versus external stressors in your life. This will clarify the types of stressors in your life. As defined by the University of Maryland's Medical Center (2013),"external stressors include adverse physical stimulus (such as pain or hot or cold temperatures) or stressful psychological environments (such as poor working conditions or abusive relationships). Internal stressors can also be physical (infections and other illnesses, inflammation) or psychological (such as intense worry about an event that may or may not occur). As far as anyone can tell, internal psychological stressors are rare or absent in most animals except humans" (http://umm.edu/health/medical/reports/articles/stress). As my past patient, Jen actually wrote about her symptoms in a table format when she was feeling at her best and worst each day along with what she was doing at those times. She did not know if it related or not but wrote about it anyway. If she would have only written about some of the times she was feeling bad or good along with what she was doing at those times it would have made it harder for me to see trends in her symptoms. She wrote freely and I was able to modify my treatment program along with making recommendations for her ergonomic factors such as propping papers on a stack of books while grading them to allow her to become pain-free. Writing can lead to healing!

Writing can also be used as a way to vent. Goldberg (2007) explains, "you can develop the right compass to reach emotional truths inside your own life without having to fabricate your experience. Your life is good – or bad – enough. Your suffering is real" (p. 111). Sometimes writing is all people need to do so they don't store everything inside of them. Sometimes people don't want others to see how they truly feel about things. Writing can solve this problem. Writing does not always need to be shown to others. It can be used strictly as a stress relief tactic. Sometimes emotional writing can be the best type of writing to read. It allows you to look back in the past, see how you felt during a situation, and what you did to correct it. Writing could also remind you that you need to correct something for your own benefit. As Goldberg (2007) states, "we are finishing the circle, closing the gap, making sense of the senseless" (p. 299). Whatever the case, you may be surprised with the feeling of empowerment you develop through writing.

SEE MOUNTAIN AND CLIMB

We began our research by designing an original survey called *The Wanner Bird Healing Survey for Pain Recovery* that included short answer writing questions. We gave the survey to physical therapy patients at Eric's clinic, and thirteen patients completed the survey. After finishing data collection at the physical therapy clinic, we met with one of Eric's former professors, Dr. Claudia Jayne Brahler, in a Skype session to discuss the results. Her expertise in both the fields of research and physical therapy would help us with our research.

Jen

For almost six months while we collected surveys from patients at the physical therapy clinic where Eric worked, I spent part of one day a week at the clinic to score surveys. I found it interesting to see the clinic from the perspective of a researcher and not a patient. Clandinin and Connelly (2000) write, "when narrative inquirers are in the field, they are never there as disembodied recorders of someone else's experience. They too are having an experience, the experience of the inquiry that entails the experience they set out to explore" (p. 81). Due to medical HIPPA regulations, I didn't know the histories of the patients from their medical charts; all I knew were the stories they chose to tell me when writing answers to the questions on the survey. I designed the written subjective questions to be scored similar to the rubrics I used in my writing classes. I enjoyed adapting my knowledge from teaching writing to help patients in a medical clinic.

Graves (2001) believes, "teaching is an emotional roller coaster" (p. 1). Research can feel like an emotional roller coaster too. It involves moments of triumph and moments of trials. No matter what obstacle Eric and I encountered during the research and writing process, we both became determined to make the project work.

Complete numerous documents for the IRB (Institutional Research Board)? Done.

Convince the university and physical therapy clinic to work together? Not a problem.

Enlist the help of both our families for proofreading articles, brainstorming ideas for recruitment flyers, and moral support? We'll figure it out.

During a trip to Indiana to visit my dad and stepmom, I took a detour to my Ohio hometown and met with Dr. Claudia Jayne Brahler, one of Eric's former professors in the DPT (Doctor of Physical Therapy) Program at the University of Dayton, who showed an interest in our project. She said our research demonstrated potential and represented a unique collaboration since English professors and physical therapists don't usually work together. Eric and I felt excited about the possibility of our research being groundbreaking and changing the future of patient education, so we encouraged each other to keep researching and writing. The good news about research being a roller coaster is that valleys such as a low number of people who wanted to participate in our study could soon be followed by peaks such as a top expert in the physical therapy field being impressed by our work. There were also individual moments when I felt discouraged and I'm sure Eric had them too, but both of us became determined to find a discovery that would make a positive difference in patients' lives.

Eric

I believe that perseverance is what makes people strong. Doing research was not an easy task, as Jen discussed. Not only did we have to go through what Jen just mentioned, but initially we had to develop an idea that could tie our two fields together in hopes of sharing new possibilities for recovery. We were both aware of the possibility for a correlation between writing and success in recovery, but needed to have research to prove it. If it wasn't for Dr. Claudia Jayne Brahler pushing Jen when they met to use her strengths as a writing teacher and stop worrying about what physical therapists might think, or our refusal to fail, this research would have failed. The three of us working together brought phenomenal insight on how patients can be treated in physical therapy (along with everything else). I now realize more than ever the importance of the vast amount of contributing factors for someone's physical health. Our goal is to share this information with the public so people can use it on top of the other recommendations by their physician or physical therapist.

Jen had to get out of her comfort zone and I had to get out of mine to make this a success. I previously hated writing and it gave me nightmares just thinking about it. I was one that chose to take Calculus 2 instead of a basic English class when obtaining my bachelor's degree at The Ohio State University. I never understood why anyone would take English over a math class. Jen loved writing and was the exact opposite of me. The one thing that brought this research idea together was how much we both enjoyed research. Sharing that enthusiasm in a topic allowed us to venture outside our comfort zones and develop a survey that included writing and numerical sections on patients throughout their physical therapy sessions called *The Wanner-Bird Healing Survey for Pain Recovery.* This survey led to publications and potential medical alterations in the future. Staying in your comfort zone eliminates possibilities you may have in your future. Breaking these barriers can lead to miraculous results and achievements.

DATA TELLS A STORY

Voice is the concept that drives writing. It means having a conversation with the writer when the writer isn't even in the room because the words reflect the writer's personality. Lamott (1994) describes writing voice as, "and the truth of your experience can only come through in your own voice" (p. 199). When Jen was a grad student in Tom Romano's class at Miami University, he stressed the importance of two dimensions of writing, artistic and technical. Romano (2013) describes the scoring process and elaborates, "to arrive at a holistic grade, I read the paper through without making a mark on the rubric, without any interruption of my reading. I relied upon my experience as a teacher, writer, and reader, on my judgment of the paper's demonstration of writing craft" (p. 160). Writing craft focuses on voice and the way the writer's personality becomes reflected through writing.

When scoring voice in writing, here's the secret: Don't think, just score. Trust the first impression. As Conner (2008) writes, "first thought is a precious gift. It is an impetus from deep within your soul that wants to be seen and heard. Honor it" (pp. 92-93). For once Jen didn't overthink things; she got into a zone where it was just her listening to the voices of the patients through their writing. She handed the numbers over to Jayne; the numbers fit with the numbers Eric converted from the objective physical therapy measures to achieve research significance. While the writing rubric for *The Wanner Bird Healing Survey for Pain Recovery* focused on both the technical and artistic dimensions of writing, the holistic, or artistic component, provided the correlations with existing objective surveys. We proved our hypothesis: patients who demonstrated a strong positive outlook and positive writing voice experienced greater healing gains on existing objective physical therapy measures.

Jen

Even if we don't find anything, I have no regrets about this journey. I thought this when Eric and I initially reviewed our research. The numbers didn't show any patterns! We decided to go over the data again. That was Eric's idea. I wanted to throw the surveys across the room. The best part of being on a team is that team members can encourage each other when someone has a bad day. We spread out the surveys on a conference table and Eric read numbers while I recorded them. Clandinin and Connelly (2000) discuss, "narrative inquiry has the compelling, sometimes confounding, quality of merging overall life experiences with specific research experience, realms of experience often separated in inquiry" (p. 115). We faced this dilemma during our research. We both knew intuitively our survey showed something, but what? We needed to support our intuition with concrete evidence. Wheelan (2013) explains of statistics, "we are now awash in data. For the most part, that is a good thing" (p. 241). We needed to discover the story the data we collected told us.

SPSS (the computer statistics program) should make data analysis easy. It can also make a researcher crazy. Running test after test happens in a matter of minutes. Finally we found a significant correlation between the written and numeric parts of our survey. Patients who clearly articulated their goals also had a high numeric confidence level they would achieve their goals. In other words, clearly stating a goal led to more confidence in achieving it. Life coaches frequently say this, such as when Beck (2001) advises, "forming a goal, especially if you write it down and visualize it, creates a search image that programs your brain to focus on anything resembling or leading to that objective" (p. 303). But what implications did our study have for the field of health education?

Eric suggested that we ask his former professor, Dr. Claudia Jayne Brahler, to join our study. We initially met with her during a Skype session. Sometimes humorous moments happen during research. To securely send the data to Jayne, I needed to add a layer of additional coding to the data. So I named each research subject after a literary character and named the file "Marilyn's Noodle Casserole" in honor of my mom's specialty. Jayne said she thought I had gone batty. I wasn't crazy, just crazy dedicated to this research.

While we waited for Jayne at the computer, Eric and I debated the book *The Age of Innocence* because we had different perspectives about the main character's decisions. I thought I learned the most about a new field during my time at the physical therapy clinic and my conversations with Eric about medicine. I never realized until then how much he learned about literature and writing from the same conversations. Our willingness to each explore a different field resulted in our survey becoming a bridge between the fields of writing and medicine. And interestingly, my students liked Eric's perspective on the novel better than mine!

During our Skype session, Jayne found initial promising results with our data. The three of us realized this could lead to more research, more clinics adopting our survey, and changing the way medical practitioners think about treating patients.

Jayne wanted to spend more time with the data, but the three of us knew Skype presented obstacles to all of us looking at numbers simultaneously. So the surveys (tucked in my carry on bag because there was no way I was letting them out of my sight) and I took a trip to Dayton. Eric checked in with Jayne and me frequently during conference calls. His quick conversion of the existing objective physical therapy instruments into a common scale impressed me. While he and Jayne discussed the instruments of DASH (Disabilities of the Arm, Shoulder and Hand), LEFS (Lower Extremity Functional Scale), NDI (Neck Disability Index), and Modified Oswestry (for back pain), I felt proud of myself for keeping up with the conversation.

Even if we don't find anything, I have no regrets about this journey. I thought this when after a couple days of work, the data didn't reveal much of significance. An outlier skewed our original significant correlation. But we had to find something! All our hard work cannot end like this! I intuitively knew I missed something, but what? Jayne looked at me and told me to think like an English teacher, not like a physical therapist. And then I knew. One of my former professors at Miami University, Dr. Tom Romano, literally wrote the book on voice in writing. How many times had I heard Romano (2004) say, “voice is the writer’s presence on the page” (p. 5). Any decent English teacher knows to score writing on two dimensions, artistic and technical. The technical part of writing focuses on the specificity of a statement; on the other side of the coin, the artistic part of writing focuses on the tone or voice of a statement. In scoring the patients’ writing, even though both the technical and artistic parts of writing existed in the rubric, I recorded only the technical score. In making the scoring easier for future physical therapists who might one day use our surveys in their clinics, I almost stole the patients’ voices from them.

I grabbed a different color pen, curled up on a couch outside Jayne’s office, and added a second number to the patients’ surveys. When Jayne compared that second score for artistic writing to Eric’s scores of percent healing gains on the objective physical therapy measurements, we confirmed our initial research hypothesis: Patients who have a higher positive outlook will demonstrate higher objective improvements. Jayne, Eric, and I found a trend showing patients who use more positive language on our survey’s short answer questions showed higher healing gains on the objective physical therapy measurements. Our preliminary findings paved the way for possible follow up studies. We accomplished our goal.

My memories gave me everything I needed. My education gave me the knowledge I needed. My resilience would not let me quit. All of this happened in my hometown where I drove past the cemetery to see my mom’s grave on the way to campus. It was a magical day when everything fit together perfectly. Heard (1995) believes, “memories darkened by ages of forgetting are still inside somewhere hiding, waiting for the right smell or touch to unlock them” (p. 86). I unlocked each piece of information at the precise moment I needed it.

Later, I learned I should not have worried about how physical therapists would score the writing questions using the rubrics I designed. Eric and I had a 91% inter-rater reliability rating when scoring the technical part of the writing and a 94% inter-reliability rating when scoring the artistic part of the writing. This further confirmed the success of our survey design.

Eric

The inter-rater reliability results surprised me as well. This showed how easy it would be for other physical therapists to use the rubric as Jen designed it. This could be used in other clinics without us having to be present! Jen knew how to adapt the scoring rubric to allow people in other professions to properly use it. She didn't have to be a physical therapist, but she learned to make modifications while thinking like one.

Jen was so dedicated to our project she flew to Dayton, Ohio to meet with Dr. Claudia Jayne Brahler. She didn't wonder if she should do that, she just did it. Sometimes the best things in life happen when you just go for something and not look back. It's always better to try than to never try and have regrets. By trying you at least have a chance to achieve your dream, while not trying you will never know what you could have done. We believed this research would work and didn't want to stop until it did. This trip she took allowed us to learn from Jayne's expertise to see the relationship of our data between artistic writing and objective gains in physical therapy. We always knew there had to be some relationship but couldn't put the pieces together prior to that.

Jen ended up performing her best when she didn't try to think like a physical therapist and solely thought as the English professor she is. The ironic thing is that this is when we saw the correlation with our data and everything came together. The collaboration of an English professor, physical therapist, and research professor ended up being key factors in this research. When we each added in our knowledge from our different fields we came up with the best approach. Very few physical therapists collaborate with English professors and vice versa. Perhaps they should change their ways.

ADDITIONAL RESEARCH

When discussing how outlook influences healing, Tindle (2013) discovered, "how we manage our responses to the world influences our health, both in the short and long term" (p. 17). The answer? Ask them to write it! The idea of managing responses to the world connected to the philosophy by writing teacher Cameron (1998) because, "writing gives us a place to say what we need to say, but also to hear what we need to hear" (p. 83). Except for innovative programs at the medical schools at Columbia University and Duke University, writing teachers usually don't work with doctors, so it made sense that the connection wouldn't be common knowledge. Writing in a journal provides a place for people to manage their responses to the world and say what needs to be said. This became a beautiful connection between the fields of writing and medicine. Rankin (2013) feels, "if it's true that the mind's positive beliefs can heal the body, everyone has an equal chance of benefitting from this phenomenon" (p. 10). In order for writing to become healing, it helps to acknowledge the words of Brown (2012), who provides the reminder, "vulnerability is the core, the heart, the center, of meaningful human experiences" (p. 12). Because Jen found the courage to share her neck pain journal with Eric, we designed research that helped more people.

Having a positive artistic writing voice not only helps physical therapy patients, but also college students. Research by Pennebaker (1997) that led to the second research study we designed revealed, "not only are there benefits to health, but writing about emotional topics has been found to reduce anxiety and depression, improve grades in college, and, as we have seen, aid people in securing new jobs" (p. 40). Jen teaches college students who write in journals every semester and are part of a class community of writers just like Erin Gruwell and the Freedom Writers. It was possible to create a new version of this classic study. Every college classroom needs a strong writing community like the one described by Gruwell and the Freedom Writers (1999) where "the students continued to write and began to forge stronger identities and to create a sense of community and an outlet for expression" (p. 275). Community means we are not alone and we have a place to share our stories.

Jen designed a writing survey and connected it to the HRQOL (Health Related Quality of Life) Survey Eric recommended and we implemented another research study using writing, this one with Jen's college students instead of Eric's physical therapy patients. This research project led to an unexpected twist. Since the surveys were anonymous and the sixty-four students who completed them didn't put their names on the surveys, the students felt they could be honest about their experiences. On the HRQOL, most students reported high anxiety. But why did they feel stressed? Eric reminded Jen to look at every question on the surveys. As she did, she had writing teacher Natalie Goldberg's voice stuck in her head. In writing, first thoughts and impressions are the truest ones; most writers tend to censor themselves if they have too much time to think about what they write. When we write our stories, we need to trust the value of first flashes of insight in writing. Writing teacher Goldberg (2013) tells writers, "say what you want to say, not what you think you should say" (p. 22). In order to write what is truly on our minds and in our hearts, Goldberg gives the advice, "in the face of all inner – and outer – resistance and opposition, just write. Pick up the pen and face yourself" (p. 179). And in facing ourselves through writing we find our voices.

Once again, voice was the answer. Just like with the physical therapy patients, the key became listening to the stories students wanted to tell. Jen scored the word students used to describe their first writing topic and the correlation became clear. Students who demonstrated a more positive writing voice showed lower anxiety. We shared the information from a stress management presentation we designed and it helped students. Helping college students reduce anxiety became an unexpected detour on this research road, but it is one worth following. Zimmermann (2002) believes, "the soul knows what it needs to heal. Through writing, it will lead you where you need to go" (p. 18). Jen wants writing to take her students where they need to go and she wants to be a role model for them as they write. Many students feel like DeSalvo (1999) who writes, "I use my writing as a way of fixing things, of making them better, of healing myself" (p. 7). Writing gives students time in class to write and process their thoughts, which can lead to insights about their lives.

In two separate research studies, we discovered that a strong positive writing voice, indicating positive attitude, can help people heal both physically and emotionally. Physical therapy patients using a positive writing voice throughout their treatment interventions demonstrated higher recovery gains. College students using a positive writing voice during journal writing demonstrated lower anxiety. It's amazing that the two studies dovetailed together beautifully. We learned from Eric's physical therapy patients that people who write with a strong artistic voice have greater healing gains, and we learned from Jen's college students that people who write with a strong artistic voice have less anxiety.

Jen

In her research about outlook and aging, Tindle (2013) discusses, "our outlook is the lens through which we view the world" (p. 5). She discovered a connection between positive outlook and health and elaborates, "a positive outlook is good medicine." (p. 6). Tindle determined that positive outlook influences the one percent of patients who achieve ideal cardiac health, but wanted to know more about the script inside the patients' heads. When I read that, I felt like jumping up and down while screaming, much like I did when I was younger and attended a 98 Degrees concert. English teachers have used writing for years to know the script in students' heads, usually in the form of prompts that require students to write responses in journals. Cameron (1998) explains, "when a writer writes from the heart of what matters to him personally, the writing is often both personal and powerful" (p. 218). Writing from the heart reveals the writer's thoughts and emotions. Since English teachers and doctors typically don't work in the same circles, bridging the fields of writing and medicine can lead to the sharing of knowledge and conversations that can lead to new discoveries.

Rankin (2013) provides additional insight from a doctor's perspective and elaborates, "there's something powerful that gets set in motion when we believe, without a doubt, that we will get well and are supported by clinicians who share our optimism" (p. 17). I felt motivated to complete my physical therapy exercises, but also felt grateful for the help of a caring clinician. Eric took the time to read my writing and support me on my journey to healing. If I had worked with a physical therapist who ignored my writing, this research and its potential to make a positive difference in the lives of numerous other patients never would have happened. Now we have the opportunity to help patients rewrite their stories and challenge clinicians to think outside the box when listening to the stories patients tell.

In her research about vulnerability, Brown (2012) used a form of qualitative research called grounded theory and explains, "stories are data with a soul and no methodology honors that more than grounded theory" (p. 252). Clandinin and Connelly (2000) acknowledge the similarities between grounded theory and narrative inquiry and elaborate, "narrative inquirers tend to begin with experience as lived and told in stories" (p. 128). As a teacher, I know my story influences the lives of my students; however, I never imagined my story as a patient could lead to the idea of using writing as healing.

I relate to the words of Gruwell and the Freedom Writers (1999) who wrote, "maybe the end of our journey is really just the beginning" (p. 277). I feel the same way about this research journey. Since then Eric and I have published book chapters, presented our findings at conferences, and discussed ideas for future writing and research. I don't know how the next chapter in this research and writing story will unfold, but I'm looking forward to the possibilities.

As a writing teacher and a writer, I have experienced for myself and witnessed in most of my students the emotional healing power of writing. I learned from this research that writing can also lead to physical healing. Pennebaker (1997) describes his research study where college students who wrote about thoughts and feelings related to a trauma had fewer visits to the health center and reports, "I'll never forget the initial thrill of finding that writing about traumas affected physical health" (p. 35). The college students in my classroom and the patients in Eric's clinic wrote about topics other than traumas, leading me to wonder about additional intersections of the tone of writing (artistic voice) as well as the topic (technical specificity), and how both contribute to health and healing. DeSalvo (1999) believes, "for our writing to be healing, we must encounter something that puzzles, confuses, troubles, or pains us" (p. 93). I agree that writing helps people heal from trauma; I used writing to help me heal emotionally from my mom's death and heal physically from my neck pain. However, I've also written about less serious topics and find I'm in a better mood than the times in my life when I don't write. Some of my students say the same thing. Gruwell (2007) writes, "writing in my diary was one of the ways I found strength. I thought if my students saw that everyone has a story – even their teacher – maybe the writing process could be cathartic for them too" (p. 148). She became a writing role model for her students, just as I am for my students, and because she shared her story with them it "seemed to intensify my desire for my students to write what needed to be written" (p. 148). I learned from this research that the topic of writing tells only part of the story. The tone of writing and the audience for the writing matter too. DeSalvo (1999) explains, "the writing process, no matter how much time we devote to it, contains a tremendous potential for healing" (p. 73). I want to continue to explore methods of using writing as healing. I want students in every classroom and patients in every physical therapy clinic to have a journal to write their stories and I want them to have understanding clinicians and teachers to listen to their stories. I want to continue asking questions, finding answers and sharing my ideas through writing. Whatever I experience in my journey as a lifelong learner, it will usually result in me writing what I feel needs to be written.

In fact, writing these words inspired me to design a new research project, one where I will give the college students in my classroom both a writing survey and a health survey. The writing survey I designed will ask students if they wrote about emotional or neutral topics in the journals they keep for class. The health survey, the HRQOL survey (Health Related Quality of Life) is a survey in the public domain that contains general questions about health. It will be interesting determining if the writing process, regardless of topic, influences health. It seemed unbelievable that I went from an idea to a finished research design in less than a week, but it speaks to how much I care about the research that even though it was time consuming, the work didn't seem like work at all. I asked Eric to help me interpret the health results of the

HRQOL, so I don't miss anything because he has more medical knowledge than I do. When you find someone with whom you work well, you want to keep that person on your team!

Eric

We continued to investigate our findings and wrote about what we found. We never knew how much our findings meant and the significance of it until we started this process. Yes, we knew it was great insight we could share, but I don't think we realized how great it truly was until later. Writing about our findings helped us investigate other possibilities our research may have brought out as well as new directions for future research. Sometimes in life if there feels like there is no path, you should just create your own and keep moving forward. If you are not sure what to do next, write about it. That's what we did with our roadblock and are continuing to find helpful information for people other than just my patients. It could be beneficial to you!

Like Jen mentioned, writing down her words allowed her to come up with a new research design that continues to look at an in-depth analysis of writing. Writing brought increased awareness to her on the importance of research. I can see that this is truly Jen's passion and I will help her along the way to fulfill her goal. It will be neat to see where the research leads. Our goal is to continue to use writing to enhance healing and to make alterations that could lead to a completely new outlook for physical healing and coping. This has the potential to lead to many more publications along the way allowing us to share what we learn with everyone.

FINDING FAITH AND FEARLESSNESS

Multigenre writing provides a writer with an opportunity to write a personal story in his or her own writing voice and support it with academic research. As Zimmermann (2002) discusses, "write about ways you can light a candle. You can learn from your sorrow and somehow help others to better endure their own. You can grow from the pain you have experienced and share with others what you've learned" (p. 180). On the first day of every new class Jen teaches, she gives each student a candle and reminds them they can be the light in the lives of others and if they are going through a difficult time a little bit of light is all they need until life gets better. Sometimes everyone needs that reminder. Handler (2013) also uses the light metaphor and writes, "many writers have gone across that bridge before you. Their experiences and the ways in which they chose to write about their loss shine a light on your path" (p. 5). Through research, we can use our experiences to reach back across the bridge and light the way for others to follow.

Since this chapter highlights Godwinks and the concept of voice led to discoveries for both research studies, one additional Godwink occurred when reading a passage by Conner (2008) who believes, "pick up a pen with the intention of connecting with that extraordinary Voice within, and your life will start rumbling, shifting, and moving" (p. 9). For her, the word voice is capitalized because it not only represents writing voice, but also connection with the Voice, or God, through writing as prayer. And another piece of this research, this work that has purpose and meaning, clicks into place. Beck (2001) writes that the word synchronicity "is sometimes used to mean a coincidence so remarkable it seems beyond chance" (p. 234). So just remember the next time something happens in your life that seems like a coincidence, consider seeing such moments of synchronicity as Godwinks.

Jen

For me, the work I do with this research represents part of my life's purpose. Spirituality feels as much a part of my life as breathing and contributes to my overall health and wellness. Rushnell (2012) writes, "I have a thesis that Divine Alignment, as well as godwinks, occur with greater frequency when you are actively involved in tasks that you believe God wants you to be doing: when you are stepping out in faith heading for what you believe to be your destiny" (p. 129). Faith helped me through the difficult times in my life, but I also possessed the fearlessness to use the pain I felt to inspire others when giving up would have seemed easier. Beck (2012) writes, "count on it: whatever you're suffering is leading you toward your life's purpose." (p. 243). I want to use my experiences to help other people with their journeys. As a teacher, I always want to make my students' lives better because their paths crossed mine. Now, my research with Eric and Jayne as well as my new knowledge about the medical field means I want to make patients' lives better too. Romano (1995) writes, "to write words that stick with readers you must have – or develop – faith in the validity of your feelings. You must be fearless in writing the words that emerge in your mind when you focus to compose" (p. 31). This research taught me to have faith in my ideas and be fearless when sharing them. My team believed in me, so I needed to believe in myself too.

I also feel amazed each time one of the puzzle pieces of this research journey connects with another puzzle piece. My knowledge and skills made those moments happen, but my religious beliefs also mean I see these moments as affirmations I reached the right place at the right time to achieve my mission of using writing to help people heal. Romano (2013) believes, “we can gain strength through giving words to the pain, through crafting language around it” (p. 176). I found this to be true as I wrote through both physical and emotional pain in my life, and I want to help other people do the same.

Clandinin and Connelly (2000) believe, “narrative inquiry, from this point of view, is one of trying to make sense of life as lived” (p. 78). Writing helps me make sense of my life, and if I can use writing to help others make sense of their lives, either students in my classroom or patients at Eric’s clinic, I will have hopefully done something meaningful by the end of my lifetime.

I accomplished significant things on my own before this research project, but working with Eric and Jayne helped me accomplish more than I ever thought I could. Working with others who always do their best work encourages me to do my best work too. Romano (2008) writes, “I tell students and teachers I work with today to have faith and fearlessness” (p. 70). Reflecting on this research experience, I always had faith that no matter the obstacles encountered, there was a way to make the pieces of this study to fall into place. I also amazed myself with my fearlessness, whether it meant relearning statistics, taking a plane trip, or telling people how much I believed in this project every step of the way. I continue to have the faith that this research will lead to more exciting discoveries in the future, as well as the fearlessness to take the steps needed to use this research to transform health education.

Tindle (2013) writes, “aspects of outlook can be contagious, and just as one person can serve as ground zero for the spread of disease, a single person with a healthy attitude can have a halo effect on friends, family, neighbors, and coworkers…and you see where it can go from there.” (p. 217). I would love for the research ideas Eric and I designed to continue to make a positive difference in the lives of his patients and my students. We added Jayne to our team, and hopefully others will join us along the way as we continue researching and writing. Clandinin and Connelly (2000) discuss, “living, telling, retelling, and reliving mark the qualities of a life” (p. 187). I like to think I stand at the beginning of a new path for research and discovery that will lead to many more stories to live, tell, retell, and relive.

I echo the sentiment of DeSalvo (1999) that "writing has helped me heal. Writing has changed my life. Writing has saved my life" (p. 3). Whether it is teaching a class or writing a book chapter, I share my ideas and hope they have a positive ripple effect on the world. Romano (2013) observes, "the work is the writing. The writing can be healing" (p. 176). Indeed it can.

Eric

As a physical therapist myself, I also want to share the gift of writing with my patients and show them an additional catalyst to their recovery process. I didn't realize until after our research how much of an effect writing could have on patients' recovery in physical therapy. I believe this can be utilized in all medical settings as an additional piece in modern medicine.

It is humbling to think that Jen and I have the ability to help others past our lifetimes. We want to help as many people in a positive way as possible while alive and after. We want this idea to last and lead to more innovative ideas in helping people recover not just while rehabilitating but also in life. Hopefully our idea will continue to spark more interest in professionals collaborating with people of different fields to change the world in a positive way.

Working with a team can lead to significantly more gains than by oneself. It brings other ideas to the table. It challenges you to be the best you can be. If the three of us did not work together, this research would not have worked out and we would not have been able to find the key elements that we needed. If we all decided to stay strictly in our fields and didn't collaborate as a team this research wouldn't have worked out as well as it did. We wouldn't have been able to come up with the combined knowledge from our different fields to find these correlations from our research. We wouldn't have had the chance to share what we learned with other professions, including sharing what we learned with you as readers. Teamwork has no limit to its potential!

GODWINK LESSONS

In completing narrative inquiries such as the one you just read in this chapter, researchers look back and reflect on the narratives of past experiences while looking forward to make plans for future projects. Business executive Sandberg (2013) started a movement encouraging women to lean in and pursue goals. She shares an example from her own life and writes, "writing this book is not just me encouraging others to lean in. This is me leaning in. Writing this book is what I would do if I weren't afraid" (p. 26). Both women and men can benefit from the advice of following dreams and goals without fear. Writing can help you process your past experiences and stay healthy while you set your future goals. DeSalvo (1999) writes, "after I became ill, I began, as many writers with wounded bodies do, to keep a record of my illness in diary form, largely because no matter how sick I was, I could always manage to scratch out ten minutes of writing while propped up on pillows" (p. 200). Whether you keep a pain journal of physical pain to share with a medical professional or a personal journal of emotional pain that no one sees except yourself, your writing leads to decreased stress and increased health. Gruwell (2009) writes of her students, "they realized that everyone has a story; they just needed the opportunity to be heard and an entrée to the healing power of writing" (p. xviii). Know that you also have a story waiting for others to hear. Members of the community can also provide a supportive audience to listen to your stories. Goldberg (2005) writes, "I don't think everyone wants to create the great American novel, but we all have a dream of telling our stories – of realizing what we think, feel, and see before we die" (p. xii). We hope this narrative inquiry of our research motivates you to write the next chapter in your story.

Sometimes we get lost in life. Even if you program your route into your GPS, you still find yourself in a different location. Detours become part of life, both when literally driving down an actual road or metaphorically driving down the road of life. Maybe you didn't get the thing you thought you wanted, but that detour can lead you to something better. One of our research studies began with the intent of adding to the literature discussing the connections between writing and health with college students. We accomplished that goal, but also discovered that the same students shared high levels of stress and anxiety. So a detour developed into successful stress management presentations. The other research study began when an English professor took a detour from the world of literature and learned about medicine, while a physical therapist learned how to score writing rubrics. When faced with a detour in life, enjoy the scenery and take some pictures. What may seem like the wrong road at the time can take you to the right place or lead to new dreams.

ACKNOWLEDGMENT

The preceding chapter contains excerpts from the following previous IGI publications:

Wanner, E.T., & Bird, J.L. (2015). Strength from spirituality. In J.L. Bird (Ed.), *Innovative collaborative practice and reflection in patient education* (pp. 218-232). Hershey, PA: Information Science Reference.

Bird, J.L., & Wanner, E.T. (2014). Educational research narratives of healing. In V.C.X. Wang (Ed.), *Adult and community health education: Tools, trends and methodologies* (pp. 264-280). Hershey, PA: Information Science Reference.

REFERENCES

Allen, C. A. (2001). *The multigenre research paper*. Portsmouth, NH: Heinemann.

American Institute of Stress. (2013). Stress statistics. *American Psychological Association*. Retrieved from http://www.statisticbrain.com/stress-statistics/

Beck, M. (2001). *Finding your own North Star*. New York, NY: Three Rivers Press.

Beck, M. (2012). *Finding your way in a wild new world*. New York, NY: Free Press.

Brown, B. (2007). *I thought it was just me*. New York, NY: Gotham Books.

Brown, B. (2012). *Daring greatly*. New York, NY: Gotham Books.

Cameron, J. (1998). *The right to write*. New York, NY: Tarcher/Putnam.

Centers for Disease Control and Prevention. (2011). Health Related Quality of Life. *Health Related Quality of Life Surveillance Program*. Retrieved from http://www.cdc.gov/hrqol/hrqol14_measure.htm

Clandinin, D. J., & Connelly, F. M. (2000). *Narrative inquiry*. San Francisco, CA: Jossey-Bass.

Conner, J. (2008). *Writing down your soul*. San Francisco, CA: Conari.

DeSalvo, L. (1999). *Writing as a way of healing*. Boston, MA: Beacon Press.

Fitzgerald, F. S. (1925). *The great Gatsby*. New York, NY: Scribner.

Goldberg, N. (1986). *Writing down the bones*. Boston, MA: Shambhala.

Goldberg, N. (2000). *Thunder and lightning*. New York, NY: Bantam.

Goldberg, N. (2005). *Writing down the bones* (2nd ed.). Boston, MA: Shambhala.

Goldberg, N. (2007). *Old friend from far away*. New York, NY: Free Press.

Goldberg, N. (2013). *The true secret of writing*. New York, NY: Atria.

Graves, D. (2001). *The energy to teach*. Portsmouth, NH: Heinemann.

Gruwell, E. (2007). Teach with your heart. New York, NY: Broadway.

Gruwell, E. (2009). Teaching hope. New York, NY: Broadway.

Gruwell, E., & the The Freedom Writers. (1999). The Freedom Writers diary. New York, NY: Broadway.

Hale, M. (2013). *The single woman*. Nashville, TN: Thomas Nelson.

Hale, M. (2014). *I've never been to Vegas but my luggage has*. Nashville, TN: Thomas Nelson.

Handler, J. (2013). *Braving the fire*. New York, NY: St. Martin's Griffin.

Heard, G. (1995). *Writing toward home*. Portsmouth, NH: Heinemann.

Kepler, H. B. (1973). *Basic graphical kinematics* (2nd ed.). New York, NY: McGraw Hill.

Kinsella, W. P. (1982). *Shoeless Joe*. New York, NY: Ballantine.

Lamott, A. (1994). *Bird by bird*. New York: Anchor Books.

Murray, D. (1996). *Crafting a life*. Portsmouth, NH: Heinemann.

Pennebaker, J. W. (1997). *Opening up: The healing power of expressing emotions*. New York, NY: The Guilford press.

Putz, M. (2006). *A teacher's guide to the multigenre research project*. Portsmouth, NH: Heinemann.

Rankin, L. (2013). *Mind over medicine*. Carlsbad, CA: Hay House.

Romano, T. (1995). *Writing with passion*. Portsmouth, NH: Heinemann.

Romano, T. (2004). *Crafting authentic voice*. Portsmouth, NH: Heinemann.

Romano, T. (2008). *Zigzag*. Portsmouth, NH: Heinemann.

Romano, T. (2013). *Fearless writing*. Portsmouth, NH: Heinemann.

Rushnell, S. (2012). *Divine alignment*. New York, NY: Howard Books.

Sandberg, S. (2013). *Lean in*. New York, NY: Alfred A. Knopf.

Schunk, D.H. (1990). Goal setting and self-efficacy during self-regulated learning. *Educational Psychologist*, *25*(1), 71–86. doi:10.120715326985ep2501_6

Tindle, H. (2013). *Up: How positive outlook can transform our health and aging*. New York, NY: Hudson Street Press.

University of Maryland Medical Center Staff. (2013). Stress. *University of Maryland Medical Center*. Retrieved from http://umm.edu/health/medical/reports/articles/stress

Wanner, E.T., & Bird, J.L. (2013). *The Wanner Bird healing survey for pain recovery*. Academic Press.

Warren, R. (2012). *The purpose driven life: What on Earth am I here for?* Grand Rapids, MI: Zondervan.

Wharton, E. (1920). *The age of innocence*. New York, NY: Collier.

Wheelan, C. (2013). *Naked statistics*. New York, NY: W.W. Norton.

Zimmermann, S. (2002). *Writing to heal the soul*. New York, NY: Three Rivers Press.

KEY TERMS AND DEFINITIONS

Artistic and Technical Writing: Artistic writing focuses on the writer's tone of word choice, also known as voice, while technical writing focuses on the writer's specificity of word choice. English teachers design rubrics that incorporate both artistic and technical writing.

Godwink: A moment where synchronicity occurs in the form of a coincidence; instead of being interpreted as a coincidence, the event is perceived as a message from God.

Journal Writing: The process of a person responding to prompts and writing about his or her thoughts and feelings. While journal writing is typically associated with writing classrooms, writing teachers including Julia Cameron, Natalie Goldberg, and Donald Murray advocate that journal writing can be done by anyone, anywhere. Journal writing can be adapted to create pain journals, where patients record the level of pain felt and the actions which caused the pain. Pain journals can subsequently be shared with medical professionals to enhance the healing process. Students in an English classroom, patients in a physical therapy clinic, and readers of this chapter in their living rooms can pick up a pen, paper, and just write.

Multigenre Writing: Discussed in the field of education by Tom Romano, a multigenre paper consists of two parts: creative writing in multiple genres and the writer's analysis of the genres.

Multigenre Healing Project: Jen and Eric designed a multigenre project where Jen wrote about her neck pain and Eric provided the end notes analysis. This different perspective on multigenre projects connects the fields of education and medicine and leads to greater patient awareness.

Narrative Inquiry: Discussed in the field of research by F. Michael Connelly and D. Jean Clandinin, narrative inquiry is a qualitative interpretative form of research that focuses on the telling, retelling, and sharing of stories. Researchers who complete narrative inquiries interpret stories and search for common threads to find patterns. They are encouraged to tell their research stories in first person as they look back to find meaning in past stories and look forward to set future goals.

Narrative Medicine: The field of medicine, used by programs such as the ones at Duke University and Columbia University, which encourages medical practitioners to use theories from the fields of literature and composition to enhance comprehension of the stories patients share.

Neck Pain Journal: Jen created a journal of what she was doing when her neck felt pain. Eric read the journal and adjusted Jen's treatment plan to make her neck feel better.

Physical Therapy Outcome Measures: Tests used by physical therapists to measure the progress a patient makes, such as such as the DASH (Disabilities of the Arm Shoulder Hand), LEFS (Lower Extremity Functional Scale), NDI (Neck Disability Index), and Modified Oswestry (for back pain). Physical therapists choose which outcome measure to use based on the body part where the patient experiences pain.

Spirituality: Regardless of religion, spirituality and a belief in a higher power can lead to increased health and provide both hope and strength for patients.

Thinking Like a Turtle: This philosophy means taking on one task at a time, which can lead to less stress.

Wanner-Bird Healing Survey for Pain Recovery: An original survey designed by Dr. Eric Wanner and Dr. Jennifer Bird. This survey features both numerical subjective questions, where patients are asked to respond to statements by circling a number from 1-5, and written subjective questions that score patients' written responses on a rubric with a score of 1, 3, or 5. The rubric incorporates both the technical and artistic dimensions of writing.

Writing Voice: Voice in writing describes how a writer uses word choice and tone to compose a journal entry or other written composition that reflects the personality of the writer. Just like each person has a unique speaking voice, each writer has a unique writing voice.

APPENDIX

Jen's Neck Pain Journal

Table 1.

Date	Pain Level 1=Low, 10=High	Observations
Summary	Left side pain is gone and I have my range of motion back. The right side pain has been a roller coaster this week. The numbers below are the average for each day; there are moments when it is better or worse but neither lasts very long.	I'm doing my exercises twice a day. I added meditation, more laughter, and a turtle necklace as my personal symbol to slow down. I checked in with a therapist to talk about my mom's death. I love my life and am peaceful with it. Okay, neck, what more do you want from me?!
Mon 4/2	Right Side Pain Level = 3	Better after physical therapy. No rehearsal tonight so time off and rest helped.
Tues 4/3	Right Side Pain Level = 1	High stress day at work with student registration for new semester and lots of stressed out students and colleagues. Doing what feels like 100 things per hour but my neck is better. Scary that neck likes stress!!
Wed 4/4	Right Side Pain Level = 4	Two days of constant stress = neck pain worse. That's kind of a no brainer. Still doing my exercises but feeling frustrated that the pain is worse today. Sleep on my side and know I'm not helping myself but I'm physically and emotionally exhausted.
Thurs 4/5	Right Side Pain Level = 5	Today is the day I wonder if I can live with pain. That lasts for about 10 minutes before I tell myself that I'm not giving up and Eric is not going to let me give up. See news story that meditation helps with pain. Motivate self to keep going.
Fri 4/6	Right Side Pain Level = 2	Feeling better today. Leave work early and hang out at the nursing home with Grandma, who feels that since she is almost 90 she no longer needs to censor anything she says. She always makes me laugh.

Chapter 2
Narratives of Research Design

Jennifer Lynne Bird
Oxbridge Academy, USA

Eric T. Wanner
Palm Beach Sports Medicine and Orthopaedic Center, USA

ABSTRACT

The authors explain the design of a survey that provides a new technology for physical therapy clinicians to use while treating patients. The survey dovetails knowledge from the fields of writing and medicine to provide a resource for patient education. In a medical clinic, a patient is asked to numerically rate how he or she feels; however, the new survey discussed not only looks at how patients feel numerically, but also how they subjectively feel using writing. This survey is a new tool that encourages communication between patients and clinicians, makes patients more aware of what they are feeling when they write down responses, and helps clinicians adjust treatment plans when they read what the patients write. Through writing, patients become accountable for their actions and increase their education. The authors focus on the connections among writing, positive outlook, and healing, as well as the lessons they learned from working together and discussing their fields of expertise.

DOI: 10.4018/978-1-7998-1931-8.ch002

INTRODUCTION TO A SYNERGISTIC COLLABORATION

When writing meets medicine, exciting possibilities occur in the fields of patient education and teacher education. Dr. Jennifer Bird is an English professor and Dr. Eric Wanner is a physical therapist. We learned a significant amount about each other's fields through a research and writing project we designed together. Patients at Eric's physical therapy clinic used strategies from Jen's writing classroom as we studied how writing about emotions affected physical health. We want our research and writing to continue to help the patients at Eric's clinic and the students in Jen's classroom.

Change takes courage. Most people live their lives never leaving their comfort zones. Johnson (2005) observes, "teaching superbly is like running a marathon by yourself in the dark. Few people even notice what you're doing, and those who notice don't pay much attention – but their oblivion doesn't slow you down. You still enjoy the thrill and satisfaction of finishing the race, and you are definitely a winner" (p. 5). But education doesn't have to be each teacher alone in a classroom, especially with technology that makes collaboration only an email away. Teachers tend to stay in their own classrooms; every once in a while they might venture down the hall to have a conversation with a colleague, but then they lock themselves back in the world of literary criticism. People often choose the safe route or the path of least resistance with their lives and with their health, even with new information, technology, and resources that could make their lives easier. At first glance it may seem unlikely that an English professor and a physical therapist would want to work together to create positive change in the lives of patients and students. Despite our divergent backgrounds, both of us share passion for research and compassion for people. We used this common ground to learn from each other and find trends between emotional writing and physical healing.

Each person has a story. Eben Alexander and Hilary Tindle are both medical doctors who advocate awareness of thoughts and feelings. Alexander (2012), a neurosurgeon, believes, "true thought is pre-physical. This is the thinking-behind-the-thinking responsible for all the genuinely consequential choices we make in the world" (p. 84). He elaborates that it is "the subliminal thinking that is always there, when we really need it, but that we have all too often lost the ability both to access and to believe in" (pp. 84-85). Tindle (2013), a doctor of internal medicine, also refers to mindfulness and explains, "this is called the triangle of awareness, in which we remain mentally centered in the midst of our thoughts, feelings, and physical sensations, each of which represents a point on the triangle" (p. 104). In her medical research, Tindle discovered that simple behavior changes could lead to better health, but most people never make changes. Tindle wondered what the script might be in the heads of the one percent of people who achieve ideal cardiac health.

To answer such questions, thinking outside one's field can prove beneficial. Writing teachers advocate for students to reflect on the script in their heads by writing about their thoughts and feelings. Cameron, a writing teacher, (1998) explains, "when we write about our lives we respond to them " (p. 94).

However, the domains of the writing classroom and the medical clinic don't typically collide. One exception is the story Rasminsky (2012) presents of Rita Charon, a medical internist who also earned a PhD in literature and explains how "Charon is the founding director of the Program in Narrative Medicine at Columbia University, where future MDs participate in writing workshops" (p. 88). We also designed a collaboration between writing and medicine and learned lessons in working together that you can apply to your life, either when sharing ideas with colleagues from different subject areas or motivating a class of students to work together.

NARRATIVE OF A SURVEY

This chapter uses the theory of narrative inquiry and the process of multigenre writing to discuss the development and implementation of a new survey. Clandinin and Connelly (2000) introduce the theory of narrative inquiry by explaining, "for us, life – as we come to it and as it comes to others – is filled with narrative fragments, enacted in storied moments of time and space, and reflected upon and understood in terms of narrative unities and discontinuities" (p. 17). They continue, "in narrative inquiry, people are looked at as embodiments of lived stories" (p. 43). Since the authors of this chapter are also the designers of the survey, instead of referring to ourselves as "the researchers," at times in our writing we choose to use first person to tell the story of our thought process as we developed our research idea. Connelly and Clandinin (1988) elaborate, "narrative is the study of how humans make meaning of experience by endlessly telling and retelling stories about themselves that both reconfigure the past and create purpose in the future" (p. 24). We use narrative to reflect on our past survey design while simultaneously setting goals for using this new technology to influence the future of patient education.

In reporting our research process by using narrative, we use the practice of multigenre writing. In describing multigenre writing, Romano (2013) explains, "multigenre places students in a situation that demands narrative thinking. It's risky. Readers might not 'get' the writer's intentions. Writers must work hard on the writing. They must craft it" (p. 22). Multigenre writing encourages writers to look beyond traditional expository writing when discussing research. Romano adds, "our students can extend that practice, incorporating traditional genres, as well as employing other means of communication they have come to know in the twenty-first century" (p. 26). In our modern society where technology surrounds us, we used technology to implement our ideas. Numerous exchanges between the authors took place over email; consequently, we use multigenre writing to replicate the original email exchanges and provide insight into our thought process.

METHODS OF DECREASING STRESS LEVELS AND IMPROVING OVERALL HEALTH

Technology leads to increased education with the ease of transmitting information, but it also leads to increased stress levels when the increased information becomes overwhelming. Look around and observe people attached to their phones while complaining they don't have enough hours in the day to accomplish everything that needs to be done. Brown (2012) argues, "one of the most universal numbing strategies is what I call crazy-busy. I often say that when they start having twelve-step meetings for busy-aholics, they'll need to rent out football stadiums. We are a culture of people who've bought into the idea that if we stay busy enough, the truth of our lives won't catch up with us" (p. 137). With the world at a rapidly increasing level of stress demands there are ways of decreasing stress levels with one of the main ones being exercise. Compare the benefits of exercise to putting air in tires on your car. You can always drive with flat tires, but won't get too far until the car breaks down. If you drive with full tires, the car will last much longer and be able to tolerate different forces that are placed on it, just like when you exercise. Why would you exercise since it takes time away from your day? Exercise has a vast number of health benefits overall. The Mayo Clinic (2011) shows that exercise can: decrease weight gain or promote weight loss as well as "prevent or manage a wide range of health problems and concerns, including stroke, metabolic syndrome, type 2 diabetes, depression, certain types of cancer, arthritis, and falls" (http://www.mayoclinic.com/health/exercise/HQ01676).

Furthermore, according to the Mayo Clinic, exercise can: improve your self-esteem and confidence, increase your muscle strength, boost your endurance, and help you fall asleep faster (http://www.mayoclinic.com/health/exercise/HQ01676).

How often should you exercise? Garber, Blissmer, Deschenes, Franklin, Lamonte, Lee, Nieman, and Swain (2011) report that the American College of Sports Medicine recommends, "most adults engage in moderate-intensity cardiorespiratory exercise training for ≥30 minutes per day on ≥5 days per week for a total of ≥150 minutes per week, vigorous-intensity cardiorespiratory exercise training for ≥20 minutes per day on ≥3 days per week (≥75 minutes per week), or a combination of moderate- and vigorous-intensity exercise to achieve a total energy expenditure of ≥500-1000 MET minimum per week. On 2-3 days per week, adults should also perform resistance exercises for each of the major muscle groups, and nueromotor exercise involving balance, agility, and coordination. Crucial to maintaining joint range of movement, completing a series of flexibility exercises for each the major muscle-tendon groups (a total of 60 seconds per exercise) on ≥2 days per week is recommended" (p. 1334). If you are sedentary, you should gradually build up to these minutes of exercise slowly ideally while being monitored by a specialist such as a physical therapist, cardiologist, sports medicine physician, or exercise physiologist. He or she should monitor symptoms and start with closer to ten minutes a day of low intensity exercise and gradually build up from there. Also if you are injured, you should see a physical therapist or physician first to get on a proper treatment intervention based upon your symptoms. It is never good to exercise through pain. Fatigue and a good burning of the muscles while working out are different than a sharp pain or any pain limiting activities of daily living. Once you get on the right track with exercising the amount as recommended, expect to see positive life changes while keeping a positive outlook on everything.

As a physical therapist myself, I (Eric) am well aware of all of these health benefits, but I kept an open mind to see what could happen if I combined this knowledge with Jen's knowledge, using writing to decrease stress levels. You will see where this collaboration has led, and how it is going to lead to life changing events.

INITIAL DISCOVERIES

What if we told you that filling out a survey while writing down goals has the potential to help you heal faster in physical therapy? Would you do it? The authors of this chapter created a survey that uses writing to assist the healing process. The survey features both numerical subjective questions, where patients are asked to rate how they feel by circling a number, and written subjective questions, where patients are asked to respond to a prompt by providing a short written answer. The writing prompts are scored using a rubric similar to the rubrics used by writing teachers when evaluating students' papers.

In designing our research and implementing our survey, we wanted to answer the question if there was a relationship between a patient's positive outlook when writing down his or her feelings and the patient's recovery process. As of this writing our research remains ongoing and we plan to study this topic further, but our initial study revealed that patients who used more positive language when responding to short answer writing prompts on the survey we designed showed higher objective improvements on existing physical therapy measurements such as the DASH (Disabilities of the Arm Shoulder Hand), LEFS (Lower Extremity Functional Scale), NDI (Neck Disability Index), and Modified Oswestry (for back pain). We hope that after more studies strengthening the validity and reliability of the survey, it will become a new technology medical practitioners can add to their tool kit of patient education resources.

ALL ABOUT GOALS

We explain our rationale for designing the survey, our thought process as we developed it, and our goals for additional research using the survey. We know that technology can lead to innovations; however, designing new technology does not mean abandoning old ideas that work well. Sharp (2000) argues, "in this day of computers and superfast information and increasingly dehumanized communication, I believe that the writer is more important to society than ever. Someone who takes the time to sit down, perhaps with pen or pencil in hand, and express themselves in their own words – this is a person with something to say and a commitment to say it" (p. 133). Furthermore, as Goldberg (2005) adds about writing, "and it's inexpensive. All you need is pen, paper (of course computer, if you are so inclined), and the human mind" (p. xii). Obviously writing does not take the place of following the treatment plan prescribed by a physical therapist, but it can make patients more aware of how their thoughts influence their actions. Cameron (2002) believes, "as mental-health experts are quick to point out, in order to move through loss and beyond it, we must acknowledge it and share it" (p. 129). Writing teachers such as Cameron use writing to help with emotional losses, so we wondered if writing could also assist physical therapy patients who suffered physical losses as a result of injuries.

Tindle (2013) saw things from a different perspective when she as a doctor became a patient. She reflects, "my upbeat attitude made me an easier patient to treat, someone willing to adhere to his medical advice and do my part to attain the best possible outcome" (p. 3). She adds, "our outlook affects our health and our aging both directly and indirectly in myriad ways" (p. 25).

Our survey takes into account several different aspects patients should be aware of during their recovery process in physical therapy. We observed that patients seem to do the best when they make strong goals. When people make a goal it motivates them to work harder at what they do. As Chua (2009) quotes Bill Copeland, "If you don't have a goal in life, you are spending your life running around and not achieving anything for yourself" (http://personalexcellence.co/blog/6-important-reasons-why-you-should-set-goals/). Cameron (2002) concurs, "each of us has an inner dream that we can unfold if we will just have the courage to admit what it is. And the faith to trust our own admission. The admitting is often very difficult. A clearing affirmation can often open the channel" (p. 193). Often, patients rely on their medical practitioners to help them with setting goals for recovery.

Rankin (2013) speaks from her perspective as a doctor and believes, "when health care professionals hold space with nurturing care, we create the ideal environment for patients to heal themselves" (p. 51). Research was performed by Younger, Gandhi, Hubbard, and Mackey (2012) that looked at the expectation patients had in physical therapy (whether positive and negative) called the SETS (Stanford Expectations of Treatment Scale). It showed that patients that had a more positive expectancy did better than patients with negative expectancy (p. 767). With this mentality, patients will be willing to do all of their exercises in physical therapy and have a better chance for a full recovery. Even if one falls just short of the goal, that patient may get to a place he or she never dreamed. In the clinic used for this research, people who do their home exercises on a routine basis seem to have better results on average for their full recovery than patients that do not. As stated by Bradley, Bogardus, Tinetti, and Inouye (1999) "the process of setting goals for medical care in the context of chronic disease has received little attention in the medical literature, despite the importance of goal-setting in the achievement of desired outcomes" (p. 267). Whether or not a patient had chronic pain, we decided it would be beneficial to address setting goals as a building block to help patients during their recovery process.

Beck (2001) states, "miracles really can and will occur when you connect with your dreams, but they're both more likely and less necessary if you do everything in your power to reach your goals" (p. 306). Writing down goals and envisioning them happening is common practice for life coaches like Beck, but because of the hectic pace in modern medical settings, medical practitioners often need to hurry from one patient to the next. Rasminsky (2012) reports the story of Rita Charon, the doctor who also earned a degree in literature to understand the power of storytelling, and now when talking to patients, "she sits with her hands in her lap – no notes, no typing – and lets the patient tell her story" (p. 88). As ideal as this sounds, due to the amount of documentation required in the physical therapy profession (or any profession in the medical field) we are unable to sit, listen, and not write down any notes. Because of this, we need to utilize a technology such as our survey that can help the patient truly express feelings without feeling under a time constraint.

Unfortunately the way the medical field is being driven, clinicians do not have as much time as desired with their patients as they once had. Doctors need to see multiple patients in a day. New technology such as electronic medical records can sometimes make a conversation between a patient and medical practitioner even more impersonal as a doctor looks at the computer instead of looking at the patient. Patients may feel like the doctor doesn't have enough time to spend with them. Rankin (2013) explains things from a doctor's perspective and states, "nobody intends for this to happen. Health-care providers have often sacrificed so much for their patients that they stop being mindful about why they're doing what they were called to do" (p. 48). She continues, "it's time to put the care back in health care" (p. 48).

How can each patient still find a way to get better to his or her full potential? Patients need to take ownership of their actions and be held accountable for doing their homework. Increasing self-awareness can be very beneficial to patients in physical therapy. It will help them figure out what activities increase their pain, when their symptoms are most noticeable, and what makes their symptoms decrease. This can help prevent the patient from re-irritating his or her injured body part and could speed up the recovery process. For example, if a patient hurts his or her shoulder, does physical therapy, but continues to hurt the shoulder during the recovery process by what he or she is doing during the day, it will prolong the recovery. The inflammatory phase will continue to start over for the recovery process with re-irritation and will make it hard for a speedy recovery. This is why self-awareness is more crucial than most realize. When the patient is able to do this, the physical therapist and physician will be able to make the most accurate diagnosis and come up with the most beneficial treatment for the patient.

Each patient has a story, but sometimes patients don't know how to share their stories, either with themselves or with clinicians. Barrett (2013) reports about her own experiences and elaborates, "I started to track my experience with just pen and paper. I recorded when I felt best (and worst) and began making deliberate changes to my environment and behavior" (p. 37). Writing can help patients make positive changes in their lives, whether it is describing chronic pain like Barrett or writing goals like patients who completed our survey. However, just like students in a classroom who need writing prompts to help them think of what to write, patients need similar guidance about what to write. Giving patients the numerical subjective questions in our survey to rate how they are feeling and the written subjective questions to describe their feelings provides instructions on where to begin the writing process. The survey then places the ball in their court and allows them to set their own goals and come up with ways to achieve them.

We decided to have patients complete the survey in the clinic because even if patients receive the instructions to write down their goals at home, the busy lives people lead often prevent them from having the time or the inclination to write. As Cheo (2012) states "a total of 90 percent of people do not have written goals. Writing down your goals does a number of things for you: It reinforces your commitment to them. It helps you remember them. It makes you accountable. It gives you focus" (http://www.bizjournals.com/boston/blog/mass-high-tech/2012/09/goal-setting-why-90-of-us-dont-do.html?page=all). Realizing how small of a percentage of time it takes for people to actually write down goals outside of the clinic makes even more sense to have them do it while in the clinic. The survey we designed made patients stop, write their goals, and rate their confidence in achieving their goals while still in a clinical setting.

STORIES OF SURVEY DEVELOPMENT

At this point in the chapter, we as the authors switch to a narrative multigenre format to continue the story of the survey development. You will still see the academic theory behind the practice of survey development, because as Romano (2013) writes, "I require students to incorporate research into multigenre papers, regardless of their subject, even if they write from deeply personal experience" (p. 43). But the rest of the story will be told from a first person perspective. We asked physical therapy patients to share their voices with us in their writing, so we intend to share our voices with you, the reader, in our writing. Brown (2012) believes, "rather than sitting on the sidelines and hurling judgment and advice, we must dare to show up and let ourselves be seen. This is vulnerability. This is daring greatly" (p. 2). So as writers and researchers, we intend to let ourselves be seen and own our story.

OLD FASHIONED WRITING MEETS MODERN MEDICAL TECHNOLOGY

When she went to Eric's physical therapy clinic for neck pain, Jen always did her home exercises. As a college English professor, she knew the value of homework. However, as a writer, she also needed to do more than simply assign her pain level a number during each session. She created a neck pain journal that stated a numeric value for her pain at different times during the day but also added her written commentary about what she was doing at the time of a certain pain level. Jen knew what type of pain she felt, when she felt it, and how she felt about it. She didn't know why she felt the pain, but hoped Eric did.

Audience becomes essential for a writer. Negative comments cause writers to put their pages away and never share their words with anyone except themselves; conversely, positive comments can provide a source of encouragement for the writer. Sharp (2000) explains, "you hand your work over to Person X and then wait, hating the waiting, praying for a good review, hoping that Person X will be honest and kind" (p. 136). For Jen, she wanted Eric to be an audience for her writing but also needed to be her own audience and reflect on what she was feeling.

In this way, writing is a mirror that reflects a writer's true feelings. Goldberg (2000) argues, "writing is an immediate mirror: it reports back to you. You can't fool anyone, especially yourself" (p. 218). Sharing writing takes risk. A writer never truly knows how an audience will react until the words are shared. Jen found the courage to share her neck pain journal with Eric. He not only read it but liked it and found a pattern to her neck pain. She felt better, and he encouraged her to write more while modifying his treatment plan to best help her.

Jen increased her self-awareness and Eric determined the most beneficial treatment for her. In addition to writing, Jen also designed a heart map of things she loved, such as listening to her favorite music when completing exercises. Heard (1995) discusses the value of heart maps and encourages people to do things they love "with the map you've already made in your heart. That's where the real home is: inside" (p. 2). Jen and Eric enjoyed their collaboration, and it became the first chapter in a longer narrative. Eric used Jen's writing to help her heal, and that story became a book chapter. They decided to continue to learn from each other through writing, research, and the development of a survey to help other patients.

Pipher (2006) argues, "in both therapy and writing, we want to help people see the connections between their actions and consequences of those actions" (p. 97). Often the answers to people's problems are right in front of them, but lack of self-awareness prevents this insight. What if a survey existed to serve as a mirror to reflect a patient's hopes and dreams, thoughts and feelings? As Driscoll (2012) quotes Edith Wharton, "there are two ways of spreading light: to be the candle or the mirror that reflects it" (http://www.csmonitor.com/Books/2012/0123/Edith-Wharton-10-best-quotes-on-her-150th-birthday/Giving-happiness-to-others).

By using this metaphor, Jen was the candle that went through this process during physical therapy, made a table which discussed when she felt the best or worst, and what she was doing during those times. She got one hundred percent pain-free with the help of physical therapy in addition to writing. We wondered if we could use what we learned to help other patients, and we hoped to bring that experience to others. We designed the survey to allow others to go through a similar experience for their recovery process to serve as a mirror of her success.

BACKGROUND OF A SURVEY

We spent some time emailing each other about ideas for a survey. Inventions are made all of the time, but rarely are you able to go back in time and read the entire process as it is taking place. We structured this section of our chapter in the form of a conversation using excerpts from our email conversations followed by our reflections after rereading our original ideas.

Jen: How do pain journals/heart maps/other creative forms of expression enhance healing for patients?

Eric: I wonder if we would be able to make the heart map into some type of survey that patients could fill out before, during, and after therapy sessions. With that we might be able to determine their success they had objectively to the amount of success they had subjectively. Or, maybe we could make a "heart survey" and compare it to something that has clinically significant research behind it (such as the Oswestry for low back pain, or LEFS for leg pain, DASH for shoulder pain, etc.). I would assume there is a correlation, but only research could tell.

Jen: I love the idea of a before, during, and after survey for patients to complete. My students complete B-D-A lesson plans and love the process because it helps them focus on what they are learning over time. I imagine the process would be similar for patients.

Eric: I do think this concept would be very similar and feel like it is a very good way to see the change throughout their intervention or process.

Jen: If they were asked to write something at home would they bring it back to the clinic or would it be best if they completed a survey in the clinic?

Eric: We could always try, but I think the best compliance would be a survey of some sort in the clinic.

Jen: Do we want to give patients the same survey before, during, and after treatment or a slightly different one?

Eric: I think that if we could give them the same survey before, during, and after it could increase the reliability for our study.

Jen: If the surveys are identical, would there be a recency effect, meaning if patients know they are going to get the identical question three times a session would they tell us what we want to hear?

Eric: I see what you are saying. Maybe if we did different aspects of the same questions for before, during, and after it would be a better idea because of that.

Jen: I was curious to see how some of the writing strategies I use with my students might look if I designed a survey with them, so I created some sample questions using eight writing theories and five types of subjective assessments used in education.

Eric: I just looked over everything and like the type of questions. I decided to write four questions and made them a little more relevant to what I would ask my patient as a physical therapist. I like the heart drawing idea, but feel like a lot of my patients may take a long time with it.

Jen: Good point about the time it would take to complete the heart map. I know you would rather patients do their exercises at the clinic instead of spending all their time there drawing heart maps!

Eric: I really like the outline and how you added to it. I think what might make it easier is if they did before therapy, while they are doing physical therapy (end of week two), and close to the end (end of week four).

Jen: We would have to make sure we ask the questions in a way to isolate the patient's feelings about treatment as opposed to feelings about the other events in their lives, especially since a lot can happen to a person in a month.

Eric: The reason why I was thinking of at the end of week two and four is because those are actually normal time-frames physical therapists shoot for when making goals for each patient.

Jen: I was grading student essays and realized it wouldn't take much to adapt the rubric I was using to the short answer questions of our survey.

Eric: This is going to be great for you to use when grading their subjective writing and making an analysis of it. Would it be possible to keep it as you have it to show how you analyzed it, and then possibly make conclusions with their writing styles in the research?

Jen: I like the idea of keeping the survey as is and making conclusions with the writing styles in the research. It makes sense to go off the objective scores and correlate them with existing surveys because those are established surveys and a logical correlation.

Eric: I will figure out the best objective measures for us to use.

If we give physical therapists a survey featuring short answer writing questions, we need to have a strong writing theory to support our ideas. We used the heart map discussed by Heard (1995) as a starting point with her belief that "I do all I can to clear out my life, but in the end there are obligations, distractions, and messes, and I write anyway" (p. 19). Patients who would respond to our survey would have all kinds of distractions, but we needed to know those distractions in order to identify obstacles that would prevent them from following through with their treatment plan.

Writers live their lives and then relive their lives when writing their stories. We wanted to study the stories the patients told in their own words to better understand their perspectives. Goldberg (2007) believes, "writing is an athletic activity" (p. 1). She compares writing to exercise and instructs, "begin to work those muscles. Just like you'd go to the gym every day, or at least three or four times a week, pick up the pen and do these ten-minute exercises" (p. 1). So when responding to our questions, patients at the physical therapy clinic gave their bodies a workout with exercises and their minds a workout with writing. And finally, the following advice by Goldberg (1990) can apply to both writing and exercise: "Shut up and write anyway. Don't use anything as an excuse" (p. 221). Holding back from writing can prevent one from truly showing how he or she is feeling and might not give optimal results for the patient and the physical therapist.

Cameron (1998) also compares writing to healing by stating, "writing is medicine. It is an appropriate antidote to injury. It is an appropriate companion for any difficult change" (p. 31). While it's true that new technology exists to help medical practitioners treat patients, the simple act of putting pen to paper is effective too. Lamott (1994) writes, "there was a part of me that believed that my journal could be a gift for others" (p. 188). But if writing in a journal leads to healing, it can also be a gift to the person writing it.

In addition to writing theory, strategies from the field of teacher education informed our research. We derived the before, during, and after treatment format for the survey using a format similar to the B-D-A instructional framework for teaching students strategies before, during, and after reading a text. Vacca, Vacca, and Mraz (2014) explain, "what a teacher does before reading, during reading, and after reading (B-D-A) is crucial to active and purposeful reading" (p. 140). We transferred an idea from the field of education to the field of medicine to assist patients with active and purposeful healing. The rubric designed to assess patient writing in the survey splits the writing into the technical (specificity of word choice) and artistic (tone of word choice) dimensions of writing. As discussed by Romano (2013), "I divided the rubric in half: a holistic part that was my gut reaction to the paper as a reader who longed to be informed, moved, and carried away by the power of written words" (p. 160). That describes the artistic part of writing. Romano continues, "In the second half of the rubric, I turned my attention to specific parts of the paper I wanted students to write" (p. 162). That describes the technical part of writing.

Goldberg (2000) discusses voice in writing and explains, “if I had consciously looked for a writing voice, I might have missed it” (p. 143). Voice is a concept used in teaching writing. In retelling their stories, writers use their own unique voices and if they try too hard to find a voice, their true personalities often don’t shine through. Romano (2004) defines voice as “our very personalities shape our voices and determine how and what we put on the page” (p. 6). It involves tone, word choice, and feeling. It’s the artistry involved in composing a writing piece that reflects the personality of the writer. When students have strong voice in their writing, it is like they are sitting next to the teacher having a conversation and telling their stories. Here is our story as we developed the rubric.

Jen: And then I realized it. Writing is both artistic and technical!!! In making the rubric easy for physical therapists to understand, there was only one score: The technical one. Any decent English teacher gives writing two scores: The artistic and the technical. I needed a pen of a different color for contrast and a space to work so I could hear the voices of the patients and the narratives their words were telling me. In a short amount of time I added a second score to each writing question, this one representing voice, tone and word choice. That information was always there in our rubric, but got overshadowed when there was just one number instead of two.

Eric: That’s awesome that you were able to do that! I want to say I can’t believe you were able to, but I’m not surprised.

Our research colleague, Dr. Claudia Jayne Brahler. reminded us to listen to the voices of the patients. So we scored the patients’ writing on both the artistic and technical dimensions of writing. The artistic writing scores aligned with the calculations completed on existing physical therapy surveys that demonstrated patient healing gains. We discovered a trend that patients who used more positive language according to the artistic writing scores on our survey demonstrated a higher percentage of healing on existing physical therapy measurements.

REFLECTIONS ON FIELD NOTES

By exchanging emails about our thought process, we used technology to design a new tool in the medical field. Field notes are an important part of qualitative research and rereading the original notes adds another perspective to the narrative. Connelly and Clandinin (1988) explain, "narrative unity is a continuum within a person's experience and renders life experiences meaningful through the unity they achieve for the person" (p. 74). Upon reflection, our email messages illuminate insights of our thought process as we designed the survey. In rereading the emails, we discovered patterns and narrative threads to our research. It is one thing to remember an experience, but another to read the exact words written at the time of that experience.

ERIC'S REFLECTIONS

Like I said in the last email to Jen, "I want to say I can't believe you were able to, but I'm not surprised"; this truly describes the type of passion Jen has in this and makes it easy for me to stay motivated and continue to write. It always works well when people working on something together share a strong passion in what they are doing and go through with their ideas. Using New Year's Resolutions as an example as stated from the University of Scranton (2012), there are "8% of people who are successful in achieving their resolution" (http://www.statisticbrain.com/new-years-resolution-statistics/). This puts into perspective how few people actually follow through with a goal and succeed. If you have a passion for something, follow through with it and be in that eight percent. We both plan to continue to be in that eight percent and look forward to further writing and research with this!

Looking at these emails reminds me of the eclectic approach we used to design our survey. One idea seemed to branch off to another until something beneficial to all patients was made for the medical setting. We truly reached a milestone in the medical field with this survey and I strongly believe that it will lead to much more research in the future. This survey has true potential to help others during their recovery process by getting the results that they are striving for. This survey allows others to freely write throughout their physical therapy sessions and be more self-aware of why they are feeling the way they are. It implements accountability that the patient must assume to get optimal results. It allows the patients to set goals knowing that if one strives for a very strong goal, coming just short of it could lead to miraculous results. It allows the physical therapist to look over the patient's thoughts on paper that they may not divulge to the therapist in regards to: how they are currently feeling, how close they feel they are to reaching their goals, and any barriers they may perceive which could prevent them from achieving their goals at a set time.

This survey is unique since it is the first time a physical therapist and an English professor came together and designed a survey for a physical therapy clinic in hopes that it could facilitate patients' full recovery in addition to normal physical therapy sessions. This entire process that Jen and I had to go through was time consuming, yet easily manageable with us both sharing a strong work ethic in this project and having the passion to make sure it would be a success. We both want to help as many people as possible in life. With physical therapy I help the patients regain the ability to do what they want to be able to do again, and Jen helps patients learn to conquer fragile moments in life with writing. Combining our thoughts into a survey I believe, is a very holistic approach for all patients in the physical therapy world.

I truly believe there is more to a patient than just pain and what they can do; the patient's personality and what they are going through in life must be accounted for, and I think our survey does a good job with this. We are both aware that we cannot discuss our thoughts with everyone individually in the physical therapy clinics, but knowing that the survey has the potential to help is fulfilling.

After rereading what Jen and I wrote, I always think of how I can best transfer this style into my practice. I became a better clinician doing this, realizing that if I allow a patient to truly express themselves to me, they will be more willing to listen to my advice and be more compliant with their physical therapy exercises. If patients are more compliant with their exercises for physical therapy it allows them to have a quicker recovery time and leads to elite results. Our survey allows for this to happen even when the clinic is very busy. It allows patients to be more at ease, while simultaneously assessing where they currently are and what goals they want to achieve. I believe that writing helps people express how they truly feel with less pressure put on them. Writing helps people set goals that they can strive for and achieve. Writing helps people come to realizations of certain things that could be affecting their health and their recovery process. Writing helps show one's true personality and how an individual is able to cope with different elements in life. Hopefully our survey will transfer over into all clinics for physical therapy and allow everyone to have the chance to really strive for their goals! Hopefully it will lead to several more research studies as well as showing the importance of patient goal setting in the medical field!

JEN'S REFLECTIONS

I'm proud of us and this research! We designed a survey about goal setting for patients. We also set our own goals for our research and achieved them. I hadn't reread these emails since we originally wrote them, and I enjoyed seeing how much we accomplished in less than a year. In less than a year, we had an idea for a survey, designed it, implemented a research study based on the survey, and found a connection between goal setting and healing. We also worked very well together. It was fun for me to see how we challenged each other in positive ways to do our best work. I knew Eric shared my dedication to the project, so whenever he thought of a wonderful idea it motivated me to develop my own wonderful ideas too.

I also appreciated how we listened to each other's ideas. We learned from each other. I found myself caring more about medicine because Eric felt passionate about it, and I hope my passion for writing inspired him too. I felt free to create because I always knew Eric would do his part of the work. Because I knew someone else depended on my contribution to the project, I was never going to give up on this research. We spent a lot of time working on this, but when something is fun it doesn't feel like work at all and that's the best part.

I loved it when Eric wrote that I help patients conquer fragile moments in life through writing. During the difficult times in my life, I viewed writing as a type of therapy. Writing about my experiences helped me process my thoughts and feelings. I also had the opportunity to witness my students experience the same writing process. In class, I give students writing prompts on various topics and time to write. Students enjoy the writing time, but more important to them is the sharing time, when they can choose to share what they wrote with their classmates. The sharing times built class community and provided a comfortable environment for discussion.

If I asked my students to share, I needed to share too. Sharing takes courage, but I discovered my writing meant more to me when I shared it than when I just left it in my notebook with myself as the only audience.

Eric helps his physical therapy patients return to what they want to do again not just by providing them with appropriate exercises that are well researched, high level manual skills as needed, and a treatment plan, but also by taking the time to learn their life stories. Writing is a way for people, whether they are students in my classroom or patients at Eric's clinic, to share their life stories. By writing, the authors of the stories often see events from a different perspective, just like Eric and I have a different perspective on our writing after rereading our original conversation with each other.

FUTURE PLANS FOR THE SURVEY

Our goal is for our survey to continue to be used in further research in multiple locations to explore the trend we found of writing incorporated in healing. We want to show physical therapists the importance of having their patients fill out our survey to help them keep on the right track throughout their physical therapy sessions. We want this to open new doors for research in the medical field so that the patient's true feelings will be taken into account even when they may not have as much time with the physician and physical therapist as they once did.

Every patient wants to feel like his or her voice is heard by a clinician, and that he or she is more than just an appointment time on a clinician's busy schedule. In the play *Our Town*, Wilder (1938) has the character Emily say, "It goes so fast. We don't have time to look at one another" (p. 100). Emily is describing life, but the same statement can be applied to a typical appointment between a patient and clinician. Medical practitioners want to stay on schedule, and sometimes pain prevents patients from thinking clearly or leads to a list of questions remembered after the conclusion of the appointment. Our survey helps patients share their true feelings and helps clinicians take into account the patient's perspective when adjusting treatment plans.

By continuing to do research, we hope to use our new technology in order to create change in the fields of medicine, writing, and patient education. Gruwell and the Freedom Writers (1999) discuss the power of writing by "encouraging you to pick up a pen and be a catalyst for change" (p. 277). We also want to be catalysts for change by encouraging patients to pick up their pens and write and by encouraging clinicians to read their patients' writing. This is why we think our new technology (*The Wanner-Bird Healing Survey for Pain Recovery*) possesses the potential to positively transform the entire medical profession.

LESSONS IN COLLABORATIVE INTERDISCIPLINARY SYNERGY

Educators in different fields can use their talents to create collaborations with colleagues in other disciplines. Connelly and Clandinin (1988) believe that teachers "come to know their own practices from their work with colleagues" (p. 209). New ideas occur when people venture outside their own practices and share their thoughts with others. Since we shared our research and writing ideas with each other in text message and email conversations, we structured this section in the form of a conversation and share both of our perspectives.

LESSON #1: DON'T LIMIT JOURNAL WRITING TO THE ENGLISH CLASSROOM

Jen: Our interdisciplinary collaboration began when I developed neck pain and Eric was my physical therapist. To process what I felt both physically and emotionally, I decided to write about it and complete a neck pain journal. I used journals with my students in my classroom and kept personal journals for my eyes only, but this was the first time I shared my writing with someone hoping that he could find a pattern in my words and help me heal.

Eric: While Jen was a patient of mine we not only discussed her recovery process, but also her writing and our research possibilities. Writing seemed to lighten Jen's mood throughout life and made her more aware of contributing factors to her neck pain. Writing helped Jen take some stress away and helped her learn to cope with traumatic events in her life. In her *Writing and Healing* blog, McCall (2011) discusses the research of James Pennebaker about the healing power of expressing emotions and explains, "writing was found to reduce anxiety and depression, improve grades in college, and aid people in finding jobs" (http://www.psychologytoday.com/blog/overcoming-child-abuse/201103/writing-and-healing). Writing helped me treat my patients more efficiently, and reminded me of other possible contributors to pain that can be easily passed up when treating patients.

Jen: This led to a conversation about if we could use the lessons learned from my writing experience during physical therapy to help other patients. It opened my eyes to new possibilities for journal writing.

Eric: For Jen, writing was a tool she started using to monitor her pain throughout the day. Jen made a table for the day that listed when she felt the best, and also when she felt the worst. With this, I was able to notice a pattern to her pain and altered my treatment to help her become pain-free.

Jen: Goldberg (2000) argues, "someone who edits your work – at any level – is giving you their mind, just as in your writing you have given them yours" (p. 189). When Eric read my writing, he edited his treatment plan in order to best help me. If I tried to remember everything instead of writing it, I probably would have missed something. I gave him insights about my pain through my writing, and he gave me back insights of how to help me heal.

Eric: This led us to the idea that writing could be a keystone in the medical field. We created our own survey that assessed the impact of a patient's positive outlook during his or her recovery process in physical therapy and his or her amount of objective improvement. We both believe that if patients have a positive outlook during physical therapy they will be more willing to write about how they are truly feeling and use more positive words throughout that time. We also believe that they will score higher with certain questions in regards to decreasing their amount of "barriers" that are preventing them from getting better during their recovery process. In her *Writing and Healing* blog, McCall (2011) again references the research of James Pennebaker and elaborates, "the more people described positive emotions in their writing, the more likely they were to be healthier afterward. But, describing negative emotions either excessively or very little or not at all correlated with poorer health" (http://www.psychologytoday.com/blog/overcoming-child-abuse/201103/writing-and-healing). Jen and I both feel like this same concept can be used for patients in the medical field.

In her research, Tindle (2013) discovered that positive outlook can influence healing. She focused on outlook and aging and elaborates, "my research joins the growing ranks of findings from around the world that point in the same direction: A positive outlook is good medicine" (p. 6). We want our research to become part of this growing trend in medicine and patient education, and our discovery after our initial research project revealed that patients who used more optimistic language on our original survey, *The Wanner-Bird Healing Survey for Pain Recovery*, showed higher healing gains on existing physical therapy measurements. We look forward to continuing our research on the topic of how positive outlook in writing influences healing.

LESSON #2: CARE ABOUT THE PROJECT

We both feel dedicated to our research project of studying how writing about physical and emotional issues associated with healing influences the recovery process for physical therapy patients. A mutual interest in a topic can bring people from different fields together. Sharing the work makes studying the topic and learning new things more fun. This allows people from different academic fields to come together and work on the same project. We used information from our different fields to design a survey that features a combination of numerical questions similar to other existing assessments given to physical therapy patients and written questions similar to the short answer responses given to students in a writing classroom. The result is a new survey unlike anything that currently exists because we combined the strengths of our areas of expertise. We felt proud of our accomplishment and decided to name the survey after ourselves, although patients did not know the name of the survey when they completed it. We copyrighted the survey and designed something that has the potential to help patients beyond our lifetimes.

Jen: Romano (2004) believes, "our own voices can take on strength and energy through other voices" (p. 96). Explaining my ideas about writing when developing my section of the survey strengthened my own voice and when Eric added his voice to the survey with his ideas about physical therapy patients I felt energized learning something new. I also feel free to be my most creative self because I know we share a dedication to the research and it is an equal collaboration, not one person doing all the work.

Eric: From a physical therapist's standpoint, one would love to have the patients share the same passion in believing they will get better and follow all the guidelines they are given. Every patient that does his or her home exercises routinely seems to have a significantly higher chance of getting better than those that do not in my clinic.

Jen: When working with students, all of them may not possess an equal passion for the project. After a recent group project, my students reflected that all of them did not share equal initial enthusiasm for the novel being discussed, but when they saw how much their team members cared, it

LESSON #4: BE HONEST

Jen: I took a leap of faith by asking Eric to read my neck pain journal, because I didn't know how he would react. Still, I knew I needed to be honest at all times. If I didn't tell him how I was feeling or what I did to cause my neck pain, he wouldn't know what treatment to use to help me get better.

Eric: Holding back on your feelings in writing only limits oneself and masks the true feelings the writer has. This is not good for the writer or the audience. With Jen writing down in her journal how she really felt I was able to see a pattern and develop a treatment program to eliminate her pain. If she would have just said that she felt fine when she did not, we would not have been able to get those results.

Jen: In order to keep getting results, we still have to be honest with each other. I feel I can share any idea with Eric and we'll discuss it. We may not use every idea we have in our research and writing, but I know we can always talk about things. That makes me want to think of even more ideas!

Heard (1995) explains, "the more honest I am with myself about my own needs, the better I can guide my readers into giving me the kind of help I truly need" (p. 131). Not holding back on feelings, whether a person is a patient writing in a neck pain journal or a teacher reading the journals kept by students, requires trust by both the writer and the audience. When different disciplines collide, collaborators need to make a commitment to trusting and sharing, whether informing each other about technical terms in each other's fields or artistic expression of insights and feelings. Mutual respect is also essential for trust and honesty to take place.

LESSON #5: BEING ALIKE YET DIFFERENT CAN HELP

Jen: Eric likes to use the phrase "think like a turtle" with his patients, and he applies the same philosophy to research. Slow down. It's a journey. I try my best to apply this attitude to my life. I bought a turtle necklace to remind me not to multitask. Still, sometimes my teaching training of planning lessons and unit plans for weeks and months of a schedule surfaces and I start wondering about the destination instead of the journey. What next? What if this happens instead of that? Then what?

Eric always reminds me to take one step of the project at a time when I'm thinking three steps ahead and I appreciate that.

Eric: When talking to patients in the clinic it is always helpful for them to be aware of a certain timeframe it will take to get them better. Some people will take longer than others, but it is always good for a patient that has more going on physiologically to keep a positive outlook and not get discouraged. Realizing that sometimes it can take a few weeks to get better after being in pain for several years is a better and more realistic way to view the physical therapy process than assuming you should be back to one hundred percent after the first visit. It takes several weeks for muscles to truly get stronger and start to support the structures they need to support.

Jen: Patients in a clinic and students in a classroom are not as different as you might think. Some students will take longer than others to finish reading a novel or writing a paper, and teachers have an entire year with students, not a day or a week or a month. My greatest teaching moments often occur when I'm not watching the clock and feel truly present in the moment with my students listening to what they have to say. By applying this strategy to our own lives, we model for students to be present in the moment with each other and accept the diverse abilities everyone possesses.

Eric: It is good to share the same passion as the person you are working with. Whether or not you each have the same interest in teaching or in medicine, determination and sharing a goal can become groundbreaking. Too many people become content, but it takes someone special to continually challenge themselves with others to achieve the same overall goal.

Murray (1996) describes the energizing feeling of collaboration as, "when I get a response from the members of my writing community, I hurry back to my desk, excited by the problems, the possibilities, the strengths I have discovered" (p. 123). It becomes easy to fall into a routine and become content. It often takes someone else to challenge that contentment and lead to the discovery of a new passion and a new goal. Willamette University (2001) has a similar approach for bringing diverse perspectives together with the liberal arts research collaborative (LARC). Seth Cotlar, the director of the program, states, "LARC gives students experience in working alongside others who may understand the world in a very different way. They may have disagreements, but they also have moments of illumination where they teach each other something new" (http://www.willamette.edu/people/

archives/2011/08/larc.html). Just like we had moments of illumination when one of us taught the other something, students can share similar enlightening moments when discussing ideas with classmates.

Jen: I need to talk or write about a research idea as soon as I think about it before my mind moves on to the novel I'm teaching in class or what I'm doing over the weekend. This usually results in long emails sent to Eric about my latest research idea. Some of my emails even include Roman Numerals with subheadings as I attempt to organize my thoughts before I forget whatever brilliant inspiration occurred to me. Eric always takes the time to answer my questions and can sort through my long narratives to summarize what we want to accomplish in a sentence or two.

Eric: As a physical therapist, I am one who always chose math or science classes over English classes, but I looked past this once I realized the positive impact writing could have on my patients. By sharing the same dedication in helping people whether in physical therapy or in the classroom we came together with writing.

LESSON #6: CHALLENGE EACH OTHER AND YOURSELF IN POSITIVE WAYS

Jen: I used to think I would never do anything with science or medicine other than watching television medical dramas. In high school I convinced my future doctor lab partner to do all the dissecting for Biology class and she agreed because I wrote amazing lab reports. When the high school students I taught English to came to my class straight from Biology, I felt queasy just hearing about what they did in class. But I wanted to challenge myself and try something new. I love learning new things, and the books I was teaching were never going to have new endings. After my mom died at a young age my dad found a notebook of observations she kept about her health. I have no idea if showing them to someone in the medical field would have saved her life, but since I couldn't help her I wanted to help other patients and other families. I thought I would never do that either because how could an English teacher do anything with medicine? On my last day of physical therapy Eric asked me if I wanted to work with him on research and writing and I realized opportunities I never thought possible actually existed.

Eric: Jen and I challenged each other to pursue our research idea and went through with it! We also ended up writing a chapter in a book together throughout the process. Henry Ford, as quoted on the website of the University of Oregon's Holden Leadership Center, a provider of Leadership Education for students (2009), was correct when he stated, "you can't build a reputation on what you are going to do" (http://leadership.uoregon.edu/resources/quotes). You have to be willing to follow through with your thoughts and maybe it will make a difference in someone's life in a positive way. That's what we continuously challenge each other to do!

Jen: Lamott (1994) elaborates, "there are probably a number of ways to tell your story right, and someone else may be able to tell you whether or not you've found one of these ways" (p. 163). By telling my story only to myself, I only see my perspective of it. Seeing my story from Eric's perspective enabled me to learn new insights about myself as a writer. Whenever Eric responds to my writing and writes something well, it motivates me to push myself and write better than I would without a coauthor. When he does his best work, I want to do the same.

LESSON #7: ENJOY THE JOURNEY AND KEEP AN OPEN MIND ALONG THE WAY

Interdisciplinary collaborations can lead to new insights and ideas.

Eric: So many times people in the medical field feel like they can only learn from other clinicians or whatever new research article or book gets published. Sometimes all you have to do is have an open mind for other possibilities and your possibilities are endless. For Jen and me working on research together, we were both given the opportunity to learn from each other. We are hoping that we can help clinicians in the medical field with the results from our research which focuses on the patient's outlook throughout physical therapy and the amount of objective improvements he or she makes.

Jen: Getting out of my comfort zone means being vulnerable because I'm working in a new field where I force myself to admit I don't know much. It means keeping an open mind for the possibilities that can happen. Cameron (1998) elaborates, "vulnerability requires that we contradict ourselves. It requires that we change our minds. It requires that our perspective shifts" (p. 148). Stepping out of the world of literary debates that exist in my English teaching world felt like stepping into a scary new world that made me vulnerable but also excited about new possibilities.

LESSON #8: SHARE IT

By sharing our experiences, we hope to inspire you and your students to participate in your own interdisciplinary collaborations with colleagues in your school and community. Daniels and Zemelman (2004) explain, "while more and more schools are creating smaller learning communities to enable such cooperative work, the great majority of us do not have this opportunity" (p. 220). If opportunities do not exist, we must find the courage to create them.

Jen: When I have teams of students discussing ideas, I ask them to share what they learn with the rest of the class at the conclusion of the discussion. This sharing becomes a celebration of their accomplishments and can lead to new ideas.

Eric: If Jen did not share how she felt while I was treating her at my clinic I would not have been able to modify her treatment program to help her get better. If we did not share our idea of the possible relationship of patients writing down their thoughts and keeping a positive outlook during their physical therapy process we would not have gotten a publication and be currently doing research. By keeping this mindset of sharing who knows what could happen in the future!

No matter how many times teachers discuss literature with students, the endings of novels never change. Gatsby will never get back together with Daisy. Elizabeth will always find love with Darcy. Anna Karenina always meets her fate on an unfortunate date with that train. Writing, however, changes as its authors change by unlocking the world and helping to make sense of life.

Writing can also lead to insightful ideas and collaborations. This was the story of our collaboration and the lessons we learned from it. We want our research and writing to continue to help the patients at Eric's clinic and the students in Jen's classroom. We hope it inspires you to complete your own writing, have less stress in your life with more time for things that bring you joy, and design your own narratives of interdisciplinary synergy.

ACKNOWLEDGMENT

The preceding chapter contains excerpts from the following previous IGI publications:

Wanner, E.T., & Bird, J.L. (2014). Incorporating a new technology for patient education. In V.C.X. Wang (Ed.), *Handbook of education and technology in a changing society* (pp. 162-174). Hershey, PA: Information Science Reference.

Reprinted in the IGI publication:

Wanner, E.T., & Bird, J.L. (2017). Incorporating a new technology for patient education. In Information Resources Management Association, (Ed.), *Healthcare ethics and training* (pp. 662-675). Hershey, PA: Information Science Reference.

Bird, J.L., & Wanner, E.T. (2014). Enhancing health education with collaborative narratives. In V.C.X. Wang (Ed.), *Handbook of education and technology in a changing society* (pp. 820-830). Hershey, PA: Information Science Reference.

REFERENCES

Alexander, E. (2012). *Proof of Heaven*. New York, NY: Simon and Schuster.

Austen, J. (2005). *Pride and prejudice*. New York, NY: Penguin. (Original work published 1813) doi:10.5117/9781904633013

Barrett, D. (2013). What is paintracking? *Pain Pathways*, *6*(1), 36–41.

Beck, M. (2001). *Finding your own North Star*. New York, NY: Three Rivers Press.

Bradley, E. H., Bogardus, S. T. Jr, Tinetti, M. E., & Inouye, S. K. (1999). Goal setting in clinical medicine. *Social Science & Medicine*, *49*(2), 267–278. doi:10.1016/S0277-9536(99)00107-0 PMID:10414834

Brown, B. (2012). *Daring greatly*. New York, NY: Gotham Books.

Cameron, J. (1998). *The right to write*. New York, NY: Tarcher/Putnam.

Cameron, J. (2002). *The artist's way* (2nd ed.). New York, NY: Tarcher/Putnam.

Cheo, K. (2012). Goal setting: why 90% of us don't do it effectively. *Boston Business Journal*. Retrieved from http://www.bizjournals.com/boston/blog/mass-high-tech/2012/09/goal-setting-why-90-of-us-dont-do.html?page=all

Chua, C. (2009). *6 important reasons why you should set goals*. Retrieved from http://personalexcellence.co/blog/6-important-reasons-why-you-should-set-goals

Clandinin, D. J., & Connelly, F. M. (2000). *Narrative inquiry*. San Francisco, CA: Jossey-Bass.

Connelly, F. M., & Clandinin, D. J. (1988). *Teachers as curriculum planners*. New York, NY: Teachers College press.

Daniels, H., & Zemelman, S. (2004). *Subject matters*. Portsmouth, NH: Heinemann.

Driscoll, M. (2012). *Edith Wharton: 10 best quotes on her 150th birthday.* Retrieved from http://www.csmonitor.com/Books/2012/0123/Edith-Wharton-10-best-quotes-on-her-150th-birthday/Giving-happiness-to-others

Fitzgerald, F. S. (1925). *The great Gatsby*. New York, NY: Scribner.

Garber, C. E., Blissmer, B., Deschenes, M. R., Franklin, B. A., Lamonte, M. J., Lee, I. M., ... Swain, D. P. (2011). Quantity and quality of exercise for developing and maintaining cardiorespiratory, musculoskeletal, and neuromotor fitness in apparently healthy adults: Guidance for prescribing exercise. *Medicine and Science in Sports and Exercise*, *43*(7), 1334–1359. doi:10.1249/MSS.0b013e318213fefb PMID:21694556

Goldberg, N. (1990). *Wild mind*. New York, NY: Bantam.

Goldberg, N. (2000). *Thunder and lightning*. New York, NY: Bantam.

Goldberg, N. (2005). *Writing down the bones* (2nd ed.). Boston, MA: Shambhala.

Goldberg, N. (2007). *Old friend from far away*. New York, NY: Free Press.

Graves, D. H. (2001). *The energy to teach*. Portsmouth, NH: Heinemann.

Gruwell, E., & the The Freedom Writers. (1999). The Freedom Writers diary. New York, NY: Broadway.

Heard, G. (1995). *Writing toward home*. Portsmouth, NH: Heinemann.

Holden Leadership Center. (2009). *Great leadership quotes.* Retrieved from http://leadership.uoregon.edu/resources/quotes

Johnson, L. (2005). *Teaching outside the box.* San Francisco, CA: Jossey-Bass.

Lamott, A. (1994). *Bird by bird.* New York, NY: Anchor Books.

Mayo Clinic Staff. (2011). 7 benefits of regular physical activity. *Mayo Clinic.* Retrieved from http://www.mayoclinic.com/health/exercise/HQ01676

McCall, C. (2011). *Writing and healing.* Retrieved from http://www.psychologytoday.com/blog/overcoming-child-abuse/201103/writing-and-healing

Murray, D. M. (1996). *Crafting a life.* Portsmouth, NH: Heinemann.

Pipher, M. (2006). *Writing to change the world.* New York, NY: Riverhead.

Rankin, L. (2013). *Mind over medicine.* Carlsbad, CA: Hay House.

Rasminsky, A. (2012). The Story Doc. *Oprah, 13*(7), 88.

Romano, T. (2004). *Crafting authentic voice.* Portsmouth, NH: Heinemann.

Romano, T. (2013). *Fearless writing.* Portsmouth, NH: Heinemann.

Sharp, C. (2000). *A writer's workshop.* New York, NY: St. Martin's Press.

Tindle, H. (2013). *Up: how positive outlook can transform our health and aging.* New York, NY: Hudson Street Press.

Tolstoy, L. (2000). *Anna Karenina.* New York, NY: Penguin. (Original work published 1873)

University of Scranton. (2012). New Year's resolution statistics. *Journal of Clinical Psychology.* Retrieved from http://www.statisticbrain.com/new-years-resolution-statistics/

Vacca, R. T., Vacca, J. L., & Mraz, M. (2014). *Content area reading* (11th ed.). Boston, MA: Pearson.

Wanner, E.T., & Bird, J.L. (2013). *The Wanner Bird healing survey for pain recovery.* Academic Press.

Wilder, T. (1938). *Our town.* New York, NY: HarperPerennial.

Willamette University. (2011). *Research program brings together scholars from different disciplines*. Retrieved from http://www.willamette.edu/people/archives/2011/08/larc.html

Younger, J., Gandhi, V., Hubbard, E., & Mackey, S. (2012). Development of the Stanford expectations of treatment scale (SETS): A tool for measuring patient outcome expectancy in clinical trials. *Clinical Trials*, *9*(6), 767–776. doi:10.1177/1740774512465064 PMID:23169874

KEY TERMS AND DEFINITIONS

Artistic and Technical Writing: Artistic writing focuses on the writer's tone of word choice, also known as voice, while technical writing focuses on the writer's specificity of word choice. English teachers often design rubrics that incorporate both artistic and technical writing when evaluating student essays.

Behavior Changes: Making a conscious effort to make lifestyle changes. Medical doctor Hilary Tindle researched patient outlook in medicine; some people make negative choices to deal with stress, such as the numbing strategies Brene Brown researched, while other people make positive choices to deal with stress, such as following the exercise recommendations suggested by experts at the American College of Sports Medicine. Ultimately the choice of which behavior changes to implement in order to cope with stress belongs to each individual.

Before, During, and After (B-D-A) Lessons: A lesson planning framework in the field of teacher education discussed by Richard and Jo Anne Vacca and used by teachers to evaluate student learning before, during, and after the reading of a text.

Heart Maps: Discussed in the field of writing by Georgia Heard, heart maps ask writers to draw a heart and inside the heart write things that the writer loves.

Interdisciplinary Collaboration: This describes the teamwork that occurs when colleagues from different disciplines work together in order to learn about each other's field of expertise. As a result of interdisciplinary collaboration, opportunities are created that may not have been discovered if the collaboration had not taken place.

Journal Writing: The process of a person responding to prompts and writing about his or her thoughts and feelings. While journal writing is typically associated with writing classrooms, writing teachers including Julia Cameron, Natalie Goldberg, and Donald Murray advocate that journal writing can be done by anyone, anywhere. Students in an English classroom, patients in a physical therapy clinic, and readers of this chapter in their living rooms can pick up pen, paper, and just write.

Multigenre Writing: Discussed in the field of education by Tom Romano, a multigenre paper consists of two parts: creative writing in multiple genres and the writer's analysis of the genres.

Narrative Inquiry: Discussed in the field of research by F. Michael Connelly and D. Jean Clandinin, narrative inquiry is a qualitative interpretative form of research that focuses on the telling, retelling, and sharing of stories. Researchers who complete narrative inquiries interpret stories and search for common threads to find patterns.

Narrative Medicine: The field of medicine, used by programs such as the one Rita Charon founded at Columbia University, which encourages medical practitioners to use theories from the fields of literature and composition to enhance comprehension of the stories patients share.

Neck Pain Journal: Jen created a journal of how her neck was feeling and what she was doing when her neck felt pain. Eric read the journal and diagnosed what Jen needed to do to make her neck feel better.

Physical Therapy Outcome Measures: Tests used by physical therapists to measure the progress a patient makes, such as such as the DASH (Disabilities of the Arm Shoulder Hand), LEFS (Lower Extremity Functional Scale), NDI (Neck Disability Index), and Modified Oswestry (for back pain).

Synergistic Collaboration: Adapted from the dictionary definition of "synergistic," this process describes people that work together and accomplish more than they could alone. When people of different disciplines work together toward a common goal, they achieve excellence and make a difference.

Wanner-Bird Healing Survey for Pain Recovery: An original survey designed by Dr. Eric Wanner and Dr. Jennifer Bird. This survey features both numerical subjective questions, where patients are asked to respond to statements by circling a number from 1-5, and written subjective questions that score patients' written responses on a rubric with a score of 1, 3, or 5. The rubric incorporates both the technical and artistic dimensions of writing.

Writing Voice: Voice in writing describes how a writer uses word choice and tone to compose a journal entry or other written composition that reflects the personality of the writer.

Chapter 3
Narratives of Health Coaching

Jennifer Lynne Bird
Oxbridge Academy, USA

Eric T. Wanner
Palm Beach Sports Medicine and Orthopaedic Center, USA

ABSTRACT

Health coaching, a recent addition to the field of health education, provides a missing link in the healing journeys of patients. Integrative health coaching incorporates vision and values into a person's goal setting process. While health coaches frequently work with healthy people who want to make changes in their lives such as finding time to exercise or getting more sleep, this narrative focuses on a health coach working with the emotional needs of physical therapy patients in a hospital.

BACKGROUND OF INTEGRATIVE HEALTH COACHING

Integrative health coaches (IHCs), such as the ones trained at Duke University Integrative Medicine where Jen received her training, focus on an eclectic approach to healing. The Wheel of Health from Duke Integrative Medicine (2010) encourages patients to reflect on multiple dimensions of health including movement, exercise and rest; nutrition; personal and professional development, physical environment; relationships and communication; spirituality; mind-body connection; and mindful awareness (p. 5). This makes health become a comprehensive plan that focuses on the person, not just the disease.

DOI: 10.4018/978-1-7998-1931-8.ch003

Health coaching and conversations about the responses to both written and numerical subjective questions can help patients illuminate the health stories they tell themselves. Health coaching can also build a bridge between helping patients decode complex medical terms and comprehending their treatment plan. When patients feel that their medical practitioners and health coaches earn the right to hear their stories, the sharing of narratives can become healing conversations. Health coaches are not psychologists; if a patient wants to share a painful story about the past, the health coach will make a referral to a psychologist. Instead, health coaches help patients maintain forward momentum for achieving their goals by providing encouragement, suggestions for completing a prescribed treatment plan, translation of potentially confusing medical terms, and a supportive person to listen.

Steele (2009) encourages medical teams "to develop the tools and systems needed for effective and consistent patient education and expectation setting" (p. 99). Such tools, according to Jones, Brady, and Gaunt (2009), include "a diary showing type of surgery and progress" (p. 100) and "homework sheets that contain exercises and assignments for patients outside scheduled PT sessions" (p. 100). Health coaching provides patient education for patients. Health coaches also serve as another member of the support team for both patients and clinicians. As Helldorfer and Moss (2007) explain, "one important component in the way many medical facilities measure success is by the degree of patient satisfaction. How patients feel about the care they are receiving starts with first impressions. Taking the time to look a patient in the eye, say hello, and ask them how they feel is an ongoing challenge when we are busy" (p. 275). Health coaches follow up with patients about how they are feeling and provide a continual assessment for clinicians of how important each patient feels about the treatment plan and his or her confidence in achieving it. If the treatment plan a clinician provides is not important to a patient, the patient will be less likely to want to accomplish it. It therefore becomes the job of the health coach to determine what the patient values and how the patient can align the treatment plan with his or her values to achieve improved healing gains. If the patient is not confident he or she can accomplish the treatment plan, the patient will also be less likely to comply with it. Once patients become non-compliant it is not possible for them to get satisfactory results. It therefore becomes the job of the health coach to provide a vision of past success for the patient to build momentum in order to achieve future success.

Since health coaching is a new field in medicine, there is not a large amount of previous studies to share. Simmons and Wolever (2011) report, "broadly defined, health coaching is a method of working with patients that utilizes thoughtful inquiry, accountability, goal clarification, goal setting, identification of obstacles, use of support systems, and connection to intrinsic motivation, vision, and values to improve health through positive behavior change" (p. 1). Simmons and Wolever summarize the existing research and elaborate,

Despite the infancy of the research, several studies have demonstrated that coaching does improve health outcomes. The strongest findings have been in cardiovascular health, where coaching has been shown to improve total cholesterol, body mass index, stress, exercise, diet, and smoking cessation. Studies of cancer patients have demonstrated decreased pain severity and increased pain control. Studies of coaching for patients with diabetes and related kidney disease have shown increases in health promoting behaviors like physical activity and diet, as well as decreases in fasting blood glucose, hemoglobin A1C, hospital admission rates, and amputations. A coaching intervention also improved outcomes in obese patients (BMIs >30), including decreased waist circumferences and increased functional health status (p. 1).

Due to health coaching's success in other medical fields, it has the potential to be successful with physical therapy patients.

Because health coaching is individualized for each patient, Jen will adjust the questions she asks based on the patient responses. Some questions that health coaches ask include the following:

Describe your future health vision. What does it look like to you? How does the treatment plan that your physical therapist gave you connect to that vision? Rate on a scale of 1-10 (1=low, 10=high) how important the treatment plan is to you. (Questions then diverge depending on patient responses. The purpose of the questions is to align the treatment plan with the patient's value system). Sample question for low number response: What are some things you could do to make the treatment plan more important to you (listening to music during exercises, writing in a journal, setting goals, etc.)? Sample question for high number response: Now that I know this is really important to you, tell me on a scale of 1-10 (1 = low, 10 = high) how confident you are accomplishing this treatment plan. (Questions then diverge depending on patient responses. The purpose of the questions is to provide the patient with a vision of success). Sample question for low number response: Tell me more about a past success you had when you achieved a goal. Sample question for high number response: Are there any obstacles we haven't addressed that would prevent you from achieving your goal?

At the conclusion of the health coaching session, Jen will offer suggestions for the patient based on the patient's response, but the purpose of health coaching is not to tell the patient what to do; the purpose is to empower the patient to take ownership of his or her own health. Jen will also provide resources as needed (give the patient a notebook if he or she wants to write in a journal, etc.)

HEALTH COACHING: THE MISSING LINK IN COMPASSIONATE CARE

As anyone who has ever been a patient can tell you, being a patient is not easy. Helldorfer and Moss (2007) elaborate, "patients enter a hospital with many unspoken fears. Most of the time they don't say a word either because they're not in touch with their feelings or they're embarrassed to express them. Some do not want to make waves. For the most part, they have an underlying belief in the technical proficiency of the professional taking care of them, yet most of them secretly yearn to be reassured anyway that they are in good hands and that we care as much about their well being as they do. We can take our profession to the next level by understanding our patients' needs beyond the unspoken" (pp. 50-51). As much as medical professionals such as doctors, nurses, and physical therapists want to be able to have long conversations with their patients, health care frequently has to focus on productivity with doctors needing to see a certain amount of patients in any given hour due to continual reimbursement cuts from insurance companies. Rankin (2013) reformed her own medical practice after learning the value of nurturing care instead of always having her hand on the door when talking to a patient and elaborates, "I now firmly believe that positive belief and nurturing care turn off the stress response, trigger the relaxation response, and return the body to its natural state of psychological rest so it can do what it does best – heal itself" (p. 79). While Dr. Mark Greene was a character on the medical drama *ER* and not a real life doctor, his advice to colleague Dr. John Carter describes today's real hospitals as well as fictional television ones: the staff of the hospital sets the tone for how patients feel about their treatment.

Furthermore, taking time to talk to patients is not contradictory to efficiency. Jones, Steele, and McClennan (2009) explain, "improving patient satisfaction and patient outcomes while reducing costs will create more value in our healthcare system" (p. 28). A patient feels happier when he or she feels a medical professional sees a person, not just a description on a chart. To do this, Jones, Steele, and McClennan continue, "we must tap into their values and preferences as much as possible" (p. 32). Vision and values are the additional piece of the healing process that health coaching provides. As summarized by Smith and Wroth (2011) the integrative health coaching process begins with vision and values, then proceeds with assessment, focus, readiness to change, goal setting, preparation for action, action, and maintenance (p. 59). Most treatment plans begin with a medical practitioner setting goals for patients. The patient is more likely to accomplish the goals if he or she feels ownership and that the treatment plan aligns with his or her vision and values. Jones, Steele, and McClennan (2009) add, "in addition, patients appreciate being made part of the solution" (p. 34). Health coaching encourages patients to set their own goals in addition to goals prescribed for them. While compassionate clinicians can provide patient education and empathy, health coaches become an additional person on the patient's health care team. Health coaches can assist patients by helping them frame their goals in easy to comprehend language while being an empathetic presence in the patient's life.

Health coaches provide patients with the gift of being present by practicing mindful awareness to remain focused on the present moment. Helldorfer and Moss (2007) state, "to be a healing presence, we must be genuinely present to the other person in need" (p. 170). This means the focus must be on the current patient, not on the long to do list that needs to be accomplished. Even within the fast pace of a hospital, it becomes important to slow down. Helldorfer and Moss explain, "within health care, our mission is to foster the health and healing of our patients. It is easy to forget that before we can bring a healing presence to others, we first have to slow down to be present" (p. 180). In fact, health coaches refer to the people they help as clients instead of patients to provide a different connotation to the professional relationship that implies a partnership instead of a doctor issuing a prescription. Health coaches partner with their clients to facilitate the change process. Pipher (2006) explains, "with our presence and attention, we suggest that honest exploration of issues is healing and that hiding from them is toxic" (p. 86). While not psychologists like Pipher, health coaches are trained in psychology and provide patients with a safe space to explore issues and obstacles that may prevent them from reaching their healing goals. Pipher continues, "facilitating a change process in clients or readers often involves orchestrating situations that allow for aha experiences" (p. 101). This is why health coaches listen more than they talk during a session and use reflective responses so a client can hear his or her own words and perhaps have an 'aha' moment. Health coaches partner with patients to advance their health and accomplish this by reviewing patients' health narratives, assisting patients in setting goals, promoting positivity, helping patients rewrite their health story, and supporting patients on their healing journey.

WRITING NARRATIVES

Every patient has a story. How much about a patient's story does a clinician know? In conducting research about outlook and aging, medical doctor Hilary Tindle (2013) reports, "our outlook, which colors our reaction to everything, can set in motion a physiologic chain reaction that we may not even be aware of, a process that ebbs and flows constantly. In medical terminology, this process is called the 'neuroendocrine response to stress' where stress is essentially any stimulus that engages us" (p. 15). Tindle discovered only one percent of people achieve ideal cardiac health and one of the questions she included on a list that existing research has yet to answer was, "what is the script going on inside their heads, if there is one?" (p. 24). For years, English teachers have used writing to learn about the script going on inside people's heads. Writing teacher Julia Cameron (1998) explains, "when we are telling the truth about how we feel and what we see, we find very precise language with which to do it" (p. 140). Writing provides a method for clinicians to learn about the script in patients' heads.

Pages of a notebook provide a place for patients to process their thoughts and also create a journal of symptoms. If a physical therapist reads the patient's journal, he or she can then make adjustments to the treatment plan if the patient's observations illuminate additional insights. It can also provide personal awareness and accountability to the current situation for the patient. Cameron (1998) emphasizes the importance of reflecting on feelings and states, "writing can be done the same way. It can be done by listening to how we feel rather than thinking about how we feel" (p. 156). Health coaches do not have to use journals with patients, but if the patient is willing and able to share thoughts in writing, journals can provide an additional healing resource. Writing should not be seen as a required homework assignment, but rather a chance for exploration and insight. To do this, writing teachers such as Natalie Goldberg (1986) recommend writing quickly without thinking too much about the words on the page since "the aim is to burn through to first thoughts, to the place where energy is unobstructed by social politeness or the internal censor, to the place where you are writing what your mind actually sees and feels, not what it thinks it should see or feel" (p. 8). Writing captures a writer's first impressions and truest thoughts, and although health coaches must never pressure anyone to share, often people want someone to know their story. It then becomes the decision of the writer whether or not to share the writing with the health coach, physical therapist, or anyone else.

While writing has healing value for the writer regardless of whether or not it is shared, if writing is used during health coaching, knowing a patient's perspective can provide the health coach with additional information to help with goal setting. Goldberg (2000) feels, "but there does come a time – I can't honestly tell you when – that we must step over the line of practice and speak and expect to be heard. But no one's listening, we whine. Then we have to figure out how to make them listen" (p. 180). How many times do patients think of one more question or observation after the medical practitioner has left the room? Even though medical practitioners are trained to hear sensitive health stories, patients may still feel embarrassed to share them which could actually make their situation harder to diagnose. The most eloquent person may still be rendered speechless when needing to ask a personal health question. Noppe-Brandon (2004) describes this feeling as, "everyone I know has felt either unheard or inarticulate at some time. Not everyone wants or needs to become a theatre artist, but everyone I know has some fears about and perceives limitations in their ability to articulate themselves" (p. xiv). Writing captures questions and fears on paper so patients can get the answers they need.

BE SMART AND SET GOALS

Goals provide people with something to strive for in life. Whether a teacher teaches a lesson plan, a physical therapist designs a treatment plan, or an individual sets a personal goal, the acronym SMART can be used to describe the goals. Soukup (2019) explains, "it's basically the idea that your goals should be Specific, Measurable, Attainable, Relevant, and Time Bound.

Meaning you should know exactly what you are trying to do; your goal should be quantifiable in some way; it should be something you can actually accomplish; it should be meaningful to you; and it should have a deadline" (pp. 102-103).

Health coaches trained at Duke University Integrative Medicine encourage clients to think SMART (specific, measurable, action oriented, realistic, timed) when setting goals. Professors at Florida Atlantic University encourage students training to be teachers to think SMART (specific content, measurable outcome, attainable action verb, resources, timeframe) when planning a lesson. Physical therapists use a similar goal setting procedure for their patients as well. Randall and McEwen (2000) elaborate, "we define functional goals as the individually meaningful activities that a person cannot perform as a result of an injury, illness, or congenital acquired condition, but wants to be able to accomplish as a result of physical therapy" (p. 1198). While the SMART acronym is not explicitly stated in the discussion of functional goals, the procedure is implicitly described as patients are encouraged to collaborate with their physical therapist in goal setting. Randall and McEwen advise therapists,

Often the best way to identify patient-centered functional goals is simply to ask the patient, 'What are your goals for therapy?' In our experience, patients seldom focus on impairments and rarely say, 'I'd like my range of motion to be within normal limits' or 'I'd like to have 5/5 strength.' They are likely to respond with a focus on functional limitation or disability: 'I want to return to work,' 'I need to be able to take care of myself at home,' 'I want to play in the game on Saturday,' or 'I want to do what the other kids do at my school.' These statements can become the starting point for writing measurable patient-centered functional goals (p. 1199).

Furthermore, health coaches use a similar approach as physical therapists for encouraging patients to set their goals. When talking to a health coach, patients also tend to focus on a personal vision instead of the treatment plan, such as perhaps not valuing the exercises but wanting to go on a cruise in a couple months. The health coach can help the patient make the connection that the exercises provided by the physical therapist can help accomplish the goal of going on the cruise. Health coaches encourage patients to dream big but also be realistic to avoid disappointment. Coates (1999) emphasizes, "goals must be realistic in terms of patients' situations and expectations, their likely length of contact with health professionals, the available resources motivated them to care more. The same applied to my research with Eric. I found myself caring more about medicine just because he loves it, and he cared more about writing because I love it.

Overall, bringing the two unique perspectives together creates an interesting project.

LESSON #3: IT'S ABOUT THE TEAM

Teams, whether they are working together on a sports field, in a classroom, or on a research project, find a way to work together and make the project work.

Jen: When discussing what to do next with our research, Eric and I will be debating possibilities. I usually find myself saying something like, "we'll figure it out." Perhaps I don't need to be explicit and state it. It's implicit a good team will achieve results and implied there will always be a solution to any problem that arises.

Eric: It's very important that everyone on the team makes equal contributions to achieve optimal results. So many times people work in a group and one person does a huge majority of the work. Think of how much better that project could have been if everyone used their minds together and contributed equally!

Graves (2001) believes, "I've found there is energy in preparing to help others" (p. 39). Effective teams encourage each other, support each other, and find energy in each other's ideas.

Jen: To inspire my students to use positive interdependence when working together, I use an idea from one of my former college professors and pick teams randomly by passing a deck of cards around the room and telling everyone who has the same number to work together. Some of them may never have worked with members of their team before, but by talking to someone new, they learn something new. Students comment that working with people outside of their circle of friends may be uncomfortable at first, but conversations occur that never would have taken place otherwise. Some students even admit to developing new friendships because of working together.

and the abilities of the educators" (p. 84). Goals also give patients a sense of control. Kolt (2003) discusses goal setting with athletes and explains, "by having a sense of control over their rehabilitation programs, athletes can increase commitment and adherence to the behaviors required for successful rehabilitation" (pp. 176-177). The same philosophy that applies to athletes can apply to any patient recovering from an injury or any individual looking to create change in their lives. Brown (2012), a professor of social work, believes, "hope is a combination of setting goals, having the tenacity and perseverance to pursue them, and believing in our own abilities" (p. 240). The biggest gift health coaches and physical therapists can give their patients is the gift of hope.

Health coaches, just like physical therapists, use reflective listening to identify themes in a patient's story. Croft (1980) provides the example that "because of the frequency and intensity of therapist-patient verbal and nonverbal interaction, each therapist must consider the potential therapeutic or destructive power of his every response. An effective response is one that fulfills one or more of these processes: clarification, reflection, interpretation, facilitation, or silence" (p. 1035). Such conversations lead to what Randall and McEwen (2000) call writing patient-centered functional goals because "after the therapist and the patient have decided on general outcomes of physical therapy, measurable goals leading to achievement of the outcomes should be identified" (p. 1200). With health coaching, patients set personal goals for themselves in addition to the treatment goals set by the physical therapist. The purpose is that if a patient becomes empowered to feel both extrinsic (external) motivation from the physical therapist as well as intrinsic (internal) motivation from within, there will be a stronger ownership of the goal. Randall and McEwen continue, "we also believe this approach to writing patient-centered functional goals will make therapy more effective and meaningful for patients, and perhaps for the therapist as well" (p. 1202). The encouragement from physical therapists, health coaches, and other medical practitioners on the team can lead the patient to feel supported and not alone on the healing journey.

Sometimes when patients experience pain, they can't picture what it feels like to do the things they love again; therefore, the power of visualization can help patients set goals. Beck (2001) discusses how visualization can help people achieve what she calls Wildly Improbable Goals (WIGs) and elaborates, "the thing was that, even though I didn't really think I could attain these goals, from the day I wrote them down I had something in my little brain that scientists might call a 'search image.' A search image is a subconscious alertness toward something you hope to find" (pp. 302-303). Writing a list of goals or using a form of artwork such as a dream board collage helps people picture what they wish to accomplish. Beck continues, "forming a goal, especially if you write it down and visualize it, creates a search image that programs your brain to focus on anything resembling or leading to that objective" (p. 303). Of course, simply visualizing a goal without taking any action won't lead to results. As Beck advises, "try to visualize every step you must take to realize the WIG you've got stuck on your planning board. If you don't know exactly – and I mean exactly – what you must do to achieve your WIG, your scheme still needs elaboration" (p. 309). The key to setting a successful goal means thinking about what you want to achieve, not what anyone else in your life thinks you should accomplish.

Granted, patients often have healing goals set for them, such as when a physical therapist makes a goal for a patient to be able to ambulate independently throughout the community for up to 300 feet to be able to safely get groceries after two weeks of treatment. If patients can set their own goals that align with the prescribed treatment plan, they will be more likely to comply with that plan. And if patients need help setting personal goals in addition to the treatment goals set for them by the physical therapist, a health coach can guide the patient through the goal setting process. Arturburn (2011) believes, "whether it is a physician, a health practitioner, a counselor, or a trusted friend, the need to connect during the pain-to-healing process is profound" (p. 104). When a patient feels encouraged by a strong health care team, everyone can celebrate the progress toward goals regardless of the speed at which those goals are achieved. "Thinking like a turtle," or making slow and steady progress, leads to elite results.

PROMOTING POSITIVITY

When Jones, Brady, and Gaunt (2009) speak of coaches, they are talking about family members instead of health coaches as they advise, "one of the coaches' responsibilities is to come to post-op group therapy classes, where they act as assistant physical therapists. Coaches encourage their loved ones and are shown and taught the dos and don'ts by the physical therapist. Many times, coaches are equipped with digital counters to ensure completion of the activities. If no family member is available, hospital volunteers often take up the coaching role" (p. 102). Family members as coaches can serve as an additional source of encouragement for patients as they complete their physical therapy treatment plan. Throughout the family coaching process, health coaches provide education and support for the families of patients. While family members will have the best intentions when serving as coaches for their loved ones, it is easy for the family to become emotionally involved because the outcome of the patient's progress affects the entire family. Health coaches provide encouragement, while providing objective distance often missing when family members coach their loved ones. Health coaches care about their clients, but they are not attached to the outcome like family members are and can provide observations family members are sometimes unwilling or unable to see unfolding due to being too close to the situation.

Health coaches also share resources for family members to take care of themselves as they take care of their loved ones. Most importantly, health coaches work with physical therapists to "teach the teachers," the family member who will take over the patient's care once the patient returns home. The importance of this is once the patient goes back home there will be a continuity of care for the patient while he or she is awaiting home physical therapy and then out-patient physical therapy. This can lead to quicker recoveries for patients. And if everyone, from the health coach to the family to the patient to all the members of the medical team work together, the beneficiary is the patient. Helldorfer and Moss (2007) share, "and, if we think through the domino effect of our work, the life we save or extend impacts families almost beyond comprehension" (p. 191). Health coaching can start or continue a positive ripple effect; drop a pebble into a pond and see how far the water spreads. As teachers know, students remember their words long after classes end. Brady and Vega (2009) observe, "the best way to learn is to teach" (p. 128). Nevertheless, as Brady and Vega continue, "most places lack a teaching and learning culture, because no one has organized it" (p. 128). Health coaches do not give lectures like professors in classrooms, but they can provide teachable moments for patients. Just like coaches of sports teams, health coaches intertwine education and encouragement to help patients keep a positive attitude while shifting motivation from the extrinsic of doing something just because a doctor says to the intrinsic of doing something because of a sense of personal accomplishment.

Maintaining a positive attitude helps patients heal. Medical doctor Lissa Rankin (2013) describes the medical science behind the connections between positive attitude and healing as "when our beliefs are hopeful and optimistic, the mind releases chemicals that put the body in a state of physiological rest, controlled primarily by the parasympathetic nervous system, and in this state of rest, the body's natural self-repair mechanisms are free to get to work fixing what's broken in the body" (p. 29). She elaborates, "if, however, the mind thinks negative beliefs, the brain perceives these as a threat" (p. 29). While a positive attitude can lead to healing, a negative attitude can lead to a stress response in the body. Rankin concludes, "It's not enough to focus solely on the body without taking into account the health of the mind" (p. 74). She changed her patient intake form and added questions about life issues as well as medical ones. Tindle (2013) concurs, "Why should outlook matter more for people who are medically 'down'? A big part of the answer, as we've seen, is that our outlook naturally influences the way we care for ourselves. Thus the associated benefits of looking up have to do with the fact that a brighter disposition goes hand in hand with better self-care and making healthier choices" (p. 199). Healthier choices can influence a patient's life long after a hospital stay concludes. As Helldorfer and Moss (2007) write, "that is what being a healing presence means – leaving others a little better as a result of our care" (p. 206). Health coaching means empowering patients to take ownership of their own health stories.

REWRITING A HEALTH STORY

Regardless of whether a person is a patient needing inpatient physical therapy after surgery or a mostly healthy individual looking to make a few adjustments to improve health, each person possesses the power to write his or her own health story. Connelly and Clandinin (1988) explain the value of believing in the power of our own narratives by providing the reminder, "narrative is designed to be thought of as an overall life study. As such it encompasses a person's past, his or her current state of mind, and his or her personal knowledge, which shapes teaching work in the future" (p. 34). Health coaches love narratives. Clandinin and Connelly (2000) discuss, "formalists begin inquiry in theory, whereas narrative inquirers tend to begin with experience as expressed in lived and told stories" (p. 40). Traditional narrative inquiries focus on past, present, and future, but health coaches meet the patient in the present.

While psychologists help patients process past experiences, health coaching focuses on the present moment to help clients build a vision for the future. Health coaching brings a contemporary addition to the traditional field of medicine, but in order to best serve patients, change becomes necessary. Helldorfer and Moss (2007) explain, "having the freedom to implement new ways of doing things is critical if we want to become the organization we envision" (p. 274). A hospital with a health coach adds an additional compassionate professional to its team while simultaneously being on the cutting edge of medicine.

Health coaching empowers patients to control and rewrite their narratives. Sometimes we can't control the things that happen to us, such as a scary health diagnosis. We can, however, control our reaction to the events and also control how we make meaning from the story. The advice Brown (2012) gives to herself and others is, "own the story! Don't bury it and let it fester or define me" (p. 80). No matter what has happened in the past, health coaches help their clients believe change is possible in the future. It doesn't matter where you've been or what you can't change in the past; it matters where you are going and what you can do to create a better future. Richardson (1997) reflects on the process of bringing new meaning to old stories and shares, "the process of rereading one's work and situating it in historical and biographical contexts reveals old story lines, many of which may not have been articulated. Voicing them offers the opportunity to rewrite them, to renarrativize one's life" (p. 5). Through conversations where the health coach reflects a client's words, a person can hear his or her own story and gain new insights. When people hear the stories they tell themselves, they may reflect how the meanings they give the stories can change with a different interpretation of the narrative.

Changing one's health story occurs whether a client is an overall healthy person looking to make behavior changes or a patient recovering from an illness. Arterburn (2011) believes, "every illness provides us with choices. In the context of healing, the greatest choice is the decision to pursue healing! When people make that choice, they typically improve" (p. 52). Healing can take place as a physical therapy patient follows through with a treatment plan to return to normal activity. Healing can also take place when a healthy person makes minor lifestyle changes in order to achieve major health benefits. For everyone, the future remains unwritten with opportunities for healthy decisions.

SPIRITUALITY AND HEALTH COACHING

Just like health coaches are not psychologists, they are also not ministers either and cannot take the place of a confidential spiritual counselor if a patient requests a session with hospital clergy. Health coaches often integrate their other areas of expertise into their practice; for example, Jen is also a certified English teacher of literature and writing and received Stephen Minister training at her church. However, she will always let the patient conversations lead the way. If a patient is receptive to writing or asks to pray, Jen has the expertise to provide additional resources to the patient. As a health coach, she can also make referrals to colleagues with other areas of expertise, such as consulting with colleague and physical therapist Eric if a patient requests more information about exercise or nutrition as part of the treatment plan.

While some patients may prefer to write their thoughts, others may prefer to speak them in prayer. Writing teacher Georgia Heard (1995) states, "all writing is in a sense prayer – a sending out of hope, a thanksgiving, a celebration, a song sent into the wind that we hope someone will hear" (p. 113). Regardless of a patient's religious beliefs, a sense of purpose is something health coaching has in common with spirituality. Spiritual beliefs and health coaching can help people connect the seemingly disconnected threads of their lives and find meaning in them. If patients have a sense of purpose and can mentally time travel into the future to imagine achieving their health goals, the goals they set become part of their larger life's purpose as they make the choice to heal. Arterburn (2011) explains, "though we acknowledge that there are many ways to be healed, the choice to heal, whether it is physical, spiritual, or psychological, is a personal choice each person must make" (p. 54). Healing is a journey, not a destination. Haugk (2012) states, "victories are results of many actions well executed; or in other words, victories come as a result of process" (p. 141). So celebrate the small victories; turtles make slow progress, but they eventually arrive where they need to go.

For patients, the journey to healing involves being vulnerable and finding the courage to share stories with people who can help. Brown (2012) explains, "from the field of health psychology, studies show that perceived vulnerability, meaning the ability to acknowledge our risks and exposure, greatly increases our chances of adhering to some kind of positive health regimen" (pp. 39-40). It becomes easier to share when a patient has a health coach and other compassionate clinicians who listen to a patient's hopes, dreams, and fears without judgment. Helldorfer and Moss (2007) remind practitioners, "an integral part of healing is the quality of human contact a patient experiences during the time they are with us" (p. 193). When a patient knows someone accepts his or her story, the next chapter of the story can begin to be written. To some people, this symbolizes a spiritual connection; to others, it means a stronger sense of awareness. Helldorfer and Moss continue, "the spiritual side of life is always present. The spiritual side of life is embedded within, and not separate from, the ordinariness of everyday life" (p. 295). By taking time to have a vision and values centered conversation with patients while also assessing the importance of a physical therapist's treatment plan and the confidence in achieving that plan, health coaches can help patients transform an ordinary moment in the hospital into an extraordinary moment of hope and healing. Oprah Winfrey (2014) reminds us, "the hardest experiences are often the ones that teach us the most" (p. 141). A health coach provides a supportive presence while the client walks through such experiences.

BUILDING SUCCESS

To provide resources as patients travel their healing journeys, the hospital where Eric and Jen worked opened a new building for inpatient rehabilitation. This center of innovation will enhance the patient experience by focusing on a comprehensive treatment plan for patients as well as the staff crystallizing as a cohesive team. As the research consultant, Eric used a data driven approach to promote the educational process of RICE (reflection, innovation, collaboration, evaluation) for clinicians. Eric brought together the most recent evidence-based research for acute care after a total joint or spine surgery for the physical therapy department to follow for elite results for the patients.

Even though it takes a patient time to heal from surgery, understandably a large number of hospital patients want to leap out of bed and get on with their lives. This can make things worse, as all education is a journey. Students can't expect to attend one class and be an expert, much like patients can't expect to heal overnight. Have faith and trust the process. Romano (1987) writes of the writing process, "all along the process it is imperative that the teacher-crafter demonstrates to apprentices all the stages of the writing process" (p. 58). Teachers demonstrate the writing process to students, while physical therapists demonstrate exercises to their patients. In both instances, learners have a role model.

Part of the hospital's plan to promote active knee movement for patients is a class designed to show patients the correct techniques for exercises. This provides the benefit of learning exercises as well as the group support from other patients who are students in the class. For thirty years teachers have used peer groups in classrooms. Romano (1987) describes his classroom as, "most students will risk saying more among their peers than with me. And, of course, the students can learn from each other in this close contact" (p. 70). By observing each other's learning exercises, patients in a physical therapy class can learn from each other as well as the physical therapist. Whether someone is a patient in a hospital or a student in a classroom, active participation becomes a necessity. The key becomes active learning. Walk into any teacher's classroom and notice that students learn more if they can participate in an activity instead of only talking about the strategy. Students need to work their brains just like physical therapy patients need to work their muscles. Johnson (1998) advocates, "unsuccessful students are rarely good goal setters. They blame their failure on other people, circumstances or luck. One of the most valuable lessons you can teach your students is how to set realistic goals, make a list of steps to move them forward, evaluate their progress, revise goals when necessary, and to set a new, higher goal, once a goal has been reached" (p. 137). Work = progress. You need to actively do something to get somewhere.

This hospital rehabilitation center meets the needs of patients through having physical therapists teach classes to scaffold knowledge, providing individual support through treatment sessions, and giving patients a goal to look forward to by having a graduation day celebration with a ceremony where patients spin a wheel (not the Wheel of Health) and receive a gift. Patients, whether they have surgery for their backs, necks, hips, or knees, are encouraged to journal and reflect on their personal healing goals. By promoting a community of health and wellness, the hospital will change the curriculum of health education. Greene (1995) writes of the curricular change process, "inevitably, curriculum has had to deal with ambiguities, with relationships; it has often opened the way to transformations and unexpected change" (p. 90). By designing a curriculum that will provide orthopedic excellence, the hospital's team of transformative leaders will create positive change in the lives of their patients and the patients' families.

COACHING AS RELATIONSHIP-BASED CARE

Health coaching is a type of Relationship-Based Care. Koloroutis (2004) defines, "Relationship-Based Care (RBC) is comprised of three crucial relationships: care provider's relationship with patients and families, care provider's relationship with self, and care provider's relationship with colleagues" (p. 4). While the primary focus of health coaching is on the care-receiver, it is also essential for the care provider to have strong self-care in order to help others, as well as be part of a team of colleagues working together to provide an integrative approach to medicine and healing. Koloroutis continues, "the care provider knows that each person's unique life story determines how he or she will experience an illness" (p. 5). Health coaches realize that while a person's unique life story leads to the moment when care is needed, it is possible to start from the present moment and add a new chapter where the life story does not become defined by illness. According to Koloroutis, "true healers provide the space for patients to heal themselves" (p. 249). Health coaches, like any Relationship-Based Care practitioner, provide encouragement and empowerment for people to take ownership of their health so they can heal.

Sometimes healing becomes enhanced in a group setting, also known as group coaching. In group coaching, participants sit in a circle and share their goals and dreams. Group coaching may look like group therapy, but it is not. Instead, group coaching more closely resembles a college writing seminar, where participants have the opportunity to respond in writing to a prompt, and then choose whether or not to share. The coach facilitates a safe space where participants can motivate each other and encourage each other to succeed. Personal and private health information is never revealed by the coach in group coaching, but by finding common ground participants see they are not alone. Baldwin (1998) discusses the value of calling a circle and elaborates, "the circle can act as a trustworthy group of people who mirror back to us our own unique qualities" (p. 139). Circle time creates a supportive environment for people to share their experiences with others.

FROM THEORY TO PRACTICE

Now that you've read extensive theory about health coaching, here is my (Jen's) story of practicing health coaching. I share my story because health coaching involves learning people's stories. To best help people, health coaches practice active listening and ask questions to know more about the narratives people tell themselves and others. Narrative insights can provide as much valuable information as numbers on a patient's chart. Helldorfer and Moss (2007) believe, "we are players on a hallowed stage, writing our own lines as we perform" (p. 182). If that sentiment sounds like it was written by an English teacher and not two professionals in the health care field, it serves as a reminder that sharing stories plays a valuable role in patient care. Health coaches, however, must adhere to strict guidelines of confidentiality in order to build trust with the people who share their stories. Therefore, due to the ethical issues of creating a powerful culture where patients feel safe knowing their personal stories will not be shared with a public audience, in this chapter it is not possible for you to read patient stories except in vague, generalized snapshots. In order for you as the reader to gain a deeper understanding of how recounting events drives a life story, I use my own personal example to illustrate the value of finding themes in the narratives people tell others while simultaneously protecting the information discussed with me by patients.

Stories help us find common ground, see life from a different perspective, and remind us that someone knows who we are and cares to let us know we are not alone on our journey. I'm an English professor. Analyzing writing and pulling out themes from a composition feels as natural to me as breathing. A powerful piece of writing synthesizes old ideas and sparks new ones. Health coaching pulls elements from different fields, all of which were part of my life before I ever took my first class at Duke Integrative Medicine. Health coaching requires the strength of listening to people's stories and finding themes in the narratives. Patients complete a combination of numerical subjective and written subjective questions about their current and desired states. They rank numerically on a scale of 1 (low) and 10 (high) how they feel about different aspects of health and respond to a corresponding writing prompt explaining why they assigned that number. The health coach needs to read the writing, pull together the narrative threads, and connect them into a cohesive theme. Clandinin and Connelly (2000) describe the qualitative interpretive field of narrative inquiry as, "we tell remembered stories of ourselves from earlier times as well as more current stories. All of these stories offer possible plotlines for our futures" (p. 60). As an English professor, I enjoy reading the stories of others through works of literature and encouraging my students to write their own stories. Health coaching uses the same principles of literary analysis and takes it one step further. Works of literature will always have the same ending, but health coaching encourages clients to write new endings to their stories.

One constant in writing theory, regardless of how the writing is put into practice, is a writer's desire to own his or her story. Richardson (1997) asks, "how do the specific circumstances in which we write affect what we write? How does what we write affect who we become? These are timeless and timely questions" (p. 1). As we change, our writing changes, but at the heart of an individual's writing lives a narrative of that person's wishes, hopes, dreams, and goals. Writing captures who we are in a moment of time. Richardson elaborates, "narrative displays the goals and intentions of human actors; it makes individuals, cultures, societies, and historical epochs comprehensible as wholes; it humanizes time; and it allows us to contemplate the effects of our actions and to alter the directions of our lives" (p. 27). Writing helps people comprehend the past, make sense of the present, and set goals for the future.

I once designed a curriculum board game to encourage the English teachers at the high school where I used to teach to share their ideas. During any change process, people need to believe they have a choice and a voice. In redesigning the English classes for high school juniors, I learned it becomes important to get all issues on the table. Greene (1995) explains, "I also believe we need to make it possible for writers to name not only the shapes and byways of their lived worlds but the problems and predicaments that have stopped and silenced them" (p, 108). No one wants to feel silenced when a new curriculum is planned and implemented. We must find the courage to speak. The important thing, according to Greene, is that "learning to write is a matter of learning to shatter the silences, of making meaning, of learning to learn" (p. 108). Teachers will resist change if they don't feel they are partners in the school's curriculum redesign plan, similar to the way patients will resist change if they don't feel they are partners in a medical treatment plan. Health coaches support the treatment plans designed by medical professionals such as physical therapists and don't change the plans. We do work with patients to build bridges which help them overcome resistance and feel part of the change process.

My dad is a city planner who is one of only several hundred people in the country to have the highest credential in the field. As a kid, I didn't care about my dad's credentials; I loved the field trips. Dad and I would get into the car and drive to study various pieces of land. What did the land look like? What potential did it have? Harper (1996) writes of the city planning process, "as a plan is adopted, the implementation tools must be made available, and their use must be encouraged at the right times and places" (p. 196). The same exact statements apply to health coaching. As clients adopt a plan, the tools to implement that plan must be made available in order for that plan to be successful. The city planning process of survey, analysis, plan, implement, feedback also perfectly describes the health coaching process. When planning a city or planning a person's life, trust the process.

Health coaching also relies on using multiple genres to connect with a client. One of my former college professors at Miami of Ohio, Tom Romano (2013) describes multigenre writing as "multigenre research writing shows faith in students as meaning makers who participate in creating the big world mural of writing" (p. 5). In health coaching, some clients may need to write about their feelings. Others may prefer to draw or create a collage. Others may want to create a playlist of songs that motivate them. Experiences happen to us, but we choose how we make meaning of our experiences. We also choose the genre in which we can best express ourselves. I smiled when I was at the physical therapy clinic and heard Eric use the term multigenre to describe a patient's healing. Multigenre medicine dovetails a treatment plan with a patient's interests to provide meaning to the healing journey.

My mom was a teacher, hospital volunteer, and probably would have been a health coach had the training existed when she was helping patients at an Ohio hospital. After her death, I had to write a new story for my life. I chose to find the positive in a devastating experience by helping people as a teacher and health coach. Every time I found myself getting stuck along the road of life, I reminded myself that I was doing exactly what my mom would want me to do by surpassing all of my goals and living my life as a positive person. One of my family members refers to me as a Health Sherpa; Sherpa mountain guides help climbers find their way, but the climbers still have to strap on their backpacks and do the work. It means a lot for me to serve as a health coach and help other people surpass their goals. I feel I can better walk with others on their journeys because of the journey I lived.

NEW PERSPECTIVES ON OLD NARRATIVES

At the time it happened, I never imagined a trip to a physical therapy clinic for neck pain could be life-changing. Connelly and Clandinin (1988) argue that there can always be a new perspective when a story is retold because, "it is a particular reconstruction of [an individual's] narrative, and there could be other reconstructions" (p. 39). For this reason, Clandinin and Connelly (2000) believe that "autobiography and memoir are recognized forms of research texts" (p. 101). Being a writer, I wrote about my pain experiences. In addition to assigning my pain level a number, I included a detailed narrative about why I chose that particular number. I laugh now rereading my old journal entries because Eric probably learned more about my life than he ever wanted to know, but interestingly he found common themes in my pain stories that helped him redesign my treatment plan and helped me heal.

Eric and I respected each other's work and decided to keep working together. Pennebaker and Evans (2014) discuss that expressive writing can lead to improved health and report, "across our first four writing studies, those in the expressive writing condition made forty-three percent fewer doctor visits for illness than those who were asked to write about superficial topics" (p. 2). Pennebaker's coauthor, English professor John Evans, was presenting a writing as healing seminar with a pediatrician colleague, Karen Jooste, at

Duke Integrative Medicine. When I attended the seminar, I learned about the health coach program and this English professor became part of Duke Med.

Eric became a physical therapist at a hospital and as a health coach I needed to complete coaching hours in a practicum setting at the same hospital to earn certification. Several staff members at the hospital wanted to use health coaching to enhance their physical therapy sessions, so Eric would complete a physical therapy evaluation followed by my health coach evaluation.

COMBINING PHYSICAL THERAPY WITH HEALTH COACHING

Jen's Perspective

I'm sitting in an exam room reviewing a patient's responses to short answer writing prompts while Eric completes a physical therapy evaluation on the same patient. The patient has responded to the prompts before the combined physical therapy/health coach session. As the patient answers Eric's evaluation questions, I write notes on the writing prompts. I'm studying voice and tone as well as pulling out themes from the writing in a similar manner to how I study the essays written by the college students I teach. The responses align. The diagnosis Eric makes with his medical evaluation aligns with my observations from the patient's writing responses. It's all connected.

Eric's Perspective

It is very helpful to listen to the patient during the evaluation process in take in how they are truly feeling. Most of the time they lead you down the correct path for their diagnosis. Listening to patients allows for more accurate diagnoses and better outcomes. If the patient can tell that you are truly listening to them they might be more compliant with your treatment intervention you design for them. Patients can become more motivated if they feel they are doing the right thing to get better and more enthused to reach their goals. Health coaches act as a catalyst to the patient's healing process helping them overcome barriers or obstacles in their way. They help the patient come up with ideas for how they can become more compliant with their home exercises and have them set goals to add to their accountability. I think this is a key component for all types of patients, especially ones that have had chronic pain. Those are usually the most difficult to treat since there can be many different things that developed over time, and on top of that the patient usually develops a psychological component thinking that they will never get better. This only makes things worse. Health coaches break down that barrier and let them know that they can have that ability and it might just be that staying compliant with a treatment intervention including consistency with their recommended home exercises is that missing component. This is a new thing in the health field and very exciting seeing the results.

COACHING TECHNIQUES AND OBSERVATIONS

This technique and observation section is written in general terms because as a coach, Jen is obligated to protect confidentiality. Integrative medicine health coaches provide a safe space for people to share their hopes, fears, and dreams and do not break that confidence unless a person is a danger to self or others. However, some generalizations can be reported about the results of coaching.

Visualization makes a difference. Jen led one patient through a visualization exercise while the patient completed Eric's prescribed exercises. The patient's leg lifted higher when visualizing a calm nature scene as opposed to talking about something stressful. Visualization techniques also help people imagine what they want to achieve. Hanging a picture or symbol of a past accomplishment on the wall is a method not only to celebrate past success, but also to envision future success.

People appreciate accountability. Clients who are not receiving physical evaluations but have health goals they want to work on appreciate checking in to give updates on their progress. It makes Jen smile when people find her for a quick check in to report success with their goals. While one of the purposes of health coaching is for people to feel self-empowerment, it always helps to have a health coach to celebrate progress. In sports, the coach motivates, but it is the individual or team who runs plays and scores points. The same applies to health coaching. The health coach motivates, but it is the individual who completes a personalized health journey.

There is value in making progress. As a baseball fan, Jen loves using the extended metaphor that baseball players can hit the ball a little over three out of every ten times and receive a batting average that still lands them in the hall of fame. Progress is not an all or nothing journey. If someone has what feels like a setback on one day, there is always tomorrow to make progress.

Health coaches can't wave a magic wand like a fairy godmother in a children's story and make everything go away. Change takes time, and progress, even a small amount, can eventually lead to large changes. Jen has a necklace with two charms, an elephant and a turtle. It's symbolic meaning? Always remember to slow down.

Coaching increases enthusiasm. The word excited has been mentioned frequently as people feel empowered to take control of their lives. Additionally, coaching gives people permission to take time for themselves without feeling selfish. People in helping professions often selflessly give to others without taking time for self-care. Several 'aha' moments happened when practitioners receiving coaching realized they cannot control others, such as a patient who won't get out of bed, but they can control their reactions. If practitioners feel happy, the happiness becomes a ripple effect that leads to happy patients.

FUTURE RESEARCH

For our next research study, we plan to complete a randomized controlled study that will take place at an inpatient orthopedic section of the hospital for post-surgical patients, specifically total knee arthroplasty (TKA) patients. Subjects will be randomly assigned a health coach. Half of the subjects will use a health coach along with physical therapy sessions while the other half of the subjects will not have a health coach and just participate in physical therapy sessions. Knee AROM (Active Range of Motion) measurements will be taken each day by a licensed physical therapist while the administration of the Health Related Quality of Life Survey (HRQOL) will take place on the first day and the day of discharge. The length of stay for each patient will be determined on the day of discharge and be strictly observational. To the best of our knowledge, unless another study is currently being conducted that has not yet been published or reported, this would be the first research study assessing the impact of health coaching on physical therapy patients.

Health coaching focuses on vision and values to help people build bridges and make connections between where they are now and where they want to be. Health coaches work with people who are mostly healthy but want to make lifestyle changes such as getting more sleep or eating healthier. Health coaches also work with patients by helping them align their vision and values with the treatment plan prescribed to them by a medical practitioner such as a physical therapist. Cameron (1998) believes, "we need to decide that we will, one, write no matter what and, two, share that writing no matter what" (p. 135). Health coaches frequently ask people questions to guide them to their goals, ask them to write their goals, and then share the goals to achieve ownership of the accomplishments. However, once a patient finishes a session with a health coach, it becomes his or her responsibility to take the necessary steps to achieve the goals. Family members who are willing to act as cheerleaders for their loved ones during the process serve as an additional source of support during the healing journey. Like pages being turned in a book, health coaches encourage patients to write the next chapters in their health stories.

ACKNOWLEDGMENT

The preceding chapter contains excerpts from the following previous IGI publications:

Bird, J.L., & Wanner, E.T. (2016). Narratives of integrative health coaching. In V.C.X. Wang (Ed.), *Handbook of research on advancing health education through technology* (pp. 170-189). Hershey, PA: Information Science Reference.

Reprinted in the IGI publication:

Bird, J.L., & Wanner, E.T. (2019). Narratives of integrative health coaching. In Information Resources Management Association (Ed.), *Complementary and alternative medicine: Breakthroughs in research and practice* (pp. 418-437). Hershey, PA: Information Science Reference.

Bird, J.L., & Wanner, E.T. (2016). Turning PAGES with health coaching and family involvement. In V.C.X. Wang (Ed.), *Handbook of research on advancing health education through technology* (pp. 213-233). Hershey, PA: Information Science Reference.

Bird, J.L., & Wanner, E.T. (2019). Turning PAGES with health coaching and family involvement. In Information Resources Management Association (Ed.), *Chronic illness and long-term care: Breakthroughs in research and practice* (pp. 255-276). Hershey, PA: Information Science Reference.

REFERENCES

Arterburn, S. (2011). *Healing is a choice*. Nashville, TN: Thomas Nelson.

Baldwin, C. (1998). *Calling the circle*. New York, NY: Bantam.

Beck, M. (2001). *Finding your own North Star*. New York, NY: Three Rivers Press.

Brady, L., & Vega, P. (2009). 5 keys to structural success. In Orthopedics and spine (pp. 107-132). Danvers, MA: HCPro.

Brown, B. (2012). *Daring greatly*. New York, NY: Gotham Books.

Cameron, J. (1998). *The right to write*. New York, NY: Tarcher/Putnam.

Centers for Disease Control and Prevention. (2011). Health Related Quality of Life. *Health Related Quality of Life Surveillance Program*. Retrieved from http://www.cdc.gov/hrqol/hrqol14_measure.htm

Chulack, C., Crichton, M., Wells, J., & Zabel, D. (1994-2009). *ER* [Television series]. Burbank, CA: Warner Brothers.

Clandinin, D. J., & Connelly, F. M. (2000). *Narrative inquiry*. San Francisco, CA: Jossey-Bass.

Coates, V. E. (1999). *Education for patients and clients*. New York, NY: Routledge.

Connelly, F. M., & Clandinin, D. J. (1988). *Teachers as curriculum planners*. New York, NY: Teachers College.

Croft, J. (1980). Interviewing in physical therapy. *Physical Therapy*, *60*(8), 1033–1036. doi:10.1093/ptj/60.8.1033 PMID:7403279

Duke Integrative Medicine Staff. (2010). *Personalized health plan manual*. Durham, NC: Duke Integrative Medicine.

Goldberg, N. (1986). *Writing down the bones*. Boston, MA: Shambhala.

Goldberg, N. (2000). *Thunder and lightning*. New York, NY: Bantam.

Greene, M. (1995). *Releasing the imagination*. San Francisco, CA: Jossey-Bass.

Harper, A. N. (1996). Tooling up for effective planning. In B. W. McClendon & A. J. Catanese (Eds.), *Planners on planning* (pp. 190–198). San Francisco, CA: Jossey-Bass.

Haugk, K. C. (2012). *Christian caregiving*. St. Louis, MO: Stephen Ministries.

Heard, G. (1995). *Writing toward home*. Portsmouth, NH: Heinemann.

Helldorfer, M., & Moss, T. (2007). *Healing with heart*. Orinda, CA: Moss Communications.

Johnson, L. (1998). *Two parts textbook, one part love*. New York, NY: Hyperion.

Jones, J., Brady, L., & Gaunt, R. (2009). The philosophy of patient-centric care. In Orthopedics and spine (pp. 81-105). Danvers, MA: HCPro.

Jones, J., Steele, D., & McClennan, C. (2009). Defining and pursuing excellence. In Orthopedics and spine (pp. 11-50). Danvers, MA: HCPro.

Koloroutis, M. (2004). *Relationship-based care*. Minneapolis, MN: Creative Health Care Management.

Kolt, G. S. (2003). Psychology of injury and rehabilitation. In G. S. Kolt (Ed.), *Physical therapies in sport and exercise* (pp. 165–183). London, UK: Churchill Livingstone.

Noppe-Brandon, G. (2004). *Find your voice*. Portsmouth, NH: Heinemann.

Pennebaker, J. W., & Evans, J. F. (2014). *Expressive writing: Words that heal*. Enumclaw, WA: Idyll Arbor.

Pipher, M. (2006). *Writing to change the world*. New York, NY: Riverhead.

Randall, K. E., & McEwen, I. R. (2000). Writing patient-centered functional goals. *Physical Therapy*, *80*(12), 1197–103. PMID:11087306

Rankin, L. (2013). *Mind over medicine*. Carlsbad, CA: Hay House.

Richardson, L. (1997). *Fields of play*. New Brunswick, NJ: Rutgers University Press.

Romano, T. (1987). *Clearing the way*. Portsmouth, NH: Heinemann.

Romano, T. (2013). *Fearless writing*. Portsmouth, NH: Heinemann.

Simmons, L. A., & Wolever, R. Q. (2011). *Health coaching: Research summary (report)*. Durham, NC: Duke Integrative Medicine / Duke University Health System.

Smith, L., & Wroth, S. (2011). *Duke integrative health coach professional training manual*. Durham, NC: Duke Integrative Medicine.

Soukup, R. (2019). *Do it scared*. Grand Rapids, MI: Zondervan.

Steele, M. K. (2009). Orthopedics and spine. Danvers, MA: HCPro.

Tindle, H. (2013). *Up: How positive outlook can transform our health and aging*. New York, NY: Hudson Street Press.

Wanner, E.T., & Bird, J.L. (2013). *The Wanner Bird healing survey for pain recovery*. Academic Press.

Winfrey, O. (2014). *What I know for sure*. New York, NY: Hearst Communications.

KEY TERMS AND DEFINITIONS

Behavior Changes: Behavior changes occur when people put forth a conscious effort to make lifestyle changes to improve health. While health coaches can encourage behavior changes, ultimately the choice of which behavior changes to implement belongs to each individual.

Community Development: The process of creating a place where people feel welcomed and supported, whether it is a neighborhood, a classroom, or a network of colleagues who provide support for an individual.

HRQOL (Health-Related Quality of Life) Survey: A general health survey in the public domain and able to be used by researchers without securing permission or paying copyright fees.

Integrative Health Coaching: Integrative health coaches help people make changes that support their vision and values of optimal health.

Integrative Medicine: A holistic approach to medicine that treats the whole person, not just the disease.

Journal Writing: The process of a person responding to prompts and writing about his or her thoughts and feelings. Even though journal writing is typically associated with writing classrooms, writing teachers including Julia Cameron and Natalie Goldberg advocate that journal writing can be done by anyone, anywhere, including patients in a hospital.

Physical Therapy Outcome Measures: Tests used by physical therapists to measure the progress a patient makes when a body part is injured, such as such as the DASH (Disabilities of the Arm Shoulder Hand), LEFS (Lower Extremity Functional Scale), NDI (Neck Disability Index), and Modified Oswestry (for back pain).

Planning Process: Used in the fields of city planning, curricular change, and health coaching, this process encompasses the following steps: survey, analysis, plan, implementation, and feedback.

Writing as Healing: James Pennebaker is known as the pioneer in this field that discusses the health benefits of writing. Numerous studies have been conducted investigating the influence of writing on physical and emotional health.

Writing Voice: Voice in writing highlights a writer's word choice and tone to compose a journal entry or other written composition that reflects the writer's personality. Every writer has a unique writing voice, just like each person has a unique speaking voice.

Chapter 4
Narratives of Emotional Truth

Jennifer Lynne Bird
Oxbridge Academy, USA

ABSTRACT

This narrative uses a multigenre format to discuss the writing theory of emotional truth, where writers share truth as they remember it. Factual truth focuses on facts, while emotional truth focuses on the emotions associated with a memory. The example provided uses health coaching, an addition to the medical field that encourages patients to share their stories and set goals for themselves in addition to the goals set for them by their medical team. Fictional elements combine with research in creative nonfiction.

BEYOND TRADITIONAL HORIZONS OF WRITING

As the character of Nick memorably reflects in the novel *The Great Gatsby* (Fitzgerald, 1925), "so we beat on, boats against the current, borne back ceaselessly into the past" (p. 180). Retelling our stories through writing helps the writer own them and while memories of stories often pull us back into the past, they don't define our future. This chapter illuminates the value of experiences while simultaneously adding insight into writing theory and practice. The discussion of the writing process can apply to teachers in a classroom as well as patients who want to describe their symptoms to a clinician. While writing typically exists inside the walls of English classrooms, expanding the horizons of how writing becomes implemented leads to innovative interdisciplinary

DOI: 10.4018/978-1-7998-1931-8.ch004

collaboration. The writing process provides a foundation and a scaffold for narrative inquiry, multigenre writing, emotional truth, and using narrative writing to enhance healing.

MEMORIES OF MARILYN

Winter in Kettering, Ohio was more brutal than usual this year. Marilyn Kepler Bird looked out the window of the hospital at the blizzard. She had been a patient in the hospital for some minor medical tests and felt ready to go home. However, no one was going home in this storm.

Things seemed serious. The hospital employees who had been snowed in at the hospital were on the front lines of dealing with any medical crisis. The doctors and nurses on call were snowed in at their homes and could not travel to the hospital to provide relief. In this era before cell phones, patients couldn't send a quick text home to let loved ones know they were okay. The landline looming on the desk at the nurses' station provided the only lifeline to the outside world. The phone started ringing. No nurses stayed at the station; they needed to be dispatched to various parts of the hospital to help patients. A trained hospital volunteer, Marilyn picked up the phone and reassured the frantic caller his loved one was okay. Marilyn put her hands on her hips, and her green eyes surveyed the chaos around her as she flipped her brown hair over her shoulders. Time to get to work.

During that blizzard week, Marilyn worked more volunteer hours than some of the paid hospital staff. To her, reassuring patients was not a job, but a calling. They needed her, and she was there. Trained as a high school social studies teacher, Marilyn liked teaching but loved health care. She counseled hospital patients scared by their internal medical conditions as well as the external blizzard. Before the medical field had a name for the role she played, she used the skills of listening and inquiry implemented by health coaches.

END NOTES FOR "MEMORIES OF MARILYN"

The previous scene you just read was a work of fiction based on fact. That scene happened before I was born, so of course I did not witness my mom Marilyn helping patients. I heard the story from her when I was a kid, and as

I was getting ready to begin my health coach training I discovered an article my dad wrote about my mom's heroism. Finding that article served as an affirmation that I was on the right path in my life.

Writing about emotional truth can heal people. I first explored multigenre writing as healing when I wrote my doctoral dissertation and used a fictional character to share factual information. I created a character named Jenna Kepler, who was a thinly disguised variation of me, and sent her into horrific circumstances worse than my reality in order to process some of the events in my life. I used emotional truth to capture the essence of an issue while freeing myself from being obligated to remember every single factual detail. Writing Jenna Kepler's story helped me heal. That's the real truth.

When writing fiction, Jenna the character said things Jenny the author couldn't because I was hurting too much. As DeSalvo (1999) explains, "if the emotional aftermath of our trauma is similar to O'Brien's, we, too, can use semifictional alter ego to tell our stories, to help us feel" (p. 167). After a crisis, fiction can help us find our way back to a new reality as we skate the fine line between fact and fiction. O'Brien (1990) describes this experience as, "I'm skimming across the surface of my own history, moving fast, riding the melt beneath the blades, doing loops and spins, and when I take a high leap into the dark and come down thirty years later, I realize it is as Tim trying to save Timmy's life with a story" (p. 246). Goldberg (2000) describes her reaction to reading O'Brien's words as, "tears sprang to my eyes. I, too, have attempted many times to keep my childhood safe, warding off death with a story" (p. 131). I agree with this sentiment. By writing a story about my mom's experiences volunteering in a hospital, for a few moments she is alive again and I get to spend a little more time with her.

One of my former professors, Tom Poetter (2013) describes the feeling of freedom in teaching as, "I was allowed to teach instead of sentenced to follow someone else's script" (p. 102). I felt grateful he applied the same philosophy to writing and gave me the opportunity to tell my story when he advised my doctoral dissertation. My dissertation committee encouraged me to write about my experiences as a method for helping me heal emotionally, but I couldn't write about my mom without crying. So I turned to fiction and created my character Jenna Kepler. Beck (2001) describes, "narrative therapy teaches people to literally rewrite their life stories, so that they tell themselves the happy truth, instead of the miserable truth" (p. 96). I used writing as a form of therapy to discuss my feelings while hiding behind my fictional character. But Jenna wasn't really a fictional character. Her first name was close to mine and her last name was my mom's maiden name. While I made up details about Jenna's life, I couldn't run from the emotional truth of my experiences. I could rewrite the fiction story and give it a happy ending, but I couldn't change how the story ended in real life.

My doctoral dissertation featured a narrative inquiry approach discussing how stories help people heal emotionally. I never imagined writing could also help people heal physically until years later when I completed research at a physical therapy clinic and continued research at a hospital.

FACT AND FICTION

I present a longer merger of fact and fiction, where you will read fictionalized narratives of a health coach's factual experiences. The fictional stories have their foundation in factual truth. Health coaches adhere to a code of ethics and must honor confidentiality to provide patients with a safe place to share their stories. Creating that safe space includes not sharing any real patient stories in a publication. To protect confidentiality, no real names of patients are used in the following narrative. All patients described are composites of several patients, and no patient described is based on the experiences of a single real person to add an additional layer of confidentiality. Furthermore, additional details have also been fictionalized so there is no possibility of a single patient being identified. Think of the patients in this narrative as fictional characters. While their stories were inspired by real patients, the important thing for you as a reader is to experience what the health coach felt when learning the patient narratives, and all the emotions are true. All of the patients received total knee arthroplasty (TKA) surgery and spoke to the health coach while in a hospital inpatient orthopedic setting. In addition to speaking with a health coach, the patients all received treatments from a physical therapist and an occupational therapist, as well as hospital care from nurses and physicians. The narrative is told in the first person "I" from my perspective as a health coach who is also an English teacher and Stephen Minister. End notes follow the narrative and elaborate on the concepts discussed. In the original version of this narrative, I named the patients after literary characters. Upon rereading and reflecting, that decision proved too distracting, so in the revision I named the patients in the memory of my four grandparents and two uncles. After the fictional narrative, I explain in my end notes section an additional rationale for my writing decisions.

PATIENT NARRATIVES

I sling my lanyard with my ID badge around my neck and pick up the list of patients I am scheduled to visit today, as I look forward to another day of health coaching and helping people. A gift card I received from my family enabled me to afford a stack of composition books for hospital patients. Every patient did not receive a journal due to the fact that some patients experienced surgical complications that made neither coaching nor writing possible for them. When patients in the hospital received a journal, there was a note on it that read as follows:

This is your journal!

Use it to…

1. Write questions for your medical team.
2. Write a list of your goals.
3. Freewrite about anything on your mind.
4. Draw pictures.
5. Annotate medical advice so you remember.

I refer to my first patient of the day as William. On the one hand, this William loves being surrounded by the constant visitors to his room; on the other hand, he is tired and in pain. Overall, William feels at peace with his life and very optimistic. He is telling jokes with the physical therapist and occupational therapist who are in the room when I arrive and I notice his great sense of humor. I appreciate the support for health coaching from all the members of the medical team. The physical therapist and occupational therapist tell William they think it would be good for him to talk to me before they leave to help another patient.

"What are you looking forward to the most when you go home?" I ask. Questions like this motivate patients to envision their lives after the hospital.

"Outdoors. My bike. My boat. My dog. Being pain free when going on a drive." He smiles and describes a beautiful scene of going for a drive, which I hope comes true for him after he leaves the hospital.

"Sometimes it's the little things we miss most." I try to add meaning while reflecting one of his statements. William changes the direction of the conversation.

"I'm happy, but exhausted. I love all my visitors, but they won't leave." He leans back against his pillows, signaling he would like to rest. Health coaching conversations in the hospital are usually short, since patients are on medication and need their rest between physical and occupational therapy treatment sessions. I have learned to make the most of the short time I have. We talk about ideas of how he could get some rest without being rude to his guests. As a health coach in a hospital, I have to accept that patients are in my life for only the duration of their short hospital stays; therefore, I do not have the opportunity to know the next chapters they write in their stories.

I then stop by to check on the writing of my second patient of the day. I call her Martha, and she is quiet and reluctant to talk about her feelings. I'm hoping that the composition notebook I gave her will encourage her to write what she is feeling. Martha was excited to write in her journal. I knock on the door and push it open. A nurse is in the room with Martha.

"These notebooks are a great idea," Martha says. The nurse smiles. Typically patients open up more when I am the only person in the room with them, but Martha keeps on talking. "I have no pain today."

"That's great news." I look at the journal buried under a book, a food tray, and other items on the table next to her and know she won't be reading her writing to me. That's okay; I've learned from the college students I teach and a large amount of research that it is the act of writing that helps people, regardless of whether or not the writing is shared. Writing in a journal gives patients such as Martha the opportunity to explore their thoughts on paper without worrying about staying awake to talk to a visitor in their hospital rooms.

"I need some rest," Martha says, but she is smiling and seems happy as she says it. "I'm excited to write more."

"Writing can help you remember things," I tell her. "Sometimes you think of your best questions after your medical team leaves the room." I notice the nurse nod in agreement while I mentally reprimand myself, because I've just lapsed into teaching, and health coaches are supposed to listen, not teach.

"Very true," Martha picks up on my thread of conversation anyway. "Oh. I'm starting to feel some pain now." That's my cue to leave as the nurse takes over Martha's care. I wonder how much she can focus on her future goals while she is in pain. Even if she's not sharing her feelings with me verbally, at least she is writing them in her journal. The nurse stops me before I go into the next patient's room and tells me the journals are a great idea.

My third patient of the day I refer to as Steven. His wife hovers over him like a bird that doesn't know where to land. "This machine is making too much noise," she remarks as she reaches for one of the machines.

"Let me get a nurse," I quickly tell her, not knowing much about the machine in question but suspecting that unplugging it would be bad. After the situation is resolved, I evaluate my options. The purpose of health coaching is to have individual conversations with people; family members, as well meaning as they are, can easily redirect a conversation.

"Will I ever leave this hospital?" Steven asks. I can still encourage him on his healing journey and talk to his wife about practicing self-care so she can better take care of him once he returns home from the hospital. I switch from a coaching role to that of motivational speaker and notice that Steven's wife has been writing in the journal. I am reminded that the hospital patients are receiving care from all the medical professionals, but who is taking care of the caregivers?

"I gave her the journal," Steven explains.

"That's fine." I look at his wife, wondering if she needs coaching more than her husband the hospital patient.

"Take care of yourself so you can better take care of him," I tell her.

"I will," she promises, but she is already reaching for her husband's pillows. This wasn't a coaching session, but hopefully I helped both of them. All I can do is my best, I tell myself. The good news about seeing patients one right after another is that I can't dwell too much on one conversation. I need to practice mindfulness and focus on each patient in the moment, not think about the ones I spoke to earlier or the ones I am going to speak to later.

"Get out of my room! Go away!" That is my introduction to my fourth patient of the day, who I name Mary Ann. The mystery I need to solve immediately is why Mary Ann has never met me, yet doesn't like me. "I can't watch my favorite singer in peace!" Mary Ann yells, and slumps against the pillow angrily. I glance at the television screen and see a singer typically more popular with the college students I teach than members of Mary Ann's older generation, and remind myself of the advice I tell my college students when I teach a reading diagnosis class. Interest + Area of Need = Effective Assessment. I assess I am not going to have an effective coaching session at this moment in time, especially when I see Mary Ann is not alone in the room. Her daughter is there with her.

"She's in pain. Please leave," Mary Ann's daughter orders. Concern of family members is understandable; anytime my grandma had surgery, my mom insisted on staying in the hospital room with her even after visiting hours.

"I'll be back," I tell Mary Ann, leaving her to her concert. A physical therapist and occupational therapist who heard the exchange with Mary Ann smile at me encouragingly. Don't let it get to you, I tell myself. As I walk past the patient admitting desk, the kind receptionist who I see multiple times a day asks me how much I've walked today. Thanks to my iPhone app, I already know that by the end of the day I will walk six miles and climb ten flights of stairs. I'm grateful a colleague advised me to wear comfortable shoes as I go to the cafeteria for a free cup of coffee I won't finish because it takes too long to drink and I want to return to my patients. I stop by the documentation room, greet the physical therapists and occupational therapists who are there, and quickly write my notes for the patients I have seen so far. The team is listening to a mix CD I made during a team development workshop, and I realize I am not just helping patients while I am here, but also my colleagues. By the time I don't finish my coffee and do finish my notes, Mary Ann's television concert has ended and I try talking to her again.

One of the physical therapists is in the room helping Mary Ann and suggests we work together. While the physical therapist teaches Mary Ann exercises, I ask her to visualize her ideal health. Her focus remains in the present, not in the future. She visualizes a peaceful scene while completing the exercises the physical therapist gives her. While health coaching encourages the setting of long term goals in timeframes of three to six months in the future, Mary Ann can only visualize one moment to the next. For her, that is what she needs. She mentions her love of antiques. My dad has been known to keep things for years and now has an impressive collection of antiques. I found the opening I needed to get her to trust me and talk. Once the physical therapist leaves, Mary Ann glares at me.

"I'm glad my daughter left. A three day hospital stay means a three day vacation from family. Where are my glasses? Have you seen my toothbrush?" Confusion has taken over her. The ethics of doing what is best for a patient overrule any additional coaching, so it's time for me to leave and let her sleep.

My fifth patient of the day wants to talk about Shakespeare instead of his health goals. I refer to him as Harold.

"Have you read this book?" Harold asks, holding up a popular contemporary novel.

"I have," I confirm. "My students like it too."

"You're a professor!" Harold claps his hands. "I always believe reading and writing have value. What's your favorite Shakespeare play? If I tell you a quote from a Shakespeare play, can you identify it? My son in high school needs to learn more quotes and appreciate the value of reading!" He is not doing it intentionally, but he is trying to distract me. This could easily turn into a conversation about literature, which I love, but that would put the focus on me and not on Harold.

"How would you compare your journey to the journey of a literary character?" I ask. While, as health coaches, we do self-manage our own thoughts and feelings, we are only human and sometimes patients learn parts of our stories. And just as English teachers discuss poems in the literature we teach, health coaches often use metaphors to reflect part of the stories they hear. In Harold's case, he compared himself to various characters in a Shakespeare play. He was on a quest just like they were, and his quest was to heal from his surgery. By the time I leave, I'm pleased with the session, and happy Harold now sees himself as the hero of his life story, just like his favorite Shakespeare characters.

"Please pray with me," instructs my sixth patient of the day, a happy and peaceful woman I refer to as Bobbie, and I soon learn of her strength. I find my dual roles as Stephen Minister and health coach emerging as I hold her hand and pray. Often when people pray, they don't know the words to say and that's okay. Word choice doesn't matter as much as the intent of the message; the same can be said for writing. I have learned to trust my heart with both prayer and writing and try not to overthink the words of my prayer. "That was beautiful," Bobbie wipes away a tear.

"How are you feeling?" I ask, knowing that one of the physical therapists told me she experienced complications during her surgery.

"What happens when we die?" Bobbie asks. I pause before answering. While she had complications during her surgery, they were not life threatening, but sometimes medical experiences cause patients to reflect on their lives.

"What do you think happens when we die?" I turn her question back to her, using another health coaching strategy of exploring what the patients feel instead of asking as experts answering all their questions. Both health coaches and Stephen Ministers guide others to find their own answers. Unlike teaching, we don't direct others what to do. In both of my roles, reflective listening and being present for another person becomes essential. I believe Heaven is a beautiful place with peace and love and happiness, where I will be reunited with everyone in my family who died, but I don't want to tell her what to believe if she has a different opinion. Bobbie starts telling me about a book she read where the author had a near death experience.

"I'm scared," she admits.

"It's okay to feel that way," I assure her. "What are you looking forward to the most when you go home?" I ask, bringing my day full circle by asking my last patient of the day the same question I asked the first.

"Watching football. Eating chocolate. Can we pray again?" Bobbie reaches for my hand. While we are praying, her doctor arrives. He bows his head and remains silent as I finish the prayer.

"Spirituality has value. It helps patients," the doctor remarks. Since patients have limited time with their doctors, I always leave the room when a doctor arrives. I never want patients to miss a moment of discussing their medical care. Bobbie's story will become another one to which I will never know the sequel. Spirituality is one of the dimensions of health explored by health coaches and it was the one that Bobbie wanted to discuss the most during my coaching session with her.

Before I conclude my day at the hospital, I leave the orthopedic wing of the hospital where I visited my six patients because I am asked to visit an oncology patient coping with a cancer diagnosis. I try to offer some comfort to a shocked patient immediately after the cancer treatment didn't work and there are no more medical options. For this patient, there is no setting of long term goals but reflecting on the question: What do you need to do to feel at peace with the time you have left? Health coaches don't usually make visits to the emergency room, but I am asked to sit with a patient's family until they can receive an update on their loved one's condition from someone on the medical team. Mixed with the tragedy of sad diagnoses are the triumphs, as I walk through the hospital hallways and witness a physical therapist and occupational therapist help a patient walk again against the odds. The best moments are the ones talking to patients, learning their narratives, and know that for a short moment in time, my life story intersected with theirs and I hopefully helped make a difference in their lives by being there.

END NOTES FOR "PATIENT NARRATIVES"

These notes focus primarily on the role of using health coaching with physical therapy patients since that is the setting where I worked as a health coach, but health coaching can also be used with cardiac patients, oncology patients, or even healthy patients who desire lifestyle changes. Some health coaches have medical backgrounds; for example, many health coaches are nurses.

But other health coaches bring our own unique knowledge to the field and offer different perspectives. My area of expertise is writing, so I am able to use that skill to help patients heal.

Regardless of background, all health coaches need to receive specific training in order to practice. The goal of using journaling as a health coach is not for the writing to result in publication, but to provide patients with another way to think about their progress. Germer (2009) discusses the value of journals and writes, "journaling is an opportunity to monitor habit change, to troubleshoot, and, most important, to notice new ways you might be responding to problems in your life" (p. 241). Journals can be used for recording narratives, tracking pain, setting goals, and celebrating the small victories in life. Neff (2011) believes in the power of gratitude journals and states, "after a relatively short time, keeping a gratitude journal can make a substantial contribution to your level of happiness" (p. 279). Writing in journals can contribute to the positive outlook that helps people heal. It reminds patients to take their recovery process during physical therapy one day and one step at a time, because small steps can lead to big changes.

Journal writing can also provide accountability for achieving goals. Lea Michele (2015) explains, "this might be a way for you to hold yourself accountable for achieving everything you want. Keeping a journal and asking yourself hard questions about what you really want to get out of your life is the best way, in my experience, to actually help you achieve your dreams" (p. 11). Displaying the list of goals in a prominent place is another way of remaining accountable and providing inspiration during the healing journey.

While Romano (1987) is describing a writing conference in an English classroom instead of a health coaching session, the same goal of establishing a safe environment applies to both a student in an English classroom and a patient in a health coaching session because, "once a comfortable, reassuring atmosphere is established, the conference proceeds. How it proceeds depends upon many things: where the student is in the writing process, what her attitude is toward the work, what problem is foremost in her mind at the moment, how far she has moved or been nudged in previous conferences. The teacher must listen and take cues from the student" (p. 87). The same description applies to health coaching, as the health coach must listen and take cues from the patient before proceeding with the conversation.

Health coaching is not therapy but shares similarities with solution-oriented brief therapy (SBT) in psychology. As Weiner-Davis (1995) describes, "the secret to its brevity is that, instead of taking a long introspective journey into the past, SBT helps people to envision a positive future and to identify fail-safe strategies for getting there" (p. 18). In her practice, she found that people often know what they need to do but need someone to ask them the right questions to help them get there. The difference is that psychologists use narratives to help patients understand the past, whereas health coaches use narratives to help patients set goals for the future.

In narrative therapy, Madigan (2011) draws a parallel between narratives used in literature and narratives told in therapy settings by stating, "if there was to be any interest and/or consistency between narrative therapy theory, practice, and research, the task of any research would be akin to that of the literary critic, insofar as cultural behavior can be treated only as a text that requires interpretation" (p. 140). English teachers encourage students to interpret the texts they read. Similarly, medical practitioners can help patients interpret the stories they tell themselves. The only difference is that the endings of classic works of literature will never change. People's lives, however, are not a book that has already been written; their lives contain unwritten pages waiting to be filled with new stories. Charon (2006) discusses narrative medicine and argues, "by virtue of being trained in the style appropriate to the genre of the chart, doctors learn to suppress their own authorial voice, their own I" (p. 142). Narrative medicine encourages medical practitioners to see each patient as living a story, not as only a name on a chart and a list of notes. Health coaches listen more than they talk, which opens the door for patients to reflect on their narratives and think how minor differences, like a change in routine for the day, can lead to major behavior change.

Most caregivers find joy and purpose in helping others. As Carter (2015) describes it, "it's the person. It isn't about the prestige or even the helping nature of our work. It's about the meaning we personally find in it and express through it, and the effort and commitment we give to it" (p. 241). Health coaches, physical therapists, and their medical colleagues may only have one chance to make a difference in a patient's life. While the patient must be the one to literally or metaphorically pick up the pen and do the work, it becomes comforting to be surrounded by members of the medical team who will remain a supportive presence. Brown (2015) writes, "when we decide to own our stories and live our truth, we bring our light to the darkness" (p. 75). By learning the stories of others, we continue to write our own.

END NOTES FOR HEALTH COACHING

Health coaching is still new to the field of medicine; consequently, research studying the benefits of health coaching is only emerging as of this writing. While health coaches have training in the field of psychology, they are not psychologists. While psychology encourages patients to look backward and health coaching encourages patients to look forward, both fields share the common thread of narratives providing connections. According to Caldwell, Grey, and Wolever (2013), "the major tenets of the health coaching process are patient-centeredness and patient-control focused around patient-originated health goals that guide the work within a supportive coaching partnership" (p. 48). The health coach works with the patient to explore the patient's attitude about change. What are the factors causing the patient to not be motivated to take care of his or her health, not think the treatment plan is important, not feel confidence in completing the treatment plan, or not feel ready to express why changing is not a priority? The health coach does not tell the patient what to do, but asks open ended questions while the patient finds his or her own answers. Defined by Smith, Lake, Simmons, Perlman, Wroth, and Wolever (2013) as "through techniques sourced from humanistic and positive psychology, solution-focused and mindfulness-based therapies, and leadership coaching, Integrative Health Coaching (IHC) provides a mechanism to empower patients through various stages of learning and change" (p. 66). The health coach partners with the physical therapist and any other member of the patient's medical team to not only help the patient comply with goals set by the medical team, but also any personal goals the patient may have which align with the treatment goals.

END NOTES FOR STEPHEN MINISTRY

Helping people through their experiences is a role of not only health coaches, but also Stephen Ministers. Haugk (2000) provides the definition as, "Stephen Ministers are lay Christians carefully recruited, selected, trained, commissioned, and supervised for lay caring ministry" (p. 17). Both roles are similar yet different. Health coaches use the same skills as Stephen Ministers of reflective listening, maintaining boundaries, encouraging people to express their feelings, asking open ended questions to lead to solutions, and providing a supportive presence. However, they differ in that health coaches encourage people to set goals to improve their health while Stephen Ministers provide prayers. Prayers can provide comfort to patients as they heal. Alexander (2012) demonstrates belief in the science of medicine because "I'm still a scientist. I'm still a doctor, and as such I have two essential duties: to honor truth and to help heal" (p. 171). Alexander (2014), however, also argues, "the fact is, science and faith, the two ways of knowing the world that have defined our culture, are much, much more entwined than we tend to think they are" (p. 63). While patients do need all the advantages of modern medicine, if saying a prayer or writing in a journal helps a patient feel better, such techniques effectively supplement their medical treatment.

Helldorfer and Moss (2007) believe, "in health care, we have a distinct mission to relieve suffering and restore hope" (p. 213). Helping a patient with the awareness that just because pain exists now doesn't mean it will exist in the future can provide a patient with hope and courage to rewrite an existing narrative. Adams (1990) describes the writing as healing process as journal therapy and explains, "when you move your negative emotions out of your body through exercise or writing, they aren't lurking around to cause tension or disease via tight muscles, stiff necks, headaches, ulcers, or heart attacks" (p. 39). She continues, "if there is one inviolate rule of journal writing, it is that there are simply no rules. Writing naturally means that you do what works for you and that you don't worry about what you're not doing in the journal" (p. 42). Therefore, writing can not only relieve emotional pain, but physical pain as well.

Obviously, if a patient experiences pain, no amount of journal writing will take the place of a treatment plan prescribed by a medical practitioner. However, writing can be used in conjunction with the treatment plan to enhance patient healing. Zimmermann (2002) believes, "by giving voice to fears, anger, and despair, by letting go of old dreams and hopes, our self-healing powers come into play" (p. 18). Writing can help us figure out what concerns us so we can help heal ourselves; we can then share our concerns with medical professionals so they can use that information to design a treatment plan that will best help us continue to heal.

CREATIVE WRITING AS HEALING

Research exists that supports using creative writing as a healing device. Pennebaker (1997) explains, "the mind torments itself by thinking about unresolved and confusing issues. One reason that writing about traumas can be so beneficial is that it is a powerful tool to discover meaning. Writing promotes self-understanding" (p. 93). But if reporting the facts of a trauma causes too much emotional pain for the writer, it may help for the writer to write about the event using creative writing. As Pennebaker and Evans (2014) discuss, "you can't help but wonder where personal narrative ends and fiction begins. Does writing fictionalized stories improve health as much as exploring your own experiences? Possibly" (p. 94). Lepore, Greenberg, Bruno, and Smyth (2002) discuss a study by Greenberg and her colleagues where study participants were asked to write about personal traumas, imaginary traumas, or nonemotional events and learned, "both real and imaginary trauma groups visited the student health center for illness less often at 1-month follow up relative to controls" (p. 106). In the original study, Greenberg, Wortman, and Stone (1996) reflect that "writing about a hypothetical trauma could also facilitate development of a more resilient version of self" (p. 600). In other words, we save our lives with stories.

And we can save other lives too.

NARRATIVE INQUIRY

Life takes unexpected directions. After we live our stories, we decide whether or not to share them. Too often, people don't share their stories because sharing takes courage, trust, and vulnerability. Clandinin and Connelly (2000) explain, "therefore, difficult as it may be to tell a story, the more difficult but important task is the retelling of stories that allow for growth and change" (p. 71). You may tell a story to someone as soon as that story happens and have one perspective. Years later, you may retell that same story to a different person and gain additional insight about how you changed between sharing sessions. Narrative inquiry, the discipline of research that encourages researchers to share stories as part of research, is described by Clandinin and Connelly (2000) as, "we imagine, therefore, that in the construction of narratives of experience, there is a reflexive relationship between living a life story, telling a life story, retelling a life story, and reliving a life story" (p. 71). In retelling a story, you relive the moments once experienced and see them from a new perspective. It helps us see where our lives are heading and opens our eyes to things we may want to adjust or keep the same.

Our stories evolve as we evolve. Clandinin and Connelly (2000) continue, "narrative inquiry carries more of a sense of continual reformulation of an inquiry than it does a sense of problem definition and solution" (p. 124). We live our stories, tell our stories, and in the reliving and retelling of our stories we often find new answers and think of new questions. Whether it is in a classroom, a clinic, or in life, we take the theories we learn and transform them in to practical strategies. Connelly and Clandinin (1988) believe, "we may think of our own education through curriculum situations in terms of theory and practice" (p. 89). In the field of narrative inquiry, a research project may end, but the stories of the participants continue. Students continue their lives long after they leave a teacher's classroom, just as patients continue their lives long after they leave a doctor's clinic.

Stories of people's lives remain ongoing, and the addition of new narratives can change a story. Cameron (1998) believes, "valuing our experience is not narcissism. It is not endless self-involvement. It is, rather, the act of paying active witness to ourselves and to our world" (p. 50). By writing, we witness our experiences as we retell them and thus relive them. We learn from our past experiences so we can move forward. Connelly and Clandinin (1988) explain, "teaching provides little opportunity for reflection. 'Doing things' is such a significant part of our daily pressures that we have little occasion to sit back and ask ourselves 'what am I doing?' We move forward but we find it hard to think back" (p. 33). People learn from an experience, but gain more insight from reflecting on the experience.

Welcome to the world of narrative inquiry. The theory of narrative inquiry supports the practice of multigenre writing.

MULTIGENRE WRITING

Multigenre writing, as defined by Dr. Tom Romano (2013), is as follows:

A multigenre paper arises from research, experience, and imagination. It is not an uninterrupted, expository monolog nor a seamless narrative. A multigenre paper is composed of many genres and subgenres, each piece self-contained, making a point of its own, yet connected to other pieces by theme and content and sometimes by repeated language, images, and genres. A multigenre paper may also contain many voices, not just the author's. The craft then – the challenge for the writer – is to make such a paper hang together as one unified whole (p. 8).

In the following section, I use multigenre writing to describe multigenre writing in the form of a found poem definition using Tom Romano's quotes. Tom Romano, one of my former professors at Miami University in Oxford, Ohio, inspired his students to use multigenre writing. For the past two school years, he inspired the high school students I teach in Skype sessions with them.

Writing is learned only through participation. Teachers who write and share their words assume a humane, participatory stance toward learning and teaching the craft of writing (1987, p. 43). The multigenre research paper I've described in this chapter requires that creativity and imagination be part of research (1995, p. 130). Multigenre papers defy most readers' expectations. Multigenre writers, therefore, must be doubly careful to orient readers quickly and supply information that will help them build meaning the further they read (2000, p. 33). I'm a narrative creature. Through telling stories I experience the power of my voice and come to understand what the stories mean (2004, p. 29). Could they learn facts about their topic and combine those facts with imagination to render intellectual and emotional truths? (2008, p. 183). I want to know the ins-and-outs of students' learning and creative journeys. I want students to be academically responsible and practice the habit of scholarly integrity. So I ask them to include endnotes (2013, p. 153).

Multigenre writing provides authors the opportunity to tell their narratives using creative and unique perspectives. The practice of multigenre writing originated in the field of English Education, where Romano (2008) provides the definition as, "instead of producing one long expository paper, students wrote about their topics in many genres. Although each piece was self-contained, making a point of its own, taken together, all the writing created a unified whole. I called the assignment a multigenre research paper" (p. 180). Multigenre writing helps writers surprise the reader and let creativity shine through traditional reporting of research. Romano (2004) elaborates, "it isn't simply one expository or narrative monolog. In multigenre papers, writers put together information from many perspectives, angles, and voices" (p. 34). Of course, as with all research papers, all the facts reported in a multigenre paper must be accurate. The most important thing with multigenre writing, however, becomes for the author to use the research to tell a compelling story.

Multigenre writing means looking at a topic from multiple perspectives, with narratives becoming the driving force. As Romano (2013) explains, "while expository forms like clear explanations, succinct position statements, and tight arguments surely have a place in multigenre papers, genres of narrative thinking carry the cognitive load" (p. 20). Multigenre writing opens up additional dimensions for research by giving the author of a multigenre paper the opportunity to present findings using innovative formats such as artwork, creative writing, and fictionalized interpretations of stories.

For example, in the practice of both health coaching and Stephen Ministry, specific accounts of patient conversations cannot be repeated in order to protect confidentiality. Consequently, sometimes the best method to present facts is by using fiction. The essence of the story remains true, but details have been changed to maintain confidentiality for participants. Romano (2000) advises teachers, "whether your students are doing secondary research and writing multigenre papers out of that or whether they are exploring aspects of their lives, urge them to use the techniques of fiction" (p. 72). Fictionalized experiences protect details confidential to people involved in the narrative while retaining the emotional truth of a story. It becomes possible for readers to feel what the author felt without needing to know names or identifying details of other participants in the story. Romano (1995) believes, "by creating fictional dreams peopled with fully realized characters driven by tension amid enough detail of setting to create atmosphere, students can create truths that show what they know" (p. 8). Fiction frees the writer of having to remember factual details, or in this case, allows for the reader to gain a better comprehension of health coaching without the author compromising confidential information unable to be shared in a publication. The goal becomes to tell a captivating story while simultaneously honoring the lives of the patients who made the story possible.

EMOTIONAL TRUTH

While writers quote factual truth, the emotional truth will always be told from the perspective of each individual writer. Examples of emotional truth include a clinician fictionalizing part of a patient's story to change identifying details or a teacher not remembering the exact clothes worn during a class but remembering perfectly the emotional resonance of the lesson taught that day.

Here is a good description of emotional truth from an author with the same last name but no relation to my research teammate Eric. Wanner (1994) says, "stories may claim to be factual truth at one end of the spectrum or metaphoric truth at the other, with all shadings in between. A story's 'truth' depends more upon its coherence than upon its faithfulness to actual events" (p. 18). So I maintain my responsibility to my readers by informing them that not every detail may be true, but the message of the piece becomes its emotional resonance. As Handler (2013) states, "what's emotionally true for you may not have the ring of truth for others who were present in the same situation" (p. 63). This is because "emotional truth isn't always provable truth" (p. 155). If the emotional truth of the story resonates with you, do the details really matter? For example, a medical practitioner can share the essence of a patient's story to provide life lessons for readers while simultaneously changing personal details to protect the patient's confidentiality. That enables the reader to comprehend the emotional truth of the experience regardless of the modification of specific details of the story.

Most fiction has some foundation in factual experiences. Even if they are not writing a fictional novel, authors of multigenre writing borrow elements from fiction to present their research as creative nonfiction, poetry, journal entries, or other genres. For example, a conversation as presented by the author is based on subjective memory and not objective facts, and therefore may not be presented in this book as exactly as it originally occurred. However, the emotional resonance of the conversation is true. As fiction writer Cleaver (2002) writes, "when you deepen the connection to your character, you deepen your connection to yourself" (p. 85). In research methods such as narrative inquiry, the lines between fact and fiction often become blurred. Clandinin and Connelly (2000) elaborate, "when pressed, what seemed like fact appears more and more as memory reconstruction, either ours or participants'. Are these reconstructions best thought of as fiction? (p. 179). As Romano (2000) says when teaching multigenre writing, " I encourage students not just to report fact in a multitude of genres but also to fictionalize what they cannot know in order to create what could or should have happened" (p. 68). Fiction, as well as other creative writing, gives writers the opportunity to present the emotional truth of a story while experiencing freedom from details either too trivial or painful to remember.

One notable example of an author reconstructing fact as fiction is *The Things They Carried*, where O'Brien (1990) writes, "I'm forty-three years old, true, and I'm a writer now, and a long time ago I walked through Quang Ngai Province as a foot soldier. Almost everything else is invented. But it's not a game. It's a form" (p. 179). As Goldberg (2000) writes when discussing *The Things They Carried*, "as I read I knew the book was all true, but he's also saying what is truth?" (p. 129). DeSalvo (1999) provides another insight about the book by stating, "but he says too, that to tell truthfully what happened to him as a foot soldier in Quang Ngai Province in Vietnam, he has had to resort to invention" (p. 165). The important thing about all stories that use fiction or other forms of creative writing to present facts is that the reader comprehends the emotional truth of the story.

Clandinin and Connelly (2000) observe, "in narrative inquiry, the distinction between fact and fiction is muddled" (p. 179). Sometimes when remembering a story in preparation for retelling it, details blur together. Lamott (1994) believes, "a writer paradoxically seeks the truth and tells lies every step of the way. It's a lie if you make something up. But you make it up in the name of the truth, and then you give your heart to expressing it clearly" (p. 52). Sometimes the emotional truth of a story resonates more than the happening truth when the emotions the writer felt mean more than specifics such as the name of a street or the color of a sweater. In *The Things They Carried*, O'Brien (1990) needed a method to provide the emotional truth of his war experiences in Vietnam while freeing himself of specific details; he explains, "I want you to feel what I felt. I want you to know why story-truth is truer sometimes than happening truth" (p. 179). The story-truth of fiction helps a writer focus on an experience without feeling confined by specific details that exist in happening-truth life. In fact, fiction helps writers focus on the facts. Goldberg (2000) describes her perspective on *The Things They Carried* and elaborates, "so O'Brien walks out into the land of fiction and looks back and tells the story from that perspective. Maybe then he can get a handle on it. Sometimes the more fictional a writer becomes, the closer he actually gets to dead center. Fiction lets us unhinge from facts and unleashes the soul of a thing" (p. 129). DeSalvo (1999) concurs that *The Things They Carried* "brilliantly solves many problems inherent in writing about extreme trauma. In the novel he writes what is, ostensibly, a memoir. But then he tells the reader the only way to tell the truth about his life is to make it up, to use "story-truth." He does this, in part, he says, because all memory is fictive" (p. 165). She continues, "we can write, not to express feelings we don't have, but to discover what we might have felt if we hadn't been terrified. This is best done, O'Brien believes, when we strive for 'story truth' rather than literal truth, when we describe semifictional stand-ins for ourselves" (p. 166). Or as O'Brien (1990) states, "what stories can do, I guess, is make things present" (p. 180). Sometimes the happening-truth feels too painful for a writer to explore in writing, so the only way for the writer to share the experience becomes to use story-truth and share the soul of the story without reliving the trauma during the retelling of events.

I experienced the converging of story-truth and happening-truth during the writing of my doctoral dissertation. With the story-truth of fiction, I felt free to focus on the emotional truth of experiences without feeling confined by specific details that existed in my happening-truth life.

While fiction writing helped me heal from emotional pain, I had to leave story-truth behind and share the happening-truth of my life in order to help me heal from physical pain. In my neck pain journal, I needed to be specific in order to help my physical therapist help me heal. I needed to be honest and share my story. When using writing to heal from emotional pain, the form, such as fiction, poetry. or personal essay, doesn't matter as much as the processing of emotional truth. Conversely, when using writing to heal from physical pain, the essential thing is telling the specific truth of events as they happen and sharing them with a medical professional who can help.

NARRATIVE MEDICINE

Since it values narratives, narrative medicine provides the foundation for presenting a patient's story using a multigenre format. Rasminsky (2012) tells the story of Dr. Rita Charon, "the founding director of the Program in Narrative Medicine at Columbia University, where future MDs participate in writing workshops and examine texts by authors" (p. 88). Charon uses information about writing and literature typically found in an English teacher's classroom to inform her practice because she "realized that the clues she needed weren't confined to lab results and diagnostic scans. They were hidden in her patients' habits, fears, beliefs, family circumstances, even their insurance battles" (p. 88). Writing can provide subjective qualitative information often missing in quantitative objective measures.

Narrative medicine presents an integrative approach to medicine that focuses on the patient's story. Patients can benefit from focusing on what Duke Integrative Medicine (2010) at Duke University calls the Wheel of Health. By asking patients to reflect on movement, exercise and rest; nutrition; personal and professional development, physical environment; relationships and communication; spirituality; mind-body connection; and mindful awareness, "the Wheel of Health represents a comprehensive perspective of well-being and it addresses all the resources available to you to optimize your health" (pp. 5-6). Integrative medicine provides patients with the opportunity to take ownership of their health, frequently by partnering with a health coach, and set wellness goals to achieve.

DIALOGUE JOURNALS

One method patients and their medical practitioners can use writing as healing is through dialogue journals. Unlike a private journal intended to be seen by only the individual writing in it, a dialogue journal is meant to be a written conversation between two or more people. It looks like an email conversation, only on notebook paper. The value of writing conversations is that it gives both authors time to reflect on ideas. Patients and family members can write their questions in a notebook so they do not forget them. The physical therapist or other medical practitioner can use the questions and any other observations to modify the treatment plan if necessary. The patient could benefit from writing down their questions between treatment sessions so they don't forget what they what to ask once the therapist arrives. Vacca, Vacca, and Mraz (2014) provide the definition, "as is the case with response and double-entry journals, students keep an ongoing record of learning as it happens in a notebook" (p. 299). Patients are therefore able to track their learning as it takes place so the medical practitioner has a record of progress and family members have a record of insights to help them care for their loved one. As Romano (1987) writes, "readers peer into the writer's very soul" (p. 41). Some people express themselves better in writing instead of speaking. Dialogue journals open the door for such conversations.

Sometimes people don't want to share their writing because it makes them feel vulnerable. Noppe-Brandon (2004) asked her students if they liked to read and write and observed, "among those who raised their hands, few chose to read or write, they simply didn't mind it. As a formerly voiceless person, who had channeled many of my own thoughts and feelings into private writing, I couldn't totally understand this. It was only as I closed the gap between my private and public expressions that I began to fully appreciate the vulnerablility involved in revealing things, even to oneself" (p. 2). Reflecting on thoughts and feelings means being vulnerable. The script in a person's head may read: What if someone doesn't like the real me? What if I don't like the real me? But during the healing process, the patient needs to trust that a medical practitioner is used to discussing sensitive medical information.

Such support can lead patients and their medial practitioners to exchange ideas in writing.

Barbieri (1995) describes the writing process as, "words came onto the page that I had not intended; the whole point of what I had been trying to say became clear to me, and I knew what I needed to write next. Stunned, I thought I had discovered magic" (p. 16). When it leads to discovery, writing does seem like magic. Kearns (1997) counters, "good writing is not the result of a magic wand; it comes from hard work" (p. 16). But when that hard work falls into place it looks effortless, like magic. And teachers, whether they are in a classroom or medical facility, can help the magic happen. Cleary (1991) believes, "we need our writing curriculum to reattach students to their souls" (p. 167). Lessons from the writing curriculum typically used in high school and college classrooms can also help patients in a medical setting.

VOICE LESSONS

Usually when people think of voice lessons, music comes to mind first. Writing voice shines through when writers, whether they are patients in a clinic or students in a classroom, follow the advice Goldberg (2007) gives, which is, "say what you want to say, not what you think you should say" (p. 2). Voice also influences how the writers share their stories. As Goldberg (2013) advises writers, "you have to find the entry into what you know inside, the way to bring it out so people will listen" (p. 26). Sometimes this means sharing information through expository writing that you are used to reading in academic textbooks. Other times, however, it involves sharing information through narratives.

In this chapter, I alternate between third person academic writing and first person narrative writing. Heard (2002) believes, "the more you include yourself in the piece and are able to tell your unique story, including your particular details, the more we, as readers, can experience it too" (p. 54). I use the pronoun "I" to own my stories and share my writing personality. Fletcher (2013) explains, "voice in writing has to do with a unique personality-on-paper" (p. 78). It becomes possible to write first person narratives while simultaneously including research and the citation of sources as part of the stories; therefore, you are reading narratives with a scaffold of research as the objective research frames the subjective narratives. This type of research is called narrative inquiry. Clandinin and Connelly (2000) explain, "voice, and dilemmas created by the consideration of it, are always sorted out by the exercise of judgment" (p. 147). Each writer makes the judgment call of how to present his or her story. We skate a thin line on the ice between artistic and technical and have research to support us as we let our voices sing.

ACKNOWLEDGMENT

The preceding chapter contains excerpts from the following previous IGI publications:

Bird, J.L., & Wanner, E.T. (2019). Turning PAGES with health coaching and family involvement. In Information Resources Management Association (Ed.), *Chronic illness and long-term care: Breakthroughs in research and practice* (pp. 255-276). Hershey, PA: Information Science Reference.

Bird, J.L. (2017). Writing healing narratives. In V.C. Bryan & J.L. Bird (Eds.), *Healthcare community synergism between patients, practitioners, and researchers*. Hershey, PA: Information Science Reference.

Bird, J.L., & Wanner, E.T. (2016). Turning PAGES with health coaching and family involvement. In V.C.X. Wang (Ed.), *Handbook of research on advancing health education through technology* (pp. 213-233). Hershey, PA: Information Science Reference.

Bird, J.L. (2015). Preface. In J.L. Bird (Ed.), *Innovative collaborative practice and reflection in patient education* (pp. xiv-xxi). Hershey, PA: Information Science Reference.

Bird, J.L., Wanner, E.T., Urenda, R., & Perry, R. (2015). Multigenre medicine. In J.L. Bird (Ed.), *Innovative collaborative practice and reflection in patient education* (pp. 1-19). Hershey, PA: Information Science Reference.

Bird, J.L., & Wanner, E.T. (2014). Educational research narratives of healing. In V.C.X. Wang (Ed.), *Adult and community health education: Tools, trends and methodologies* (pp. 264-280). Hershey, PA: Information Science Reference.

REFERENCES

Adams, K. (1990). *Journal to the Self*. New York, NY: Warner Books.

Alexander, E. (2012). *Proof of Heaven*. New York, NY: Simon and Schuster.

Alexander, E. (2014). *The map of Heaven*. New York, NY: Simon and Schuster.

Barbieri, M. (1995). *Sounds from the heart*. Portsmouth, NH: Heinemann.

Beck, M. (2001). *Finding your own North Star*. New York, NY: Three Rivers Press.

Brown, B. (2015). *Rising strong*. New York, NY: Spiegel & Grau.

Caldwell, K., Gray, J., & Wolever, R. Q. (2013). The process of patient empowerment in integrative health coaching: How does it happen? *Global Advances in Health and Medicine: Improving Healthcare Outcomes Worldwide*, *2*(3), 48–57. doi:10.7453/gahmj.2013.026 PMID:24416672

Cameron, J. (1998). *The right to write*. New York: Tarcher/Putnam.

Carter, C. (2015). *The sweet spot*. New York, NY: Ballantine.

Charon, R. (2006). *Narrative medicine: honoring the stories of illness*. New York, NY: Oxford University Press.

Clandinin, D. J., & Connelly, F. M. (2000). *Narrative inquiry*. San Francisco, CA: Jossey-Bass.

Cleary, L. M. (1991). *From the other side of the desk*. Portsmouth, NH: Heinemann.

Cleaver, J. (2002). *Immediate fiction*. New York, NY: St. Martin's Press.

Connelly, F. M., & Clandinin, D. J. (1988). *Teachers as curriculum planners*. New York, NY: Teachers College.

DeSalvo, L. (1999). *Writing as a way of healing*. Boston, MA: Beacon Press.

Duke Integrative Medicine Staff. (2010). *Personalized health plan manual*. Durham, NC: Duke Integrative Medicine.

Fitzgerald, F. S. (1925). *The great Gatsby*. New York, NY: Scribner.

Fletcher, R. (2013). *What a writer needs* (2nd ed.). Portsmouth, NH: Heinemann.

Germer, C. K. (2009). *The Mindful path to self-compassion*. New York, NY: The Guilford Press.

Goldberg, N. (2000). *Thunder and lightning*. New York, NY: Bantam.

Goldberg, N. (2007). *Old friend from far away*. New York, NY: Free Press.

Goldberg, N. (2013). *The true secret of writing*. New York, NY: Atria.

Greenberg, M. A., Wortman, C. B., & Stone, A. A. (1996). Emotional expression and physical health: Revising traumatic memories or fostering self-regulation. *Journal of Personality and Social Psychology*, *71*(3), 588–602. doi:10.1037/0022-3514.71.3.588 PMID:8831163

Handler, J. (2013). *Braving the fire*. New York, NY: St. Martin's Griffin.

Haugk, K. C. (2000). *When and how to use mental health resources*. St. Louis, MO: Stephen Ministries.

Heard, G. (2002). *The revision toolbox*. Portsmouth, NH: Heinemann.

Helldorfer, M., & Moss, T. (2007). *Healing with heart*. Orinda, CA: Moss Communications.

Kearns, J. (1997). *Where to begin: a guide to teaching secondary English*. Portsmouth, NH: Heinemann.

Lamott, A. (1994). *Bird by bird*. New York: Anchor Books.

Lepore, S. J., Greenberg, M. A., Bruno, M., & Smyth, J. M. (2002). Expressive writing and health: self-regulation of emotion-related experience, physiology, and behavior. In S. J. Lepore & J. M. Smyth (Eds.), *The writing cure* (pp. 99–117). Washington, DC: American Psychological Association. doi:10.1037/10451-005

Madigan, S. (2011). *Narrative therapy*. Washington, DC: American Psychological Association.

Michele, L. (2015). *You first: journal your way to your best life*. New York, NY: Crown Archetype.

Neff, K. (2011). *Self compassion: the proven power of being kind to yourself*. New York, NY: HarperCollins.

Noppe-Brandon, G. (2004). *Find your voice*. Portsmouth, NH: Heinemann.

O'Brien, T. (1990). *The things they carried*. New York, NY: Broadway Books.

Pennebaker, J. W. (1997). *Opening up: the healing power of expressing emotions*. New York, NY: The Guilford Press.

Pennebaker, J. W., & Evans, J. F. (2014). *Expressive writing: words that heal*. Enumclaw, WA: Idyll Arbor.

Poetter, T. S. (2013). Stemming the tide. *Kappa Delta Pi Record, 49*(3), 100–104. doi:10.1080/00228958.2013.819195

Rasminsky, A. (2012). The story doc. *Oprah, 13*(7), 88.

Romano, T. (1987). *Clearing the way*. Portsmouth, NH: Heinemann.

Romano, T. (1995). *Writing with passion*. Portsmouth, NH: Heinemann.

Romano, T. (2000). *Blending genre, altering style*. Portsmouth, NH: Heinemann.

Romano, T. (2004). *Crafting authentic voice*. Portsmouth, NH: Heinemann.

Romano, T. (2008). *Zigzag*. Portsmouth, NH: Heinemann.

Romano, T. (2013). *Fearless writing*. Portsmouth, NH: Heinemann.

Smith, L. L., Lake, N. H., Simmons, L. A., Perlman, A., Wroth, S., & Wolever, R. Q. (2013). Integrative health coach training: A model for shifting the paradigm toward patient-centricity and meeting new national prevention goals. *Global Advances in Health and Medicine: Improving Healthcare Outcomes Worldwide*, *2*(3), 66–74. doi:10.7453/gahmj.2013.034 PMID:24416674

Vacca, R. T., Vacca, J. L., & Mraz, M. (2014). *Content area reading* (11th ed.). Boston, MA: Pearson.

Wanner, S. Y. (1994). *On with the story*. Portsmouth, NH: Heinemann.

Weiner-Davis, M. (1995). *Fire your shrink*. New York, NY: Simon & Schuster.

Zimmermann, S. (2002). *Writing to heal the soul*. New York, NY: Three Rivers Press.

KEY TERMS AND DEFINITIONS

Journal Writing: The process of a person responding to prompts and writing about his or her thoughts and feelings. While journal writing is typically associated with writing classrooms, writing teachers including Julia Cameron, Natalie Goldberg, and Donald Murray advocate that journal writing can be done by anyone, anywhere. Students in an English classroom, patients in a physical therapy clinic, and readers of this chapter in their living rooms can pick up pen, paper, and just write.

Multigenre Writing: Discussed in the field of education by Tom Romano, a multigenre paper consists of two parts: creative writing in multiple genres and the writer's analysis of the genres.

Narrative Inquiry: Discussed in the field of research by F. Michael Connelly and D. Jean Clandinin, narrative inquiry is a qualitative interpretative form of research that focuses on the telling, retelling, and sharing of stories.

Researchers who complete narrative inquiries interpret stories and search for common threads to find patterns. They are encouraged to tell their research stories in first person as they look back to find meaning in past stories and look forward to set future goals.

Story-Truth and Happening-Truth: Happening-truth is an objective factual account of events which occurred. Story-truth, sometimes referred to as emotional truth, is a subjective reflection of a person's thoughts and feelings about the same event when retelling that story. Writers such as Tim O'Brien, Natalie Goldberg, and Anne Lamott believe in the power of emotional truth that enables writers to switch back and forth from objective observations to subjective emotions when sharing a story.

Writing Voice: Voice in writing describes how a writer uses word choice and tone to compose a journal entry or other written composition that reflects the personality of the writer. Just like each person has a unique speaking voice, each writer has a unique writing voice.

Chapter 5
Narratives of Curriculum Design

Jennifer Lynne Bird
Oxbridge Academy, USA

ABSTRACT

This narrative provides a foundation for the PAGES program. PAGES is an acronym for practice patience, accept the present, gather information, encourage, and self-care. Each part of the acronym represents advice that people can implement into their lives. The two primary examples focus on families of physical therapy patients in a hospital and advisors of students in a school. The PAGES program presents a new initiative as well as reflections on applying the information to a variety of settings.

DESIGNING PAGES

PAGES, the program described in this writing, happened because of a large foundation of writing. Rarely does any single piece of writing happen in isolation. Program development and new learning opportunities occur because of the outcomes of previous writing and research. Often different pieces of writing fit together like puzzle pieces to form a larger picture. Heard (1995) confirms, "the obstacles I face – lack of time, too many projects at once – as well as the obstacles all writers face – rejection, criticism, doubts and insecurities, unfinished poems and stories – are impossible to avoid and can be valuable teachers" (pp. 38-39). Writers consistently overcome obstacles to develop new ideas. Jen, an English teacher and health coach, completed

DOI: 10.4018/978-1-7998-1931-8.ch005

extensive writing and research with Eric, a physical therapist and research consultant, which provided a foundation upon which to scaffold this new idea. Family involvement becomes the heart and soul of PAGES. While physical therapists, health coaches, and other medical professionals can offer support to a hospital patient, when the patient goes home from the hospital, the relay baton of care gets passed to the family member caregiver. Similarly, while teachers, academic advisors, and other education professionals can offer support to a student, when the student goes home from the school, the relay baton of care gets passed to the family member caregiver.

This narrative provides a foundation for the PAGES program. While the program was originally designed for the families of hospital patients, the same strategy was later adapted to help the families of high school students. It can also be adapted to other fields as you as the reader view appropriate. PAGES is an acronym that serves as a reminder for families of hospital patients to reflect on what they need to do to help their loved ones recover after surgery. It also serves as a reminder for families of students to reflect on what they need to do to help their loved ones achieve success in school. The designers used expertise in health coaching, curriculum design, teaching, writing, and research in a physical therapy clinic to create the PAGES program with the intent it will make a difference to people who apply the strategy to their lives.

THE PAGES FAMILY COACHING PROGRAM

Helping patients turn new pages and write new chapters in their healing journeys

To help your loved one who is a patient:

- **Practice Patience:** Healing is a journey. No one can wave a magic wand and provide an immediate cure. Celebrate progress, no matter how small.
- **Accept the Present:** Feelings of guilt, anger, and frustration are normal, but are not helpful when coaching. No matter what happened in the past, this is where you are now. Worrying about the future only causes additional stress. Try your best to remain in the present moment. Consider writing in a journal to sort through your feelings.
- **Gather Information:** The medical professionals such as doctors, physical therapists, occupational therapists, nurses, and speech therapists are here to help you. Ask questions, and listen to their

instructions. Consider bringing a notebook with you to write down information so you don't have to remember it.

- **Encourage:** During the healing journey, patients need cheerleaders. You are a source of hope and light during this process and a little support can make a large difference.
- **Self-Care:** In order to take care of your loved one, take care of yourself too. You can better help someone else when your own needs, such as hunger and sleep, are met too.

PAGES CURRICULUM

In 2015, Jen completed a health coaching internship at a hospital, where she served as a member of the inpatient physical therapy team and helped patients with the emotional side of healing. While they both worked at the hospital, Jen and Eric designed a family coaching program called PAGES. Due to the changing needs of programs at the hospital, the program never reached the implementation stage. In a serendipitous moment, Jen joined the advisory committee at the high school where she works with the goal of designing mentoring strategies to enhance the lives of high school students. The PAGES program, which incorporates strategies from a variety of relationship based leadership curricula, can easily adapt to fit the needs of high school students.

- **Practice Patience:** As high school students continue their journeys through life, they need supportive adults as role models. Often, the most significant goals cannot happen overnight. Empower students by celebrating progress, no matter how small. Students have numerous people giving them advice, so active listening proves valuable in a role as advisor.
- **Accept the Present:** Try to remain in the present moment. It becomes easy for both teachers and students to think of the myriad of tasks to accomplish in a day, but advisory time provides a break for students from past mistakes and future worries. Journal writing also helps students sort through their feelings.
- **Gather Information:** Ask open ended questions, and listen to student answers. As an advisor, use reflective statements to acknowledge student feelings. If students need additional assistance, refer them to the appropriate resource such as college counseling or the school psychologist.

- **Encourage:** During the high school journey, students need support. As an advisor, you provide a source of hope, which makes a difference.
- **Self-Care:** In order to take care of your students, take care of yourself too. You can better help someone else when your own needs, such as hunger and sleep, are met.

Skills such as being in the present moment, practicing active listening, asking open ended questions, and using reflective statements to acknowledge the feelings of others appear in several training programs. Kenneth Haugk (2000) and the team at Stephen Ministries designed a program to prepare lay caregivers to assist ministers in helping members of a congregation who experience losses. For people looking to improve or maintain health, the team at Duke University Integrative Medicine (2010) designed a health coaching program. To promote care of self and others, the team at Creative Health Care Management (2003) designed a relationship based care model for showing compassion in the workplace. The PAGES program combines elements from all of these programs, as well as the theory and practice of curriculum design in schools, to meet the needs of high school students.

Some educators may feel concern that advisory represents time away from classes. However, teacher Graves (2001) argues, "curriculum is the sum total of the content of human experience from the time we arise until we go to bed in the evening" (p. 47). Hence, curriculum does not only represent the lesson plans and textbooks teachers use in their classrooms; curriculum also represents life and lived experiences. Johnson (1998) explains, "life is magnified and feelings are intensified for children" (p. 173). Advisory represents a place where students can discuss topics with an adult mentor, or write about feelings in a journal to process emotions on the page. English professor Romano (2000) describes the value of students writing in journals and elaborates, "when we write expressively in a journal, we imprint ideas, information, and experience deeply within us. We live topics by re-creating them with words on paper, by pulling images and dialog from the flow of our lives" (p. 138). When students explore their thoughts and feelings in writing or through conversation, it becomes important for both teachers and students to remember that, while teachers may serve as mentors and advisors, teachers cannot play the role of counselor. Brown (2018) explains, "if struggle is being down in a hole, empathy is not jumping into the hole with someone who is struggling and taking on their emotions, or owning their struggle as yours to fix. If their issues become yours, now you have two people stuck in a hole. Not helpful. Boundaries are important here" (p. 142). If teachers see signs of depression, anxiety, or any other emotional distress in students, the teacher should refer the student to the school psychologist.

With an advisory curriculum, it becomes essential to give students a voice in their learning experiences. Beane (1997) believes, "since curriculum integration is tied to the larger concept of democratic education, the matter of student participation in planning their own experiences must eventually become a crucial aspect of the design" (p. 9). Therefore, even though teachers may develop a plan for advisory, student experiences should play a role in an advisory session. Connelly and Clandinin (1988) advise teachers to use reflection when learning student narratives because, "it is their curriculum, their personal practical knowledge and narratives of experience that fall within your guidance" (p. 197). In order for students to feel comfortable sharing their stories, teachers need to provide a safe space for such conversations. Brown (2018) advises teachers, "we must be guardians of a space that allows students to breathe and be curious and explore the world and be who they are without suffocation. They deserve one place where they can rumble with vulnerability and their hearts can exhale" (p. 13). Small advisory groups can provide such a place for students. Sandberg and Grant (2017) describe the launch of "Lean In Circles, small groups of peers who meet regularly to support and encourage one another" (p. 134). Like a Lean In Circle for adults, a high school advisory represents a place where peers encourage and support each other.

PAGES, the acronym for this program, symbolizes the idea of turning new pages in life. The skills of practicing patience, accepting the present, gathering information, encouragement, and self-care provide the foundations of a supportive learning community. Through a regular advisory meeting, advisors can help students turn the pages of their own life stories and write new chapters of success.

FOUNDATION FOR PAGES

This idea for the PAGES program began once Jen began working as a health coach at a hospital. During her time at the hospital she worked with staff members who wanted to make health adjustments to their lives. Eric, a physical therapist, and Jen also worked with staff members who had a physical health issue such as back pain, knee pain, or neck pain. Eric gave the patients specific exercises to complete or performed appropriate manual techniques after diagnosing their condition, while Jen talked with them to assess the importance of the treatment plan to them and their confidence in completing the treatment plan. This helped us see the patient's barriers to the recovery process so we could help the person overcome those barriers. This process made a positive difference in patients' healing and has been very rewarding for us as practitioners.

TURNING PAGES FOR NEW POSSIBILITIES

Since the foundation for PAGES exists in curriculum development, which usually takes place in a school, it became easy to modify the strategy from a group classroom environment in a hospital to a classroom environment in a school. Regardless of whether a hospital patient experiences recovery from a surgical procedure or a high school student experiences a difficult day at school, family support provides a foundation for success. Havrilesky (2018) describes how people can create change as, "we are called to plant these seeds in our world: to dare to tell every living soul that they already matter, that their seemingly mundane lives are a slowly unfolding mystery, that their small choices and acts of generosity are vitally important" (p. 217). Lee (2018) provides a similar description of change as, "the lesson of renewal is that from small seeds big things grow" (p. 298). She continues, "it's not far-fetched to believe that from the seeds of our own joy, a whole world can be reborn" (p. 298). Every person needs to know that he or she matters to other people; therefore, a support network provides the necessary environment to demonstrate care and community.

CREATING A CARING CURRICULUM

If energy is put into the curriculum design and lesson plans, the energy will be reflected in the teacher as the lesson is taught and the students will subsequently benefit from it. Graves (2001) states, "the energy of the curriculum lies in the making, learning, and planning of what is ahead" (p. 49). Sometimes, however, the curriculum is not explicitly stated but implicitly implied. This is called the hidden curriculum. As Connelly and Clandinin (1988) define, "generally speaking, people think of the hidden curriculum as falling in the area of attitudes and values" (p. 154). In a classroom or physical therapy clinic, the hidden curriculum can encompass everything from the posters hanging on the walls to the smiles on the instructors' faces. Patients also bring their own hidden curriculum to their treatment sessions. A patient may not want to complete exercises as part of a treatment plan, but may want to achieve the goal of being pain free for a vacation. Health coaches can build bridges to link the information in the patient's mind to illuminate the fact that doing the exercises will lead to a pain free vacation. Health coaches can also enlist the support of family members to offer additional encouragement during the healing journey.

Similarly, students bring their own hidden curriculum to a classroom. A student may not want to complete an assignment as part of a lesson plan, but may want to achieve the goal of earning a high grade in the class. Advisors for a student play more of a coaching role than a teaching role; therefore, advisors can build bridges to link the information in the student's mind to illuminate the fact that studying will lead to a high grade.

Both health coaches and teacher advisors may choose to use writing as a method of managing the myriad emotions experienced in a coaching setting. Cameron (1998) believes, "every time I put my hand to the page, I am altering the energy that flows through my life" (p. 201). Whether writing encourages the venting of frustrations or the setting of goals, it brings clarity to the writer and eases anxiety. Clark (2018) explains, "both in writing and in speech, embracing a narrative of healing can be powerful in constructing a present and a future not at the mercy of the past" (p. 325). However, before writing takes place in any type of coaching setting, the coach must establish a safe environment. People often serve as their own worst critics. Neff (2011) confirms it helps "to treat ourselves with the same kindness, caring, and compassion we would show to a good friend, or even a stranger for that matter. Sadly, however, there's almost no one whom we treat as badly as ourselves" (p. 6). A safe environment creates space for members of a community to honestly speak their feelings.

Whether a person has a goal of a pain free vacation or a high grade in a class, emotions make a difference in the achievement of the goal. Medical doctor Tindle (2013) explains, "the evidence shows that people with a high degree of anger do worse healthwise" (p. 29). Medical doctor Rankin (2013) agrees that, "when you make efforts to increase your happiness, the health of the body tends to follow" (p. 142). Hope creates a desire to achieve goals, leads to increased motivation, and paves the way for a possible shorter road to achieve a goal; conversely; anger creates obstacles or adds to existing obstacles, leads to decreased motivation, and paves the way for possible longer road to achieve a goal.

Encouragement provided by supportive communities can transform the emotions of participants. Social worker Brown (2015) discovered, "in my work, I've found that moving out of powerlessness, and even despair, requires hope" (p. 202). Brown (2017) advocates turning negative emotions into positive ones because "anger is a catalyst. Holding on to it will make us exhausted and sick" (p. 67). She continues, "it's an emotion that we need to transform into something life-giving: courage, love, change, compassion, justice" (p. 68). Even if people want to transform their emotions, such a change requires trust and vulnerability. Brown (2018) explains, "trust is the stacking and layering of small moments and reciprocal vulnerability over time. Trust and vulnerability grow together, and to betray one is to destroy both" (p. 34). Change may not immediately occur, but over time a supportive community creates the environment for participants to trust each other and feel vulnerable with each other.

While the theory described in the subsequent sections focuses on hospital patients and schools, the practice of PAGES can adapt to multiple learning environments. Use the examples as inspiration to fill unwritten pages in an organization's future with new ideas and possibilities.

ASSESSMENT REVELATIONS

When implementing a program, assessment occurs to ensure the program meets its goals. Jen illustrates the similarities between assessment in the education and medical fields.

When I became the Director of the Writing and Reading Center (WRC) at Oxbridge Academy, I inherited the twenty-five high school student peer tutors who worked in the WRC during their study hall. We used the book *The Longman Guide to Peer Tutoring* to inspire us to practice the strategies of non-judging, open-ended questions, presencing, reflective statements, and active listening during peer tutoring conferences. In my role as WRC Director, I need to reflect on how teachers assessed student assessments. Reflection led to revelations about assessment.

What if I evaluated students at the beginning of the class instead of the end?

What if I approached evaluation like a physical therapist does?

I thought about how Eric, a physical therapist, evaluates patients. I arrive at the clinic and he asks me to rate on a number scale how I am feeling (numeric evaluation) and why (narrative evaluation). For example, my pain might be a 5 (on a scale of 10) because I looked down too long when reading a book. While I do my initial stretches (warm up), he takes his exercise plan (lesson plan) and adjusts it based on the information I just told him (differentiation). I leave the clinic feeling better (what learning should be).

So here is how this could work in my classroom. Instead of exit slips, where students answer questions as they leave, I use entrance slips. Students arrive with a post-it note (ideally completed for homework, but I can have post-its by the door if they forget). Students have to tell me how they would rank their comprehension numerically and give me a reason why. Students would then have to write their responses on the board so their classmates can see. For example, after reading a scene in *The Great Gatsby*, one student might give comprehension a 3 because he did not understand why Gatsby received a strange phone call. Another student might give comprehension a 7 because she loved the romantic scene where Daisy and Gatsby were staring at the green light.

While students write in journals (warm ups, I would quickly use their numbers and narratives to modify my lesson plans to inform my teaching for the day (differentiation). For example, if I have high numbers, I can ask higher level learning questions or have a Socratic seminar where students share their opinions. If I have low numbers, I may ask students to complete a double-entry journal where they choose a confusing quote and write what they think it means. If I have numbers all over the scale, I may break students into small groups and ask them to share their thoughts with each other. Then (hopefully), students leave the classroom feeling better about the text (what learning should be).

Assessment for a program such as PAGES does not have to look identical to this example, but should demonstrate thought and reflection to ensure the program meets its objectives.

GREATER HEALING GAINS THROUGH FAMILY INVOLVEMENT

Similar to how family support can lead to educational success for a child, evidence exists that family involvement leads to greater healing for patients. Ryan, Wade, Nice, Shenefelt, and Shepard (1996) discovered, "family involvement was found to be a significant aspect of a patient's rehabilitation"

(p. 159). Through a series of interviews with forty physical therapists, the researchers learned, "the shift from hospital to home care increases the effect on the family unit and significantly expands the role of the physical therapist in involving the family in the rehabilitation process. Such trends in healthcare require that physical therapists have effective, time-efficient strategies for involving family members in a way that ensures the highest potential for optimal recovery of the patient" (p. 160). However, some family members may have barriers in their family dynamics to work thorough while attempting to provide support for their loved one who is a physical therapy patient going through an exercise treatment plan.

Physical therapists can expertly inform family members about the patient's at home treatment plan. Nevertheless, due to demands by insurance companies and the health care system for clinicians to consistently demonstrate increased productivity, a physical therapist may not be able to have a lengthy conversation with a patient's family about how the family is navigating the crisis of the patient's surgery and how everyone can move forward together as a family unit. This is where health coaches can provide much needed assistance for both physical therapists and families. The authors of the family involvement research study observed, "the success with which a family adapts to crisis depends on a variety of factors from financial resources to the family's expectations and knowledge of the patient's condition" (p. 160). Health coaches are trained in psychology but are not psychologists; if a family wants to have a lengthy session about past issues in the family dynamics the health coach will make a referral to a psychologist. The role of the health coach is to help the patient, and therefore also the family members, to focus on the present situation and offer strategies and resources for breaking down barriers and overcoming obstacles, that help maintain forward momentum. The researchers concluded that "the physical therapist's knowledge of what the family is experiencing is crucial in guiding the family towards appropriate goal setting" (p. 175). The emerging field of health coaching did not exist when this research study was conducted, but health coaches, physical therapists, and families can all work together to ensure elite results for the patient.

DESIGNING A CURRICULUM OF FAMILY INVOLVEMENT

Creating a new curriculum, whether it is at a school or a hospital, takes thought and effort. A teacher can't just walk into a classroom, wave a copy of *The Great Gatsby* at students, and teach without a lesson plan or a curriculum to support that lesson plan. Similarly, it helps the families of patients to know the expectations of the physical therapist for the exercise plan. As Marshall, Sears, and Schubert (2000) explain, "we believe that the essence of curriculum studies lies in the way each educator internalizes fundamental questions of what curriculum is and should be – and the attendant whys, whens, and whereas of its enactment" (p. 3). Anyone designing a new curriculum needs to ask the questions of why a lesson is being taught, when the lesson is going to be taught, and how it is going to be presented.

In one example, when family members coach patients, the why is that as the primary caregivers, a family member will have to take over supervision of the patient's home exercise plan once the patient leaves the hospital and help the patient remember to do the exercises. The when begins when the family member attends group physical therapy classes with the patient and learns instructions about the exercises from the physical therapist. And the how happens when family members offer encouragement and support to become an extra member on the team that helps motivate the patient to achieve success.

In another example, when teachers coach students, the why is that as the educator, a teacher will use a variety of instructional techniques to inspire students to learn. The when begins when the students step into the classroom and the teacher sets the tone for learning. And the how happens when the teacher offers encouragement and support to become an extra member on the team that helps motivate the students to achieve success.

To be successful, a curriculum also needs to incorporate goal setting. Beane (1997) explains, "curriculum integration centers the curriculum on life itself rather than on the mastery of fragmented information within the boundaries of subject areas. It works off a view of learning as the continuous integration of new knowledge and experience so as to deepen and broaden our understanding of ourselves and our world" (p. 18). Curriculum integration encourages democratic education and active learning, where participants have ownership of the curriculum instead of having someone else tell it to them. The goals of a curriculum often evolve from evidence based practice, such as action research. Action research occurs when a teacher develops a new idea and tries it in a classroom setting. Or as Connelly and Clandinin (1988) explain, "action research is, therefore, a deliberate way of creating new situations and of telling the story of who we are" (p. 153). If an idea is implemented and succeeds, it often becomes adapted into the curriculum. While action research has its foundation in the field of education, it can be modified for use in other fields. Part of health coaching involves encouraging people to set goals to take ownership of their healing. In this instance, the goal setting process becomes collaborative. A curriculum that provides the foundation of effective information that sets people up for success enhances the goal setting process. Clandinin and Connelly (2000) elaborate, "the teacher is part of the curriculum and therefore part of the establishment of the goals in the first place and part of the ensuing achievement" (p. 29). Just as teachers celebrate their student's successes in a classroom, physical therapists celebrate their patient's successes in a clinic. The creation of SMART (specific, measurable, action oriented, realistic, timed) goals in both settings means that learning becomes a collaborative team effort, with the successful outcome of one goal leading to the setting of a new goal. Connelly and Clandinin (1988) continue, "administering the curriculum meant the narrative living out of a personal philosophy of education" (p. 196). The best teachers combine the artistic and technical when teaching. They teach the required elements of the curriculum using methods that make the lessons come alive for students. The execution of an effective lesson resembles a beautiful figure skating or dance routine. Skaters and dancers must complete required technical elements, but also infuse their performance with artistic interpretation and passion.

Every curriculum also needs a solid theoretical foundation to support the practice of teaching. The next sections highlight the dimensions of PAGES and why they are important. Teachers, family members of hospital patients, physical therapists, health coaches, other medical practitioners, other educators, and readers interested in learning something new can all benefit from the following information.

PRACTICE PATIENCE

In children's stories, a fairy godmother frequently shows up to save the day. There is a literary term for this too, called "Deus ex machina," Latin for God from a machine, meaning unexpected rescue. It can be seen in superhero stories too, when characters are rescued from a seemingly impossible situation. Real life doesn't work that way, and people must do the work to reach their goals. Having a positive attitude can help make everything easier. Tindle (2013) believes that if one person has a positive attitude it can influence an entire community because, "when we learn to see the interconnectedness of things in this way, we understand how a positive attitude in one person can benefit countless others, because every person who is able to look up to mental and physical health gives herself maximal opportunity to develop her unique talents. Whenever even one of us can accomplish this feat, it not only stokes the enthusiasm of the entire group but also adds to our collective resources. To this end, cultivating a healthy outlook may perhaps be society's ultimate return on investment" (p. 218). Therefore, if everyone involved in the patient's healing journey (such as doctors, nurses, physical therapists, health coaches, and family members) promotes positivity the patient will know it is okay to take the time needed to heal. Comparatively, if everyone involved in a student's educational journey (such as teachers, advisors, counselors, and family members) promotes positivity the student will know it is okay to take the time needed to learn.

Promoting positivity can help patients not only emotionally, but also physically. Rankin (2013) discusses the connection between mind and body and asks, "so what happens to the body when the mind is in a dark place? Emotional suffering might start in the mind, but it is ultimately an embodied experience. You don't just experience unhappiness in your mind. You feel it in your body, as suffering cascades through your body via the stress response" (p. 132-133). If a patient feels upset about the length of time it is taking to heal, it is possible that the emotional stress will manifest itself as additional physical symptoms.

Studies show that a positive outlook leads to greater healing gains. Younger, Gandhi, Hubbard, and Mackey (2012) studied the positive or negative expectations patients had in physical therapy with the SETS (Stanford Expectations of Treatment Scale) and learned patients with a more positive expectancy did better than patients with negative expectancy (p. 767). Our own research led to the design of a new survey, *The Wanner Bird Healing Survey for Pain Recovery* (2013) and the conclusion that patients in a physical therapy clinic who used more positive language when responding to short writing prompts performed better on existing objective physical therapy measures.

In order to have a positive attitude, patients need to feel they are in a safe environment. It takes time and patience to establish trust. Advice given by Johnson (1998) can apply to hospitals as well as schools because, as is true with anyone being taught, "they need time to see that we sincerely care about them, have something valuable to teach them, and will not embarrass them when they make mistakes. We need time to get to know their personalities and maturity levels, as well as their intellectual abilities and academic needs. It also takes time to create an environment in our classrooms that is comfortable and secure, so students can relax and concentrate on their lessons" (p. 101). Physical therapists collaborate with health coaches and family members to establish a supportive environment for the patient during group physical therapy classes just like teachers collaborate with advisors and family members to establish a supportive environment for students.

ACCEPT THE PRESENT

When a loved one needs surgery and physical therapy, family members experience a myriad of emotions. They may feel anger at the circumstances that landed the patient in the hospital, or frustrated that the patient is not healing faster. They may feel guilty if their actions contributed to the patient's condition or helpless because they can't take away the pain. All of these feelings are normal, but do not help the patient. Therefore, it is important for family members to deal with their feelings by writing in a journal or talking to someone such as a supportive friend or professional counselor if additional help is needed. While writing in a journal can help patients heal, journals can also help family members sort through their feelings.

Zimmermann (2002) explains, "there is now extensive research that shows writing – the simple act of putting down your deepest thoughts and feelings on paper – is one of the most powerful and effective means to ease and ultimately heal sorrow" (p. 18). Anyone visiting the English Department at a high school or college will most likely hear discussion of research studies illustrating how writing improves emotional health. Writing helps caregivers process their emotions so they can better help their family members who are patients. Caregivers can choose to keep their writing to themselves or share it with a health coach or other professional if they need to discuss their feelings.

Health coaching meets people where they are in the present moment. Health coaches can help family members accept that they cannot change the past, so they must work with the patient in the present situation to set goals for the future. Health coaches can help a patient see the importance of a treatment plan and increase the patient's confidence in completing the treatment plan by connecting the treatment plan to the patient's vision and values. Pipher (2006) explains, "in both therapy and writing, we want to help people see the connections between their actions and consequences of those actions" (p. 97). It is also important for family members to realize they cannot force change on their loved one. In order for a person to make a change, he or she needs to reach the conclusion that change is necessary. Pipher continues, "people do not change unless they have a powerful emotional turning. This may be thorough epiphanies, insights, or deep connecting moments between the people in the room" (p. 100). While one person cannot make another person change, showing acceptance and being a supportive presence can set the stage for powerful insights by the patient to occur. The same process occurs in classrooms. If a teacher, advisor, or family member serves as a supportive presence the safe environment creates insightful student learning moments.

Another part of the health coaching process is accountability. Health coaches work with people to set goals and make connections, but they also ask the people they are coaching to be accountable for their actions. With family members, sometimes emotions get in the way when trying to hold a loved one accountable for his or her actions. As Brown (2010) explains, "it's hard for us to understand that we can be compassionate and accepting while we hold people accountable for their behaviors" (p. 18). Sometimes when coaching a family member, emotions take over when the patient is not demonstrating accountability for complying with the treatment plan. Since health coaches have an objective distance from the patient that family members do not, health coaches can remind family coaches to continue to show compassion and acceptance during the patient's healing journey.

With family relationships, dynamics can get complicated. Beck (2008) elaborates, "you may be one of the lucky people whose loved ones and associates are all delighted and inspired when you set out to live your right life. More likely, though, you'll encounter some level of resistance. After all, the most common reason we stray from our best lives is that we're socialized to behave in ways that aren't right for us. Our social groups, almost by definition, tend to disapprove when we drop those behaviors" (p. 191). Regardless of what has happened between family members in the past, it is important for family members to put any issues aside when coaching the patient. If the family member has felt disappointed in the patient's behavior in the past, bringing those emotions into a group physical therapy class does not help the patient heal in the present moment. Change can be difficult for everyone, especially family members who did not ask for their lives to be disrupted by the patient's surgery. However, as Nick tells Gatsby in *The Great Gatsby* by Fitzgerald (1925), "you can't repeat the past" (p. 116). This quote from literature is powerful advice for families too.

In addition to family members demonstrating acceptance for the patient's current medical reality, the patient has to accept that even when the family is accepting and supportive, the patient still has to do the work to reach his or her healing goals. Beck (2001) states, " people whose families were accepting and supportive have to face the fact that familial love can't take them all the way to their right lives" (p. 70). Beck continues with the reminder, "but you will still have to do the physical therapy to get your bones and muscles to work again. The same thing is true of psychological wounds" (p. 70). No matter how many people are cheering in the audience, the patient still needs to stand on the metaphorical stage of the physical therapy clinic and perform the exercises.

GATHER INFORMATION

The more information a patient knows, the more empowered he or she feels while on the healing journey. Family members can help the patient by being another person to listen to the advice and instructions given by the medical professionals treating the patient. Medical professionals such as physical therapists want the patient to succeed and will provide helpful suggestions for how to complete the treatment intervention and make lifestyle adjustments during the healing process. By continuing to be a supportive presence, family members can make this gathering of information a team effort to ensure the comprehension of all information.

Sometimes when patients are in pain they have a hard time remembering important information given to them by the therapist or information they want to share with the therapist. Family members can help make sure patients fully understand the important information once they get home or ask the important questions to the therapist. Knowing a patient's initial thoughts about factors causing pain can assist clinicians in developing a treatment plan. Juhan (1998) explains, "this missing link of conscious, active engagement is of enormous importance when it comes to strategies of therapeutic intervention. Some of the habits I am unconsciously perpetuating are reinforcing – sometimes even creating – my current difficulties" (p. 350). Writing can illuminate such habits for both the patient and the clinician so ineffective old habits can be replaced by effective new ones. English teachers use journals and writing conferences with students to discover patterns in student writing. Family members can use journals to record information stated by the clinician so it is remembered, and patients can use journals to track their pain so the clinician can see patterns. By doing this, patients can provide an additional dimension of information for the clinician, and family members can make sure they have all information correctly written down for when the patient arrives home. Barrett (2013) writes about her own experiences with chronic pain and describes, "I started to track my experience with just pen and paper. I recorded when I felt best (and worst) and began making deliberate changes to my environment and behavior. One at a time, I assessed the factors in my life" (p. 37). Not all patients demonstrate the same initiative Barrett did in writing about pain, so writing prompts and surveys such as *The Wanner-Bird Healing Survey for Pain Recovery* assist patients in writing their thoughts. Nevertheless, asking a patient to write becomes only half the story. The other half involves a supportive clinician willing to read the writing.

ENCOURAGE

If patients know their loved ones will walk with them on their healing journey and be a source of comfort and support, they know they are not alone and part of a supportive community while they heal. If a patient is completing a set of exercises and looks across the room to see a health coach or family member offering words of encouragement, the patient will most likely experience increased motivation to comply with the treatment plan. By celebrating accomplishments and providing the reassurance that mistakes and setbacks are part of the healing journey, the best possible environment can be created for the patient. Likewise, when teachers give students the reassurance that mistakes are part of the learning journey, the best possible environment can be created for the student.

No one needs to be alone while on a healing journey. Graves (2001) believes, "emotional and intellectual isolation is terribly draining. We have to make the energy investment ourselves to improve the emotional climate around us. A strong collegial relationship is too important personally and professionally for us to wait for others to come to us. Rather, we have to initiate contact with others because of its energy-giving possibilities. The more we take risks and learn from each other, the greater the energy-giving satisfaction. Ultimately, we see beyond our own limited collegial relationship to the possibilities of an energy-given vision we can fulfill together" (p. 68). Everyone can feel more energized about a treatment plan if all the clinicians and caregivers collaborate in a climate of care to help patients heal. Helldorfer and Moss (2007) discuss the importance of a climate of care because "while our focus at work is always on our patients, we are also part of a larger community of colleagues where we care for one another, and where each person has a role to play in creating the climate" (p. 163). A climate where patients feel encouraged to achieve their goals can make a positive difference in healing.

Some communities, such as the schools children attend or the neighborhoods where families live, become permanent fixtures in people's lives. Other communities, such as the hospital community where patients spend only a few days, are temporary. Nevertheless, a supportive community of any kind, even if it is for a short amount of time, can make a lasting impact. If a patient attends a group physical therapy class to learn exercises from the physical therapist, discuss goals with the health coach, and receive encouragement from a family member, it can make the patient feel accepted. Even talking with other patients who are experiencing similar health issues can create a sense of community and belonging. Brown (2012) explains that people need to feel unconditional belonging and elaborates, "what makes that such a challenge is that most of us struggle to feel a sense of belonging – to know that we are part of something, not despite our vulnerabilities, but because of them" (p. 233). When a patient is in a hospital room after surgery, it becomes easy to feel vulnerable. A strong community that makes the patient feel part of something greater than oneself can provide encouragement for the patient. The same philosophy applies to a classroom or advisory group in a school, where a strong community provides encouragement for the student.

It becomes essential for patients to feel part of a community as they heal because loneliness can lead to additional stress. Rankin (2013) discovered, "the reality is that loneliness causes stress, while loving community relaxes you. The effects of stress and relaxation don't just affect the mind; they affect the body. When you lack supportive community and feel you must handle life alone, the daily overwhelm may trigger anxiety, which the brain perceives as a threat" (p. 86). Additional stress can influence the body's ability to heal, so it becomes important to counteract the stress response with the relaxation found in an encouraging community.

As part of her popular *Lean In* movement discussed in her book of the same title, Sandberg (2013) encourages people to create their own Lean In Circles to provide a network of colleagues for each other to share ideas, since "communication works best when we combine appropriateness with authenticity, finding that sweet spot where opinions are not brutally honest but delicately honest" (p. 78). A Lean In Circle can easily be created in a hospital where patients can talk to each other and learn from each other. The patients' families can also become part of the circle by offering encouragement to each other. If one family is having a difficult day, another family who has gone through a similar experience can be there to provide support as stories are shared. Baldwin (1998) discusses the value of calling a circle because "calling a circle doesn't have to be a huge risk or lengthy experiment. We can start small, start with one evening" (p. 14). Patients sitting in a circle sharing their stories with a health coach during a group coaching session or families sitting in a circle leaning on each other and learning from each other can become a method to lean in and start a conversation.

Advisors in a school can also call a circle for their advisory group by gathering students to sit in a circle and asking a question such as, "how did you feel about last week's assembly?" Students then respond one at a time without interrupting each other. If someone tries to interrupt, the advisor provides a reminder for that comment to wait until after each student in the circle has the opportunity to share. After each person in the circle speaks, the advisor can then lead a discussion based on the comments students shared during circle time. This process reminds students that their voices and ideas matter to others, especially their advisor.

Through their encouragement of a patient going through treatment, family members become healers. Physical therapists, health coaches, and other clinicians are drawn to healing professions because of a desire to help others. Beck (2012) describes the healers as, "every now and again, though, I've met individuals who seem to embody the whole premise of the healer's archetype. These people are walking generators of peace, hope, compassion, and restoration. The things they accomplish often seem miraculous, but they themselves are universally humble, insisting that their work is simple and pragmatic" (p. xxi). Family members can join the team and also become a source of peace, hope, compassion, and restoration for the patient.

SELF-CARE

Most people want to help others before they help themselves. However, taking care of someone else to the point where one's own needs are neglected is not healthy. There is a reason that airlines give the speech about in the event of an emergency, put on your own mask before helping others with theirs. If the caregiver collapses from exhaustion, there is no one to help the patient.

Practicing self-care also applies to teachers in a classroom. With all the students to help, reports to complete, and papers to grade, it becomes easy for teachers to neglect their personal lives. Teachers need to remind themselves to practice self-care in order to best help their students.

One way to practice self-care is to engage in mindful awareness. Tindle (2013) defines, "mindfulness is simply choosing to be aware of whatever you are thinking, feeling, and sensing right now" (p. 105). Being the caregiver for a loved one can cause stress and lead to burnout. Mindfulness means providing permission to not have to do anything for anyone for awhile and just be with one's own thoughts and feelings in the present moment. Mindfulness means simply closing your eyes for a few minutes in meditation, or practicing a more formal meditation such as a Mindfulness Based Stress Reduction (MBSR) workshop or yoga class. Kabat-Zinn (2013), one of the leading experts in the field, shares the advice, "learning how to suspend all your doing and shift over to a being mode, how to make time for yourself, how to slow down and nurture calmness and self-acceptance in yourself, learning to observe what your mind is up to from moment to moment, how to watch your thoughts and how to let go of them without getting caught up and driven by them, how to make room for new ways of seeing old problems and for perceiving the interconnectedness of things – these are some of the lessons of mindfulness" (p. 6). Reading these words cannot take the place of a yoga class or MBSR class taught by an experienced instructor, so consider taking classes in your community if you want more formal mindfulness training than just closing your eyes to meditate.

When experiencing stress from caregiving, relaxation time becomes essential for the caregiver to maintain his or her own health. Rankin (2013) suggests "other relaxing activities such as laughter, playing with pets, journaling, prayer, napping, yoga, getting a massage, reading, singing, playing a musical instrument, gardening, cooking, tai chi, going for a walk, taking a hot bath, and enjoying nature may also activate your parasympathetic nervous system and allow the body to return to a state of rest so it can go about the business of self-repair" (p. 153). Another resource can be writing in a journal. Baldwin (2006) describes how journals provide a record of our lives because "each journal's contents are eclectic: reports of the day's events, recorded feelings, dreams, dialogues, fantasies, sketches, recipes, quotes from current reading material, cartoons and clippings, photographs and four-leaf clovers – whatever writers want to leave recorded in their passage through time" (p. 5). Journals provide a resource to share any emotions experienced during an emotional day of caregiving. If you need additional resources for caregivers, visit websites such as Caregiver.com (2015) that have current articles, places to find support groups in your community, and other helpful information.

TEACHING LESSONS

Typically teachers don't set up their classrooms in a hospital but in a school, yet the same theory applies. Brady and Vega (2009) believe, "the best way to learn is to teach" (p. 128). However, as Brady and Vega observe, "most places lack a teaching and learning culture, because no one has organized it" (p. 128). The hospital will have the teaching and learning culture because it has organized group physical therapy classes for patients. Patients in the hospital will receive the same powerful learning moments as students in a classroom due to the effective educators who will teach them.

Gruwell (2009) describes such learning moments as "those priceless moments when students' faces lit up, their hands flew in the air, and I knew they 'got it,' validated all the sleepless nights and began to ease my self-doubt" (p. xix). All the effort becomes worth it when the teacher, whether it is a high school writing teacher demonstrating the craft of revision or a physical therapist demonstrating a series of exercises, makes a connection to the subject area in such a way that the students grasp the concept. Group physical therapy classes use modeling. As Johnson (2005) explains, "modeling is one of the most effective ways to teach new skills" (p. 169). When a patient sees the physical therapist or physical therapist assistant demonstrating exercises, the patient is more likely to remember the concept. Another effective educational component of the group physical therapy classes is using family members as assistant coaches. Johnson continues, "teachers tend to be nurturing souls. We like to help other people. But we also like to be in control, and many of us find it difficult to delegate any of our authority. Sharing your authority can provide huge dividends, however" (p. 95). Sharing authority with family members, especially since the family members will take over the supervision of the exercises when the patient returns home, makes everyone share the work and makes the patient's healing journey a team effort.

Granted, as every teacher who has ever stood in front of a group of students will share, teaching can be challenging. Graves (2001) believes, "yes, teaching is an emotional roller coaster because our business is the growth of human beings" (p. 149). But with modeling by an excellent physical therapist teacher, goal setting from a health coach, and support from family members, patients will experience powerful learning moments as they heal.

HEALING THROUGH WRITING

Writing has been mentioned several times in this narrative as a method for people to process their thoughts and feelings. Jen is also a writing teacher, so as part of her health coaching she uses her writing training and credentials. Other health coaches have different backgrounds that they may choose to incorporate into their coaching.

Health coaches can lead group coaching sessions and writing workshops for either patients or their family members. While a circle sharing session may look like group therapy, it is important to remember that group health coaching and writing workshops are not group therapy. Instead of focusing on past issues like group therapy, group coaching focuses on meeting the needs of people where they are in the present and finding strategies to help them move forward. Beck (2008) reminds people that it is never too late to make changes in life because, "if you feel stuck in your present life, if you feel no enthusiasm for anything, if you think you have no purpose or that you lost that purpose somewhere along the way, I guarantee you are living in a dungeon made of stories – and that none of those limiting stories are true" (p. 53). Sharing stories in a supportive environment may help people feel encouraged to regain their sense of purpose.

Sometimes people experience stress when they find themselves struggling to focus on the myriad of thoughts occupying their minds. Goldberg (2000) reports, "we don't own our thoughts, even if they are filled with all our own details. They come through us, like heartbeat and breath" (p. 30). And the more thoughts come through, the more overwhelmed a person can feel. Expressive writing helps control the chaos. Romano (2000) discusses the value of expressive writing and elaborates, "when we write expressively in a journal, we imprint ideas, information, and experience deeply within us. We live topics by re-creating them with words on paper, by pulling images and dialog from the flow of our lives" (p. 138). Expressive writing is often best completed when an individual has time to reflect. Pennebaker and Evans (2014) concur, "expressive writing can force you to deal with important emotional experiences that you may have been avoiding" (p. 27). No matter the age of a person, whether teenager or senior citizen, writing helps the author articulate emotional experiences so physical and emotional healing can begin. And no one has to read the writing or grade it.

WRITING THE NEXT CHAPTER IN THE HEALING JOURNEY

Writing practice can enhance a group coaching class led by a health coach or other medical professional. A group class provides accountability and structure for hospital patients and their families, similar to the way a school classroom provides accountability and structure for students. Students in a classroom receive advice from teachers like Rief (1992) who instruct, "we take at least thirty minutes each Monday for silent writing. I begin my writing with the students during this time" (p. 30). After attending a group physical therapy class or occupational therapy class, attending a group coaching class with writing activities can become another part of the patient's schedule. Group coaching enables people to walk through their healing journeys together, empower patients, and provide families with the educational resources they need to assist physical therapists with exercises. Murray (1996) writes, "we forge communities when we share who we are, what we feel, what we think; and writing allows a sharing beyond the room, even beyond our lifetime" (p. 7). After participating in discussion as part of the community, patients will then be encouraged to write their goals for the next day. The written goals can be displayed in a location of the patient's hospital room and later the patient's home to provide a visual reminder of goals. Patients can also celebrate any successes and vent any frustrations through writing. The same writing strategies apply to students in an English classroom or advisory group. As Johnson (2005) advises her students, "say whatever you want. Then rip up the paper into tiny shreds and throw it away" (p. 263). Patients can rip up writing if it helps them vent frustrations or save their writing as a powerful reminder of celebrating success. And know that regardless of what happened today, tomorrow is another day.

MORE CHAPTERS FOR PAGES

PAGES was chosen as an acronym for this program because it symbolizes turning a new page in life. People turn pages of a book to get to the next chapter in the story, just as people can use the PAGES program to get to the next chapter of their own life stories. Unlike a book that has already been written, life represents a series of unwritten pages for the author to narrate and experience. Clandinin and Connelly (2000) describe the study of narratives, called narrative inquiry, as, "we characterized narrative inquiry as a kind of fluid inquiry, a kind of inquiry that challenges accepted inquiry and representation assumptions. It is a kind of inquiry that necessitates ongoing reflection, what we have called wakefulness" (p. 184). Wakefulness and reflection echo the mention of mindfulness earlier in this narrative, when healing can occur by practicing patience, accepting the present, gathering information, encouragement and self-care.

We don't know other people's stories. We can, however, turn the PAGES to learn more.

ACKNOWLEDGMENT

The preceding chapter contains excerpts from the following previous IGI publications:

Bird, J.L., & Wanner, E.T. (2016). Turning PAGES with health coaching and family involvement. In V.C.X. Wang (Ed.), *Handbook of research on advancing health education through technology* (pp. 213-233). Hershey, PA: Information Science Reference.

Reprinted in the IGI publication:

Bird, J.L., & Wanner, E.T. (2019). Turning PAGES with health coaching and family involvement. In Information Resources Management Association (Ed.), *Chronic illness and long-term care: Breakthroughs in research and practice* (pp. 255-276). Hershey, PA: Information Science Reference.

REFERENCES

Baldwin, C. (1998). *Calling the circle*. New York, NY: Bantam.

Baldwin, C. (2006). *One to one*. Lanham, MD: Rowman and Littlefield.

Barrett, D. (2013). What is paintracking? *Pain Pathways*, *6*(1), 36–41.

Beane, J. A. (1997). *Curriculum integration*. New York, NY: Teachers College Press.

Beck, M. (2001). *Finding your own North Star*. New York, NY: Three Rivers Press.

Beck, M. (2008). *Steering by starlight*. New York, NY: Rodale.

Beck, M. (2012). *Finding your way in a wild new world*. New York, NY: Free Press.

Brady, L., & Vega, P. (2009). 5 keys to structural success. In Orthopedics and spine (pp. 107-132). Danvers, MA: HCPro.

Brown, B. (2010). *The gifts of imperfection*. Center City, MN: Hazelden.

Brown, B. (2012). *Daring greatly*. New York, NY: Gotham Books.

Brown, B. (2015). *Rising strong*. New York, NY: Spiegel & Grau.

Brown, B. (2017). *Braving the wilderness*. New York, NY: Random House.

Brown, B. (2018). *Dare to lead*. New York, NY: Random House.

Cameron, J. (1998). *The right to write*. New York, NY: Tarcher/Putnam.

Caregiver.com Inc. (2015). Today's caregiver. *Caregiver.com*. Retrieved from http://caregiver.com/index.htm

Clandinin, D. J., & Connelly, F. M. (2000). *Narrative inquiry*. San Francisco, CA: Jossey-Bass.

Clark, A. H. (2018). *Hack your anxiety*. Naperville, IL: Sourcebooks, Inc.

Connelly, F. M., & Clandinin, D. J. (1988). *Teachers as curriculum planners*. New York, NY: Teachers College.

Creative Health Care Management Staff. (2003). *Re-igniting the Spirit of Caring*. Minneapolis, MN: Creative Health Care Management.

Duke Integrative Medicine Staff. (2010). *Personalized Health Plan Manual*. Durham, NC: Duke Integrative Medicine.

Fitzgerald, F. S. (1925). *The great Gatsby*. New York, NY: Scribner.

Gillespie, P., & Learner, N. (2008). *The Longman guide to peer tutoring* (2nd ed.). New York, NY: Pearson.

Goldberg, N. (2000). *Thunder and lightning*. New York, NY: Bantam.

Graves, D. H. (2001). *The energy to teach*. Portsmouth, NH: Heinemann.

Gruwell, E. (2009). Teaching hope. New York, NY: Broadway.

Haugk, K. C. (2012). *Christian caregiving*. St. Louis, MO: Stephen Ministries.

Havrilesky, H. (2018). *What if this were enough?* New York: Doubleday.

Heard, G. (1995). *Writing toward home*. Portsmouth, NH: Heinemann.

Helldorfer, M., & Moss, T. (2007). *Healing with heart*. Orinda, CA: Moss Communications.

Johnson, L. (1998). *Two parts textbook, one part love*. New York, NY: Hyperion.

Johnson, L. (2005). *Teaching outside the box*. San Francisco, CA: Jossey-Bass.

Juhan, D. (1998). *Job's body* (2nd ed.). Barrytown, NY: Station Hill.

Kabat-Zinn, J. (2013). *Full catastrophe living* (2nd ed.). New York, NY: Bantam.

Lee, I. F. (2018). *Joyful*. New York, NY: Little, Brown Spark.

Marshall, J. D., Sears, J. T., & Schubert, W. H. (2000). *Turning points in curriculum*. Upper Saddle River, NJ: Merrill/Prentice Hall.

Murray, D. (1996). *Crafting a life*. Portsmouth, NH: Heinemann.

Neff, K. (2011). *Self compassion: the proven power of being kind to yourself*. New York, NY: HarperCollins.

Pennebaker, J. W., & Evans, J. F. (2014). *Expressive writing: words that heal*. Enumclaw, WA: Idyll Arbor.

Pipher, M. (2006). *Writing to change the world*. New York, NY: Riverhead.

Rankin, L. (2013). *Mind over medicine*. Carlsbad, CA: Hay House.

Rief, L. (1992). *Seeking diversity*. Portsmouth, NH: Heinemann.

Romano, T. (2000). *Blending genre, altering style*. Portsmouth, NH: Heinemann.

Ryan, N. P., Wade, J. C., Nice, A., Shenefelt, H., & Shepard, K. (1996). Physical therapists' perceptions of family involvement in the rehabilitation process. *Physiotherapy Research International*, *1*(3), 159–179. doi:10.1002/pri.56 PMID:9238732

Sandberg, S. (2013). *Lean in*. New York, NY: Alfred A. Knopf.

Sandberg, S., & Grant, A. (2017). *Option B*. New York, NY: Knopf.

Stephen Ministries Staff. (2000). *Stephen Ministry Training Manual*. St. Louis, MO: Stephen Ministries.

Tindle, H. (2013). *Up: How positive outlook can transform our health and aging*. New York, NY: Hudson Street Press.

Wanner, E.T., & Bird, J.L. (2013). *The Wanner Bird healing survey for pain recovery*. Academic Press.

Younger, J., Gandhi, V., Hubbard, E., & Mackey, S. (2012). Development of the Stanford expectations of treatment scale (SETS): A tool for measuring patient outcome expectancy in clinical trials. *Clinical Trials*, *9*(6), 767–776. doi:10.1177/1740774512465064 PMID:23169874

Zimmermann, S. (2002). *Writing to heal the soul*. New York, NY: Three Rivers Press.

KEY TERMS AND DEFINITIONS

Accept the Present: Feelings of guilt, anger, and frustration are normal, but are not helpful when coaching. No matter what happened in the past, this is where you are now. Worrying about the future only causes additional stress. Try your best to remain in the present moment. Consider writing in a journal to sort through your feelings.

Encourage: During the healing journey, patients need cheerleaders. You are a source of hope and light during this process and a little support can make a large difference.

Gather Information: The medical professionals such as doctors, physical therapists, occupational therapists, nurses, and speech therapists are here to help you. Ask questions and listen to their instructions. Consider bringing a notebook with you to write down information so you don't have to remember it.

PAGES: An acronym for the terms described below (applied to a school setting)

Practice Patience: As high school students continue their journeys through life, they need supportive adults as role models. Often, the most significant goals cannot happen overnight. Empower students by celebrating progress, no matter how small. Students have numerous people giving them advice, so active listening proves valuable in a role as advisor.

Self-Care: In order to take care of your loved one, take care of yourself too. You can better help someone else when your own needs, such as hunger and sleep, are met too.

Chapter 6
Narratives of Patient Care

Jennifer Lynne Bird
Oxbridge Academy, USA

ABSTRACT

People, including hospital patients, want someone to know their stories. Teachers in English classrooms rely on narratives to learn their students' stories. Since learning patients' narratives is an emerging trend in the field of physical therapy as well as other medical practice, connections between writing, health coaching, and physical therapy illustrate the value of patients sharing narratives with their clinicians. Keeping journals tracking pain can assist patients when providing information to their medical practitioners.

PATIENT NARRATIVES

Every patient has a story. Recent trends in physical therapy focus on patient narratives. Greenfield, Jensen, Delany, Mostrom, Knab, and Jampel (2015) explain, "an initial goal of introducing narrative, therefore, is to demonstrate how narrative can be meaningful and relevant to physical therapy practitioners" (p. 928). To learn more about writing narratives, physical therapists can borrow methods from English teachers. English teachers encourage students to write in journals because first drafts of writing capture the writer's truest thoughts. Writing teacher Goldberg (1986) explains, "first thoughts are present. They are not a cover-up of what is actually happening or being felt" (p. 10). Writing opens a window to the stories people tell themselves, which can be beneficial for helping not only students in a writing classroom but also patients

DOI: 10.4018/978-1-7998-1931-8.ch006

in a physical therapy clinic. By having insight into a patient's thoughts, the medical practitioner can learn insights about the patient's narrative that will enhance the development of a successful treatment plan.

Journal writing provides an outlet of expression, thus allowing for the emergence of writing voice. Greenfield and Jensen (2010) discuss the value of patients' voices and elaborate, "imagine what we may find out about the work of physical therapists if we developed clinical case knowledge that is based on understanding the patient's voice? How could we better hear that voice?" (p. 1195). English teachers hear their students' voices through writing as well as speaking, so writing can provide information for physical therapists that patients may forget to share during a conversation. Writing teacher Tom Romano (2004) describes, "one of the great things about writing is that by doing it, we can construct a persona. We can craft an authentic voice" (p. 218). When students share their authentic voices, writing teachers help them discuss their emotions; similarly, when patients share their authentic voices, physical therapists help them discuss their symptoms.

Research studies demonstrating that expressing emotional writing can lead to physical healing began with Pennebaker (1997), who conducted a research study that showed "people who wrote about their deepest thoughts and feelings surrounding a trauma evidenced an impressive drop in illness visits after the study compared with the other groups" (p. 34). More studies confirmed the results of the original, and Files (2016) advises, "so, patients, get out thy notebooks and heal thyselves" (p. 102). While written responses by a patient cannot cure a condition that requires physical therapy, writing does show contributing factors for the cause of the pain. A patient's narrative can provide a clinician with additional information that, connected to the data from existing objective physical therapy measures, can lead to a diagnosis. Bezner (2015) discusses the value of the emerging field of health coaching and explains, "the American Physical Therapy Association (APTA) has recently undertaken an effort to identify and create resources to support physical therapists and physical therapist assistants to incorporate approaches that promote health and enhance wellness into physical therapist practice" (p. 1436). Resources include health coaches to focus on the emotional side of healing and goal setting for patients. Journal writing, often used by health coaches, provides an additional resource for both patients and physical therapists. Journaling can also have healing benefits if a person is experiencing medical symptoms.

Patients do not need to write a long essay in a physical therapy clinic or write a significant amount of words at home in a journal to remember what to tell their physical therapist about their pain levels. Short answer response questions, whether they are on a survey used in a clinic or in a notebook to write out steps for goals, are effective in leading to the processing of emotions. Wilkerson Miller (2017) describes the recent trend of dot journals, also known as bullet journals, as, "a dot journal is a system for writing down all the things you want to remember in a single notebook" (p. 4). Patients can use this method to write down questions or information they want to remember to share with their physical therapist.

Writing does not have to be about a trauma, but for some patients the circumstances that led them to seek medical treatment can feel like a trauma, so it helps to express such thoughts and feelings in writing. Dalebout (2016) explains the most important thing in journal writing is honesty, "but sometimes letting it out is messy. And messy writing is often the most healing writing" (p. 39). Writing teachers believe the best way to write is to trust initial impressions about a topic without overthinking a response. Files (2016) encourages, "let the writing serve its true purpose: to lead you to your truths" (p. 83). Physical therapy patients can apply this method by writing quick notes or observations between sessions to share with their physical therapists of what activities they were doing when they felt pain. A patient may have a low pain level right before a physical therapy session but forget to tell the physical therapist about a higher pain level felt the previous day. A pain journal can assist the physical therapist in modifying the treatment plan as needed based on information revealed in the writing that the patient may forget to mention during a conversation about pain levels.

Keeping track of symptoms and pain levels in a journal can help patients remember information to share with their medical providers. In her medical practice, Tindle (2013) conducted research about outlook and searched for a way to capture the script her patients told themselves because "if we can briefly slow down our internal dialogue long enough to take a look at it, we gain yet another window into our current outlook in action and catch glimpses of a new outlook" (p. 111). Journal writing helps English teachers determine the stories students tell themselves; consequently, writing can provide the same benefit for professionals in the medical field. Writing teacher Cameron (1998) believes, "when there is something we are not telling ourselves, our writing points that out" (p. 140). Therefore, writing can help medical practitioners, including physical therapists, learn their patients' stories.

Learning the stories patients tell themselves can lead to behavior change and empowerment. Bernstein (2016) explains, "our own interpretation determines our perception of the reality we experience" (p. 24). For example, if a patient's writing reflects a negative attitude, a physical therapist, health coach, physician, or other medical professional can help the patient set new goals and rewrite the narrative. Writing provides an outlet to help patients discuss their narratives and help them eliminate emotional barriers that may impede physical healing.

NARRATIVE MEDICINE IN PHYSICAL THERAPY CLINICS

Experts in the medical field illustrate that narratives are not limited to the English classroom. Charon (2006) explains, "I use the term narrative medicine to mean medicine practiced with these narrative skills of recognizing, absorbing, interpreting, and being moved by the stories of illness" (p. 4). Charon studied the genre of writing in a medical chart and made the connection that, "whatever the specialty of the writer, his or her chart note carries information in its form as well as its content. As is true for novels, plays, or poetry, the news one gets from a hospital note is transmitted by the words written as well as by the formal characteristics in which it is written" (p. 142). While she acknowledges that medical practitioners need to practice clinical detachment, it also helps them to know a patient's story as well as a diagnosis.

Greenfield, Jensen, Delany, Mostrom, Knab, and Jampel (2015) advocate the use of narratives in physical therapy education and practice. They elaborate, "highlighting context, characters, and plots allows a narrative to carry meaning, to potentially counter a reliance on objective measures of practice, and to build a bridge or create dialectic that connects the objective and subjective in clinical practice experience to help therapists iteratively move between these 2 essential aspects of human experience" (p. 925). A patient's narrative can provide a clinician with additional information that, connected to the data from existing objective physical therapy measures, can lead to a diagnosis. Physical therapists use evidence from objective measures such as the DASH, LEFS, NDI, and Modified Oswestry to help categorize patient pain and design a treatment plan. While written responses by a patient cannot diagnose a patient's medical condition, writing does show contributing factors for what the diagnosis may be. Physical therapists put subjective aspects such as writing responses into the clinical prediction rule to predict what the chances are that a patient has a specific diagnosis.

In addition to traditional diagnostic reasoning, Greenfield and Jensen (2010) encourage clinicians to use narrative reasoning. They explain, "narrative reasoning involves understanding the patient's story – his or her illness experience and its context and his or her beliefs and values. This strategy involves an interpretive paradigm, similar to phenomenology, focusing on context-dependent and subjectively constructed knowledge (about phenomena)" (p. 1194). Narratives are subjective, as each patient views his or her story through the lens of experience. Clandinin and Connelly (2000) believe, "as narrative inquirers we work within the space not only with our participants but also with ourselves. Working in this space means that we become visible with our own lived and told stories" (pp. 61-62). The combination of actively telling the stories of others while reflecting on their own stories enables researchers to relate to the story. By learning the patient's story, the clinician can view the narrative from the patient's perspective.

Greenfield, Jensen, Delany, Mostrom, Knab, and Jampel (2015) reference Charon's work and elaborate, "narrative medicine provides the clinician an opportunity to listen carefully to and reflect upon a patient's experiences with illness, representing that experience in a story or narrative, and ultimately providing the clinician insights that foster a strong commitment in caring for that patient. These ideas are particularly relevant for physical therapist practice, where therapists form close bonds with their patients and depend on their patients' cooperation and active engagement in their rehabilitation" (p. 928). When a patient writes a narrative, it helps both the patient and the physical therapist.

Activities a patient engaged in to cause pain at the beginning of the week may be forgotten or misinterpreted by the time the patient tells the story to the physical therapist at the end of the week's physical therapy session; therefore, writing helps the patient remember. Greenfield, Jensen, and their colleagues (2015) continue their discussion of narratives by stating, "based on our experiences with students and clinicians, writing narratives is a skill that needs to be taught, learned, and practiced in the same way that problem solving and other forms of clinical reasoning require practice and explicit instruction" (p. 928). Patients feel more comfortable during treatment if a compassionate clinician demonstrates willingness to listen to their stories. In a study measuring communication between physical therapists and patients with back pain, Roberts and Bucksey (2007) concluded, "once the content of a physical therapy encounter is established, the next challenge is to use communication skills that maximally enhance treatment outcomes" (p. 586). While one study certainly cannot capture conversations between all physical therapists and their patients, it does raise awareness of the value of using narratives to enhance communication between therapist and patient.

INCORPORATING THE THEORY OF NARRATIVE INQUIRY AND THE PRACTICE OF HEALTH COACHING

It benefits physical therapists to know their patients' narratives that can illuminate emotional barriers to physical healing. Linton and Shaw (2011) argue, "the application of psychological knowledge in physical therapy might range from providing reassurance to setting goals or inquiring about the functional consequences of pain. However, there is an apparent lack of knowledge and tools to adequately apply this knowledge" (p. 700). Due to the large number of patients that physical therapists must see a day, even though the physical therapist may want to have a long conversation with a patient, it may not be possible due to time restrictions. This is where a health coach can help. While health coaches use conversation to learn patients' stories, they can also use journal writing methods that reflect strategies English teachers use with their students. Regardless of whether they use conversation or writing to have patients talk about their answers to questions, health coaches learn the narratives of the people they serve in order to best provide encouragement and support as a new chapter in each person's story is written. This narrative focuses on using health coaching with physical therapy patients, but health coaches benefit patients in other medical settings as well.

Asking questions and finding themes in stories involves inquiry. Narrative inquiry is the qualitative interpretive field of research where researchers find narrative threads in stories that reflect themes. Like a physical therapist finds a narrative thread in a patient's story which may help explain physical symptoms, a health coach finds narrative unity in a patient's story which may help explain emotional barriers to adhering to a treatment plan and accomplishing goals. By rereading previous writing and interpreting the narrative thread that runs through their stories, writers rewrite narratives. Medical professionals such as physical therapists can help patients rewrite narratives by reframing a negative perspective into a positive one. Connelly and Clandinin (1988) elaborate, "this ongoing reflection-on-action on a daily basis begins to provide insight into personal knowledge when you reread entries over several days and weeks. What connecting threads are apparent over time? Are there events or ideas that recur?" (p. 35). From this perspective, one narrative can be placed in a larger context to show how the puzzle pieces of a person's story fit together.

Patients bring their own vision of a healthy life as well as their personal values into their narratives of experience. Health coaching focuses on aligning a person's vision and values to goals so the person develops ownership. The goal, therefore, becomes something the person wants to do (intrinsic motivation) instead of something the person is told to do (extrinsic motivation). A supportive medical team consisting of a physical therapist, health coach, and other compassionate caregivers can provide encouragement and accountability. While some physical therapists and physical therapist assistants are also health coaches, more frequently physical therapists are partnering with health coaches so the patient has another supportive person on his or her team during the healing journey.

Often people have value conflicts which prevent them from making changes in their lives. A patient may want to complete a home exercise plan from a physical therapist, but that will take away time from watching a favorite television show with family. The strategy of motivational interviewing can help patients identify such barriers and potential solutions. Bezner (2015) believes, "applying health behavior change theories and using motivational interviewing will enable physical therapists to effectively counsel and support the patient or client to adopt healthy behaviors" (p. 1441). Or, if due to needing to see a large number of patients, the physical therapist is unable to provide the counseling, a health coach can share that responsibility. Caldwell, Gray, and Wolever (2013) discuss how health coaching is similar yet different from motivational interviewing and explain, "first, there is a more directive element in MI that is usually not seen in health coaching. Second, MI often helps patients target a social or provider-determined goal (eg, abstinence from substance use) as much as a patient-driven goal. Third, while in MI, the central focus is on overcoming ambivalence to change, the overarching aim of IHC is broader, though elements of MI may be used in the process" (p. 55). Health coaching uses motivational interviewing as one of its foundations.

In motivational interviewing, Miller and Rollnick (2002) argue, "the implication is that there are at least these three critical components of motivation: readiness, willingness, and ability" (p. 10). Are we willing to change? Do we feel we have the ability to change? Are we ready to change? Numerical subjective questions focusing on a number scale and written subjective questions featuring open ended short answer prompts assess importance, confidence, and expression of priorities to present a snapshot of patient motivation. If an exercise treatment plan is not important to a patient, if a patient is not confident in completing the plan, or if a patient expresses other emotional barriers, the health coach will partner with the patient to develop an action plan for overcoming obstacles and accomplishing goals. Increasing patient motivation through importance, confidence, and expression leads to behavior change. Behavior change and a transformation in outlook can lead to increased patient compliance of a treatment plan.

Smith, Lake, Simmons, Perlman, Wroth, and Wolever (2013) elaborate of integrative health coaching, "while coaches may have a wide knowledge base of medical issues and diverse healthcare resources, their area of expertise is not medicine – it is specifically in building motivation for behavior change" (p. 69). Health coaches don't tell people what to do; they ask questions and serve as a supportive presence until people find the solutions to their problems.

Integrative Health Coaches see the patient as a person, not just a diagnosis. While physicians, physical therapists, and other medical professionals provide a diagnosis and treatment plan, health coaches partner with both medical teams and patients to build bridges between where the patient is now and where he or she wants to be. Smith, Lake, Simmons, Perlman, Wroth, and Wolever (2013) explain, "often in collaboration with clinicians and educators who design and clarify treatment plans, IH coaches work with each patient's whole situation – from his or her spiritual beliefs to exercise aversions – to foster an environment where their plans can take hold" (p. 69-70). Health coaches have a variety of backgrounds but must receive specific training to become a certified health coach.

Health coaches work in settings such as clinics, private practice, and hospitals; their purpose is to encourage patients to envision success and set goals to accomplish results. Caldwell, Gray and Wolever (2013) elaborate, "the major tenets of the health coaching process, then, are patient-centeredness and patient control focused around patient-originated health goals that are accomplished within a supportive coaching partnership" (p. 56). While each patient will most likely have a series of treatment goals set for them, such as a plan of exercises to complete at home designed by a physical therapist, a health coach will encourage a patient to align that treatment plan to personal goals, as well as align the treatment plan to vision and values. A patient may not want to complete exercises as part of a treatment plan prescribed by the physical therapist, but the patient may want to go on a family vacation. By asking open ended questions as well as summarizing and reflecting the patient's statements, the health coach helps the patient find connections between the value of spending time with family, the vision of a pain free vacation, and the treatment plan. The patient realizes how the goals set by the physical therapist (a certain number of exercises per day) relate to the personal goal of a vacation (more quality time with family). Writing down a goal also leads to accountability. Whether they are short term goals of being pain free or long term goals about health and life, capturing them on paper and displaying them in a prominent place becomes a powerful reminder to stay motivated.

WRITING NARRATIVES

If students in an English class have the power to rewrite their narratives, so do patients in a hospital or clinic. Goldberg (1986) discusses that when writing, writers need to trust their first impressions and not censor their thoughts because "to do writing practice means to deal ultimately with your whole life" (p. 3). To deal with life means being honest with oneself. As Heard (1995) explains, "in writing, I try to tell the truth" (p. 119). Writers write about an event, but then choose how to interpret their narrative when rereading their stories. An interpretation can range from positive feelings of acknowledging the story happened and moving forward, to negative feelings of remaining stuck in the story.

Regardless of the writer's attitude, he or she must own the story and write honestly, even if no one sees the story but the writer. Lamott (1994) elaborates, "you set out to tell a story of some sort, to tell the truth as you feel it, because something is calling you to do so" (p. 31). When writers write the truth, it leads to awareness of the stories they tell themselves. Because each person views a story through the lens of experience, while a story may seem true to the author, a person's subjective interpretation may differ from objective facts. Files (2016) explains, "the details that show up when you write may not match those of any of the other players in the drama, but they are your truth" (p. 79). For example, a patient may have neck pain, which is the objective truth of a situation. The subjective truth, filtered through the lens of emotion, means the patient may interpret the pain as caused by a single traumatic event and think something is seriously wrong. When transferring thoughts from mind to paper, however, the patient realizes there could be other interpretations of the story and consults a physical therapist, who sees a pattern to the patient's behavior and can provide an additional interpretation that the patient's ongoing actions contribute to the neck pain.

In her medical practice, Rankin (2013) tells her patients that in addition to receiving care from medical providers, they need to do their part in their own healing because "you need radical self-care, not just in your health habits, but in the rest of your life" (p. 163). Writing can encourage patients to process their emotions, help patients set goals for their healing, record symptoms and identify activities that cause pain that can help physical therapists, physicians, or other medical practitioners implement the most effective treatment plan.

Seeing thoughts and feelings on paper serves the dual purpose of gaining clarity and releasing feelings. Brown (2015) believes, "writing can be an extremely powerful tool for uncovering the story we're making up" (p. 218). Sometimes people believe a story to be true because they are emotionally connected to it, but writing can help uncover the facts and strip a story down to its basic essence so a person can see if the story is really factually true or emotionally what is perceived to be true. Cameron (1998) states, "I write to tell myself the truth, the whole truth, and nothing but the truth. I write, not to make art, but to make sense" (p. 109). By trusting first impressions when writing, writers learn the truth of what is in their hearts and minds and what they may need to address before moving forward. When people own their stories, they feel more in control of their lives. Brown (2010) believes, "the willingness to tell our stories, feel the pain of others, and stay genuinely connected in this disconnected world is not something we can do halfheartedly" (p. 21). No matter what has happened to in the past, each day brings a new opportunity to write a new chapter in a life story.

Medical practitioners such as health coaches or physical therapists can use writing to help people rewrite their stories and create a next new chapter of health and hope. Tindle (2013) reports, "even the brightest bulbs sometimes flicker. Being an optimist doesn't necessarily mean you're the brightest bulb on the Christmas tree. It means you keep your bulb burning brightly and steadily enough to light up your own path – and maybe the path of others – to better physical, mental, and spiritual health" (p. 72). Rankin (2013) adds, "if you're a pessimist prone to unhappiness, don't despair. According to happiness researchers, things like optimism and happiness can be learned, and you can enjoy the physical and mental health benefits as a result" (p. 138). A positive attitude brings healing benefits and helps patients feel hopeful about their healing journeys.

If the stories patients tell themselves create stress, writing helps the author craft a new narrative. Enayati (2015) feels perspective can alleviate the stress people experience since "we may have a story of stress that does not serve us, but we have the power to choose our perceptions, to choose different stories, more aligned with reality, that do serve us better. We can choose a narrative that helps reframe the stressors that besiege and overwhelm us as catalysts that become our strengths and guides" (p. 32). Patients in pain may find themselves stuck in their stories, blaming themselves for what caused their current condition, and making themselves feel worse. Brown (2015) explains, "there's growing empirical evidence that not owning and integrating our stories affects not just our emotional health but also our physical well-being" (p. 67). It therefore becomes important to not only own the story, but demonstrate self-compassion. Brown (2012) explains, "we must also remember that our worthiness, that core belief that we are enough, comes only when we live inside our story" (p. 132). Writing allows for a story to be relived and reinterpreted in order to change the narrative's perspective.

WRITING AS HEALING

Psychologist James Pennebaker conducted significant research illustrating writing can lead to healing. According to Pennebaker and Evans (2014), "since the first expressive writing studies were published in the 1980s, at least 300 studies about the benefits of expressive writing have been published. While the first studies focused almost exclusively on physician visits for illness, the scope of benefit measures has grown exponentially" (p. 9).

Sometimes people can mentally beat themselves up and relieve a story, thinking what could have, should have, or would have been different if only another outcome occurred. Once again, writing can help. Conner (2008) believes, "writing can't change the story, but it can change how you think about it. It can change how you feel about it. It can change what it means to you" (p. 122). Writing about an experience helps people see it from a new perspective with the benefit of reflecting on the learning experience. Handler (2013) states, "you've started to accept that your story is part of you" (p. 225). Some call it intuition, others call it purpose, but writers trust the writing to process the past, accept the present, and lead them where they need to go in the future.

In order to share stories, writers need to stop the self-censor, trust themselves, and just write. As Goldberg (2007) writes, "let your mind first believe you are dedicated, that you sincerely want the truth, are willing to take what comes through. Keep moving the pen. Keep practicing" (p. 4). Stories will unfold on the page and words can lead to needed answers. Not only can words lead to needed answers we need, but they can also help people heal both physically and emotionally.

When writing, the ideas will connect as the words flow. Zimmermann (2002) believes, "writing about the same thing repeatedly from slightly different angles is a healthy part of the process. You create new dimensions. You gain distance and clarity" (p. 27). Thanks to the magic of editing and revision, writers can rearrange words into different combinations, but the original intent of the writing, the heart of the piece, often appears in the very first draft. If writers wrestle too much with words, the message they really want to say gets lost along the way. Begin by capturing the inspirations and first impressions in an initial piece of writing. There is time later for interpretation and revision. Brown (2018) believes, "writing slows the winds and calms the seas" (p. 263). The calm after the storm often results in clarity.

It may be physical pain that causes a patient to walk through the doors of a physical therapy clinic for treatment, but the patient's emotional outlook contributes to physical healing. Even though a session with a health coach cannot heal physical pain or take the place of a treatment plan prescribed by a physical therapist, it can help patients discuss their narratives and help them eliminate emotional barriers that may impede physical healing. In addition to talking to a health coach, writing encourages patients to share their narratives, which can help physical therapists make a diagnosis and adjust a treatment plan as needed.

EDUCATIONAL NARRATIVES

Each person views his or her narrative through the lens of subjective experience. Asking questions and finding themes in stories involves inquiry. Clandinin and Connelly (2000) argue, "in narrative thinking, interpretations of events can always be otherwise" (p. 31). Narrative inquiry is the qualitative interpretive field of research where researchers find narrative threads in stories that reflect themes. Connelly and Clandinin (1988) elaborate, "try to understand a narrative unity as a thread or theme that runs through the narrative of experience and that provides a way to see how the rules, principles, images, and metaphors relate one to the other as they are called out by the practical situations in which we find ourselves" (p. 75). In other words, when a person shares a story, he or she selects what details to share or not to share. Clandinin and Connelly (2000) describe the process of converting informal field texts into a formal research text by stating, "we find ourselves frequently engaged in writing a variety of different kinds of interim texts, texts situated in the spaces between field texts and final, published research texts" (p. 133). The interim texts of my journal entries don't make those texts any less worthy than the formal research projects I designed and implemented. Connelly and Clandinin (1988) argue that education, especially when it comes to narratives, does not have to take place in the classroom and elaborate, "education, in this view, is a narrative of experience that grows and strengthens a person's capabilities to cope with life" (p. 27). People view their lives through the lenses of narratives of experience, and sharing narratives enables people to own their stories. Brown (2015) discusses the value of owning stories and explains, "I know that it takes more than courage to own your story. We own our stories so we don't spend our lives being defined by them or denying them" (p. 40). When people own their stories and find the strength to share their narratives with others, they find the courage to write new chapters to their stories and change the endings of their narratives.

Furthermore, when presenting narratives, writers can choose which genres best illustrate their ideas. Romano (2000) describes this format as multigenre writing and discusses narrative as a foundation as he explains, "multigenre papers, however, as I conceive them, demand that writers think narratively. Writers must meld the cognitive with the emotional" (p. 24). Therefore, you will read my personal teaching experiences in the form of narratives.

WRITING AS HEALING RESEARCH

Research illustrates the value of writing to assist healing. Pennebaker (1997) completed a research study that showed "people who wrote about their deepest thoughts and feelings surrounding a trauma evidenced an impressive drop in illness visits after the study compared with the other groups" (p. 34). More studies confirmed the results of the original, as Enayati (2015) reports, "study after study bore out Pennebaker's thesis that putting negative experiences into words has positive physical and psychological effects" (p. 73). Brown (2015) adds, "what's important to note about Pennebaker's research is the fact that he advocates limited writing, or short spurts" (p. 87). Short answer responses effectively lead the writer to process emotions and eliminate both physical and emotional stress. Writing also does not have to be about a trauma to be beneficial to the writer. Pennebaker and Smyth (2016) conclude, "writing can be an inexpensive, simple, albeit sometimes painful way to help maintain our health" (p. 80). The pain they refer to is that sometimes people may feel worse short term after writing if they explore an emotional topic, but long term they feel better by releasing their emotions because "writing moves us to a resolution. Even if there is no meaning to an event, it becomes psychologically complete" (p. 152). Writing can also release physical tension in the body when emotional tension is released onto the page.

When writing, it becomes essential to trust initial impressions and not overthink. Goldberg (2000) describes this process as "first thoughts have their own structure, move in their own rhythm, rise full-muscled from the bottom of the mind. They appear and disappear, present themselves and fade away unless we try to smother them, frightened by their power and truth, or smash them into polite second or third thoughts" (pp. 30-31). The first response to a prompt such as "How are you feeling?" is often the truest and most honest response before a person's self-censor can reevaluate and change the perspective. Sharp (2000) suggests, "whatever it takes, don't think, don't second-guess, don't edit. This exercise must come as directly as possible from your head to the page, traveling without censorship" (p. 18). When I teach writing classes to high school and college students, sometimes I provide writing prompts to help students think about a specific topic, but other times I encourage students to write whatever is on their minds. Lamott (1994) advises writers, "you need to start somewhere. Start by getting something – anything – down on paper" (p. 25). Brown (2015) agrees, "what you write doesn't have to be a sweeping narrative. It can be a bulleted list on a Post-it note or a simple paragraph in a journal. Just get it down" (p. 86). Determining if the act of completing the writing process would have healing benefits for students regardless of the topic discussed provided the foundation for the writing as healing research.

Pennebaker (1997) conducted a significant study discussing the health benefits of writing and concludes, "as we have found in many of our studies, you may feel sad or depressed immediately after writing. These negative feelings usually dissipate within an hour or so. In rare cases, they may last a day or two. The overwhelming majority of our volunteers, however, report feelings of relief, happiness, and contentment soon after the writing studies are concluded" (p. 42). Pennebaker and Chung (2010) highlight concrete physical health benefits of Pennebaker's research and elaborate, "writing or talking about emotional experiences relative to writing about superficial control topics has been found to be associated with significant drops in physician visits from before to after writing among relatively healthy samples" (p. 16). Therefore, research demonstrates that writing can heal people not only emotionally but also physically. Evans (2010) reports, "wellness and writing are connected in ways yet to be fully researched and exploited, but the literature of several disciplines declares that for many people wellness and writing are connected in ways useful for emotional, physical, and spiritual health" (p. 3). I plan to continue research to discover additional influences of writing on emotional, physical, and spiritual healing.

After completing research on writing as healing, I included writing workshops as a daily part of the curriculum of my college classroom. The high school students I teach write in journals almost daily. During writing conferences, students tell me that writing in their journals helps relieve stress. Stress can be contagious. As Enayati (2015) observes, "we volley emotions back and forth all the time, as part of every interaction – however brief or extended – that we have with each another. We can 'catch' other people's stress, all with amazing speed" (p. 154). One student would walk into the classroom sharing concern about an upcoming exam, and soon most of the students in the classroom were worried. Each class, I attempted to shift the momentum by beginning with a reading/writing workshop. At the end of the semester, students shared with me that it helped. Students had ten minutes to write in their journals about either a topic of their choice or a quote I wrote on the board. I did not grade the writing in order to encourage students to share their feelings with the pages of their notebooks. If students didn't want to write, they could read a book of their choice. I share the belief of Gruwell and her students, The Freedom Writers (2009), who write, "the greatest lesson the Freedom Writers and I have learned is to validate that everyone has a story" (p. 283). My goal as a teacher, writer, and researcher is for students to share their stories through writing.

THE PROCESS OF WRITING NARRATIVES

Advice that follows is designed for educators interested in using writing in their classrooms, patients interested in using writing while in an inpatient or outpatient setting, and for medical professionals interested in knowing more about the healing benefits of learning patients' narratives. The subsequent sections explain writing techniques that can be adapted to a classroom as well as applied to the medical field.

So, if you are a patient who has a hospital stay for a surgery, a series of physical therapy treatments for an injury, or questions for your medical provider, consider writing your narrative in a journal. If you are a medical practitioner, consider using writing as a supplement to traditional objective clinical measures. If you are a teacher, consider using writing in your classroom. Writing our narratives and sharing them leads to numerous potential opportunities for healing.

To begin, writing doesn't have to be kept in a journal or be a long narrative. Transferring thoughts from the mind to the page becomes the most important thing, especially for hospital patients who may not have a lot of time to write because they are taking pain medication or need to rest. Also keep in mind that no English teacher is going to grade this writing, so it doesn't matter if there are incomplete thoughts, grammar mistakes, or no clear structure to the writing. English teachers can also use this strategy by encouraging students to write in journals where students feel free to make mistakes without the pressure of a grade. The important thing is to accept yourself as you are and don't judge yourself or your writing. Cameron (1998) explains, "we can either demand that we write well or we can settle more comfortably into writing down what seems to want to come through us – good, bad, or indifferent" (p. 11). Another key component of writing narratives is to trust the writing process of what Romano (1987) refers to as "percolating, drafting, revising, editing, and publication" (p. 55).

Percolating: Thinking about ideas to possibly put on paper. Goldberg (2000) discusses the value of trusting first impressions as "our ideas and intentions can mask and cover up a story; there is a life force that will declare itself if you let it. Get out of the way" (p. 42). The truest impression of what a person thinks is usually the first impression before the writer has time to second guess thoughts and question the words.

Drafting: Capturing a vision on paper, and continuing to follow initial ideas. Writing can help the writer sort through emotions and discover insights. Often people remember something more when they write it down instead of trying to memorize the information. Goldberg (1990) describes this as, "we are going to write down what we think. Right or wrong doesn't matter. We are standing up and saying who we are" (p. 139). Hence, writing benefits the writer.

Revising: Reframing ideas to allow for new perspective. Goldberg (1986) elaborates, "so while we are busy writing, all the burning life we are eager to express should come out of a place of peace" (p. 167). Writing can create such peace; the writer releases worry and stress onto the page. Rereading the words provides the opportunity to gain a new perspective.

Editing: Cleaning up a piece of writing in preparation to share with an audience. While some writing is for the writer's eyes only, in the medical field sharing writing with a trusted medical professional can bring additional healing benefits. Goldberg (2013) advises writers, "you have to find the entry into what you know inside, the way to bring it out so people will listen" (p. 26). Writing down a list of symptoms and bringing it to the attention of the physical therapist or physician can help the clinician see patterns and obtain additional insights about a patient's health to adjust the treatment plan if necessary.

Publishing: Trusting someone else enough to share the written words. As Goldberg (2007) states, "it's your call, when you write. Trust the urge inside you to lead you to the right choice" (p. 165). If we trust our words, writing will lead us where we need to go. And with the support of a strong medical team, writing becomes an additional resource in the healing process.

TRUSTING FIRST IMPRESSIONS

Journals provide a private place to explore feelings about relationships, including the relationship with oneself. But in order to write honestly, the writer has to ignore the self-censor and write from the heart. Cameron (1998) explains, "acting our way into right thinking is putting pen to the page even when the censor is shrieking" (p. 35). This means writing whatever comes to mind and trusting first thoughts and impressions before censoring anything written out of worry of what anyone else might think. Goldberg (1986) answers the question, "why else are first thoughts so energizing? Because they have to do with freshness and inspiration" (p. 10). Frequently writers ignore first thoughts because they fear what others may think if the writing is read. But not all writing needs to be for an audience.

Students in an English classroom become used to writing essays, turning them in for a grade from the teacher, and being evaluated. However, teachers also need to give students time to write in journals without requiring students to share the writing. Romano (2004) elaborates, "students need to pay attention to their deep feeling and thinking. They will waste less time if they put aside the tangential, focus on what needs to be written, and respect the words tearing through the brain. They need to respond to their emotions. They need to move on the images flashing in their minds" (p. 49). The same philosophy that applies to students completing journals in an English classroom also applies to patients completing journals in a medical clinic.

For people to write what needs to be written, they need to trust that all writing does not have to be read, that there is a time to share but also a time to write for one's eyes only. Therefore, the journal becomes an effective method for practicing patience because a notebook page doesn't talk back or judge the author. Goldberg (2013) describes the moment of first thoughts as, "a flash, a moment appears when we fall through and what we are fighting, running from, struggling with becomes open, luminous – or, even better, not a problem, just what it is" (p. 23). Such advice reflects why numerous writing teachers believe first thoughts are the truest ones and the best method of capturing writing voice. By not judging their words, writers can find the answers to life's problems and practice patience while they arrive at the answers.

FINDING VOICE THROUGH WRITING

Just like everyone has a unique speaking voice, everyone has a unique writing voice. When a writer's voice shines through in a composition, it is like the writer is in the room having a conversation with the speaker. Graves (1994) discusses voice in writing and states, "voice is the imprint of ourselves on our writing" (p. 81). He elaborates, "the writing process has a driving force called voice. Technically, voice is not a process component or a step in the journey from choice-rehearsal to final revision. Rather, it underlies every part of the process." (p. 81). Voice exists in the way a writer uses language. The tone of writing can capture mood even if the reader can't see the writer's facial expression. The way a writer writes a phrase can illustrate written expression and reflect a personality on paper. As Murray (1985) explains, "voice allows the reader to hear an individual human being speak from the page" (p. 21). He continues, "we respond to voice when we hear it. Voice gives the text individuality, energy, concern. Voice is, of course, closely allied to style or tone, but I prefer the term 'voice' for it seems more accurate and more helpful for the beginner" (p. 21). Just like people sometimes silence their speaking voices, they similarly silence their writing voices. But listening to one's voice can lead to acceptance of the present moment.

By not censoring ourselves, we illuminate what we truly need and want. We can start making plans for how to get to where we are in the present to where we want to be in the future. It can give a person hope that the present situation won't always be the way it is now.

Often writers ask themselves questions such as: What do I say? How do I say it? Heard (1995) encourages writers to speak and shares, "as I walk, I write. Words circle my head. I speak lines out loud to see how they'll sound" (p. 32). Sometimes writing happens in the mind before a writer ever puts pen to paper or fingers to computer keyboard. This prewriting process, often called percolating to capture the image of an idea brewing just like coffee before it can be shared, is valuable. Nevertheless, an idea will forever remain in the writer's mind unless he or she finds the voice to speak it. Lamott (1994) advises writers, "you need to trust yourself, especially on a first draft, where amid the anxiety and self-doubt, there should be a real sense of your imagination" (p. 112). That self-trust is how we as writers find our voices. Our writing voices always remain with us; we just need to find the courage to share them.

Teachers who give students a classroom that symbolizes a safe space for sharing provide a platform for voices to be heard. Romano (2004) reminds students, "voice will come. Voice will come when you heed passion, push forward with language, are brave on the page, everything else be damned" (p. 51). Teachers encourage students to share their voices by reminding them they have something to say. Gruwell (1999) writes about her students, "although I'm not an expert on the subject, I've always felt that all kids learned to rebel. Understanding this rebellious nature, I encouraged the Freedom Writers to use a pen as a means of revolution" (p. 276). Gruwell and her students published a book sharing their writing and provided inspiration to others who wanted to use writing as a catalyst for change in their lives.

TEACHERS SET THE TONE

While anyone, regardless of age, always has the option of picking up a pen and a blank notebook, students need guidance from their teachers, whether that teacher is in the writing classroom sharing a new writing prompt or the physical therapy clinic sharing a new exercise. Romano (1987) explains, "the teacher is the first and most convincing example of the kind of behavior she wants in her class. She writes honestly, she shares what she's written, she listens to the writing of her students and respects their voices and visions" (p. 43). An English teacher who feels willing to share his or her own writing with students sets the tone for a comfortable class community where students feel encouraged to explore their own ideas through writing. Similarly, a physical therapist who is willing to model exercises for a patient sets the tone for a comfortable learning environment where patients feel encouraged to complete their exercises.

Writing teachers who don't write are like swimming teachers who never jump into the pool; why should teenagers take them seriously? So when teaching a writing workshop for students, patients, or family members, teachers need to view themselves as writers. As Atwell (1987) argues, "teachers do not require student writers to do anything they don't do themselves as writers. They draw on their personal knowledge of writing when conferring with students" (p. 283). Kearns (1997) concurs, "students do not see teachers write enough. They see us talking, reading, viewing, reprimanding, ordering, conferencing, and sometimes listening. They need to see us writing" (p. 83). When teachers share writing with their students, it does not mean sharing personal information that will make everyone in the room uncomfortable. It means providing information and modeling a strategy so information is gathered and learning can occur.

Modeling opens the door for students to feel more confident sharing their own experiences in writing. As Gaughan (1997) explains, "sharing my struggles with writing helped create the atmosphere of trust students need to write honestly and subsequently boosted individual students' confidence" (p. 7). Too often, students feel the pressure to be perfect in school. Cleary (1991) describes this perfectionism as "students became good-grade junkies, and as they began to work for teachers, they stopped writing for themselves" (p. 67). When teachers become willing to model their writing process, with all the revisions, edits, and drafts, students learn to see writing as a process and a journey with all the risks and rewards that come with it.

Very few first drafts are the final draft of a writing composition. Barbieri (1995) believes, "all writing leads to insight and discovery, and revising offers opportunities to dig deeper, to refine thinking, to follow new trains of thought" (p. 25). Modeling can reframe setbacks as part of the learning process, not a catastrophic event. Hubbard (1996) elaborates, "when teachers write and share how they write with their students, they are able to provide more than the overt activities that make up the skill of writing – they can share their own inner processes as well" (p. 47). Gathering information means trusting the process. It means empowering the writer to set goals for himself or herself, which means the goals will be more likely to be achieved when the writer takes ownership of them instead of completing a composition just to make a teacher happy. Connelly and Clandinin (1988) believe, "life's narratives are the context for making meaning of school situations" (p. 27). We think of learning as taking place in schools, but learning also takes place in the classroom of life.

WRITING WITH PASSION

Most people can relate to the feeling of being completely absorbed in an activity and getting into the zone where time fades away. Writing helps illuminate what the writer values. Illuminating values can lead to encouragement; health coaches consistently connect a patient's goals to vision and values in order for people to see connections to the goals in their lives and feel excited about achieving them. Teachers use the same process to help students achieve goals. Romano (2013) explains, "to capture stream of consciousness, the writer has to let go of control more than usual, trust the gush of language and associations even more" (p. 117). If people trust the gush of feeling and become willing to write about things that bring joy, they start on the path to feeling encouraged to find their passion in life.

Discovering passion leads to purpose. A journal serves as a mirror reflecting goals accomplished, which encourages the patient to persevere while recovering. Pipher (2006) elaborates, "by diving into the experience of writing, you will learn what you truly think and who you really are" (p. 44). Sometimes people struggle to figure out who they are, especially if an event creates chaos in a once stable life. Writing can bring you back to yourself and remind you who you are. Romano (1995) describes seeing students find their passion and writes, "in my experience, passion in students has usually led to strong positions, critical thinking, further analysis, and stirring, often eloquent language" (p. 25). One way to find what will bring passion in the future is to remember what brought passion in the past. According to Goldberg (2007), "writing is your practice as you mow through your memories, the even chord among the highs and lows" (p. 70). Memories of past successes and remembering a time when happiness happened often sets the stage for future dreams.

Intuitively, we all know what we want to do with the one life each of us has been given, but the challenging part becomes following our hearts no matter what others think. Lamott (1994) reminds us to recapture our true desires because "you get your intuition back when you make space for it, when you stop the chattering of the rational mind" (p. 112). Writing can help process feelings and goals; a phrase on paper can make the impossible seem possible if it is broken down into steps. Goldberg (1990) describes a strategy for articulating goals and feelings and advises, "a helpful technique: right in the middle of saying nothing, right in the middle of a sentence, put a dash and write, 'What I really want to say is…' and go on writing" (p. 73).

We say what we need to say. We keep writing. We keep living. We welcome the encouragement from others as we set our goals and find the strength to encourage ourselves.

THE PERFECT PROCESS OF IMPERFECT WRITING

When a writer needs to say something, the best advice is for writing to light the way. As Heard (1995) observes when struggling with a piece of writing, "I had changed the intent of the writing, just as people move a stream by redirecting its banks, hoping the water will obey. It never does. Neither did my writing" (p. 41). A writer should not feel confined to any specific form; writing can appear as a poem, recipe, song, essay, or other creative genre depending on the writer's mood and topic. As Gaughan (2001) observes, "multiple genres act as multiple lenses" (p. 21). With writing, the journey becomes more important than the destination. Regardless of the genres we write, writing provides a moment for self-care and a reason to give a few moments to oneself. This is especially important for caregivers giving time to others.

We are all the experts of our own lives, and no one can tell our story in the exact same way we can. Vinz (1996) discusses the value of narratives and explains, "when past and present were considered as dimensions of the whole experience, these teachers authored new stories that transgressed particular moments, beliefs, or actions" (p. 92). Each person authors his or her story, regardless if they are a student in a classroom at school, a student in a group physical therapy class, or a student in the classroom of life. An author may choose for a story to remain private or choose to share it. By sharing our stories with each other, we all become teachers and students of each other's narratives of experience. Writing doesn't have a right answer, like 2+2=4. We write to find the right answers. Romano (2008) believes, "but I am a teacher. I know that the path toward accomplishment can be a zigzag one, replete with setbacks, wrong turns, and backtracking. That's why I value approximation so much: the flawed attempt, the good intentions gone awry, the achievement of approximately what you were after. For those who participate in good faith, learning is a matter of growth and development" (p. 206). We have faith in the fact writing helps us learn and grow. Writing reminds us to practice self-care.

ADDITIONAL WRITING STRATEGIES

I once sent my students on a writing field trip as part of class. They had to pick a location of their choice and write about a topic of their choice. I never asked them to share their writing with me; their only assignment was to send me an email telling how the experience made them feel. This assignment was part of my normal classroom practices and not part of any research study, but a summary of student comments provides the insight that writing felt peaceful and therapeutic for the college students who participated in the activity. Murray (1996) believes, "writers must learn to have faith in the writing act; they are led by the writing to discover what they have to say and how it may be said" (p. 25). During their writing time, my students discovered what they needed to say. I hope narratives help you find your voice as well.

ACKNOWLEDGMENT

The preceding chapter contains excerpts from the following previous IGI publications:

Bird, J.L., & Wanner, E.T. (2019). Turning PAGES with health coaching and family involvement. In Information Resources Management Association (Ed.), *Chronic illness and long-term care: Breakthroughs in research and practice* (pp. 255-276). Hershey, PA: Information Science Reference.

Bird, J.L. (2018). Constantly connected: Managing stress in today's technological times. In V.C. Bryan, A. Musgrove, & J. Powers (Eds.), *Handbook of research on human development in the digital age* (pp. 385-402). Hershey, PA: Information Science Reference.

Bird, J.L. (2017). Writing healing narratives. In V.C. Bryan & J.L. Bird (Eds.), *Healthcare community synergism between patients, practitioners, and researchers*. Hershey, PA: Information Science Reference.

Bird, J.L., & Wanner, E.T. (2016). Turning PAGES with health coaching and family involvement. In V.C.X. Wang (Ed.), *Handbook of research on advancing health education through technology* (pp. 213-233). Hershey, PA: Information Science Reference.

REFERENCES

Atwell, N. (1987). *In the middle*. Portsmouth, NH: Heinemann.

Barbieri, M. (1995). *Sounds from the heart*. Portsmouth, NH: Heinemann.

Bernstein, G. (2016). *The universe has your back*. Carlsbad, CA: Hay House.

Bezner, J. R. (2015). Promoting health and wellness: Implications for physical therapist practice. *Physical Therapy*, *95*(10), 1433–1444. doi:10.2522/ptj.20140271 PMID:25908523

Brown, B. (2010). *The gifts of imperfection*. Center City, MN: Hazelden.

Brown, B. (2012). *Daring greatly*. New York, NY: Gotham Books.

Brown, B. (2015). *Rising strong*. New York, NY: Spiegel & Grau.

Brown, B. (2018). *Dare to lead*. New York, NY: Random House.

Caldwell, K., Gray, J., & Wolever, R. Q. (2013). The process of patient empowerment in integrative health coaching: How does it happen? *Global Advances in Health and Medicine: Improving Healthcare Outcomes Worldwide*, *2*(3), 48–57. doi:10.7453/gahmj.2013.026 PMID:24416672

Cameron, J. (1998). *The right to write*. New York: Tarcher/Putnam.

Charon, R. (2006). *Narrative medicine: honoring the stories of illness*. New York, NY: Oxford University Press.

Clandinin, D. J., & Connelly, F. M. (2000). *Narrative inquiry*. San Francisco, CA: Jossey-Bass.

Cleary, L. M. (1991). *From the other side of the desk*. Portsmouth, NH: Heinemann.

Connelly, F. M., & Clandinin, D. J. (1988). *Teachers as curriculum planners*. New York, NY: Teachers College.

Conner, J. (2008). *Writing down your soul*. San Francisco, CA: Conari.

Dalebout, K. (2016). *Let it out*. Carlsbad, CA: Hay House.

Enayati, A. (2015). *Seeking serenity*. New York, NY: New American Library.

Evans, J. F. (2010). Introducing wellness & writing connections conference papers. In J. F. Evans (Ed.), *Wellness & Writing Connections* (pp. 3–10). Enumclaw, WA: Idyll Arbor, Inc.

Files, M. (2016). *Writing what you know*. New York, NY: Allworth.

Gaughan, J. (1997). *Cultural reflections*. Portsmouth, NH: Heinemann.

Gaughan, J. (2001). *Reinventing English*. Portsmouth, NH: Heinemann.

Goldberg, N. (1986). *Writing down the bones*. Boston, MA: Shambhala.

Goldberg, N. (1990). *Wild mind*. New York, NY: Bantam.

Goldberg, N. (2000). *Thunder and lightning*. New York, NY: Bantam.

Goldberg, N. (2007). *Old friend from far away*. New York, NY: Free Press.

Goldberg, N. (2013). *The true secret of writing*. New York, NY: Atria.

Graves, D. H. (1994). *A fresh look at writing*. Portsmouth, NH: Heinemann.

Greenfield, B. H., & Jensen, G. M. (2010). Understanding the lived experiences of patients: Application of a phenomenological approach to ethics. *Physical Therapy*, *90*(8), 1185–1201. doi:10.2522/ptj.20090348 PMID:20539020

Greenfield, B. H., Jensen, G. M., Delany, C. M., Mostrom, E., Knab, M., & Jampel, A. (2015). Power and promise of narrative for advancing physical therapist education and practice. *Physical Therapy*, *95*(6), 924–933. doi:10.2522/ptj.20140085 PMID:25524869

Gruwell, E., & the The Freedom Writers. (1999). The Freedom Writers diary. New York, NY: Broadway.

Gruwell, E., & the The Freedom Writers. (2009). The Freedom Writers diary (2nd ed.). New York, NY: Broadway.

Handler, J. (2013). *Braving the fire*. New York, NY: St. Martin's Griffin.

Heard, G. (1995). *Writing toward home*. Portsmouth, NH: Heinemann.

Hubbard, R. S. (1996). *A workshop of the possible*. York, ME: Stenhouse.

Kearns, J. (1997). *Where to begin: a guide to teaching secondary English*. Portsmouth, NH: Heinemann.

Lamott, A. (1994). *Bird by bird*. New York: Anchor Books.

Linton, S. J., & Shaw, W. S. (2011). Impact of psychological factors in the experience of pain. *Physical Therapy, 91*(5), 700–711. doi:10.2522/ptj.20100330 PMID:21451097

Miller, R. W. (2017). *Dot journaling*. New York, NY: The Experiment.

Miller, W. R., & Rollnick, S. (2002). *Motivational interviewing* (2nd ed.). New York, NY: The Guilford Press.

Murray, D. M. (1985). *A writer teaches writing* (2nd ed.). Boston, MA: Houghton Mifflin.

Murray, D. M. (1996). *Crafting a life*. Portsmouth, NH: Heinemann.

Pennebaker, J., & Chung, C. K. (2010). Expressive writing, emotional upheavals, and health. In J. Evans (Ed.), *Wellness and writing connections* (pp. 11–52). Enumclaw, WA: Idyll Arbor.

Pennebaker, J. W. (1997). *Opening up: the healing power of expressing emotions*. New York, NY: The Guilford Press.

Pennebaker, J. W., & Evans, J. F. (2014). *Expressive writing: words that heal.* Enumclaw, WA: Idyll Arbor.

Pennebaker, J. W., & Smyth, J. M. (2016). *Opening up by writing it down.* New York, NY: The Guilford Press.

Pipher, M. (2006). *Writing to change the world.* New York, NY: Riverhead.

Rankin, L. (2013). *Mind over medicine*. Carlsbad, CA: Hay House.

Roberts, L., & Bucksey, S. J. (2007). Communicating with patients: What happens in practice? *Physical Therapy, 87*(5), 586–594. doi:10.2522/ptj.20060077 PMID:17405807

Romano, T. (1987). *Clearing the way*. Portsmouth, NH: Heinemann.

Romano, T. (1995). *Writing with passion*. Portsmouth, NH: Heinemann.

Romano, T. (2000). *Blending genre, altering style*. Portsmouth, NH: Heinemann.

Romano, T. (2004). *Crafting authentic voice*. Portsmouth, NH: Heinemann.

Romano, T. (2008). *Zigzag*. Portsmouth, NH: Heinemann.

Romano, T. (2013). *Fearless writing*. Portsmouth, NH: Heinemann.

Sharp, C. (2000). *A writer's workbook*. New York, NY: St. Martin's Press.

Smith, L. L., Lake, N. H., Simmons, L. A., Perlman, A., Wroth, S., & Wolever, R. Q. (2013). Integrative health coach training: A model for shifting the paradigm toward patient-centricity and meeting new national prevention goals. *Global Advances in Health and Medicine: Improving Healthcare Outcomes Worldwide*, *2*(3), 66–74. doi:10.7453/gahmj.2013.034 PMID:24416674

Tindle, H. (2013). *Up: How positive outlook can transform our health and aging*. New York, NY: Hudson Street Press.

Vinz, R. (1996). *Composing a teaching life*. Portsmouth, NH: Heinemann.

Zimmermann, S. (2002). *Writing to heal the soul*. New York, NY: Three Rivers Press.

KEY TERMS AND DEFINITIONS

Expressive Writing: Writing that is exploratory and focuses on meaning and first impressions.

Narrative Inquiry: Discussed in the field of research by F. Michael Connelly and D. Jean Clandinin, narrative inquiry is a qualitative interpretative form of research that focuses on the telling, retelling, and sharing of stories. Researchers who complete narrative inquiries interpret stories and search for common threads to find patterns. They are encouraged to tell their research stories in first person as they look back to find meaning in past stories and look forward to set future goals.

Narrative Medicine: The field of medicine, used by programs such as the one Rita Charon founded at Columbia University, which encourages medical practitioners to use theories from the fields of literature and composition to enhance comprehension of the stories patients share.

Narrative Writing: Writing that shares a story. Narrative writing is frequently told from a first person perspective.

Writing as Healing: Numerous studies have been conducted investigating the influence of writing on physical and emotional health. James Pennebaker is a leader in the field which explores the health benefits of writing.

Writing Process: Composing an essay using percolating, drafting, revising, editing, and publication.

Chapter 7
Narratives of Anxiety

Jennifer Lynne Bird
Oxbridge Academy, USA

Eric T. Wanner
Palm Beach Sports Medicine and Orthopaedic Center, USA

ABSTRACT

This research project began as a study using both quantitative and qualitative methods to learn about the connections between writing and healing. College students who wrote in journals throughout the semester as part of normal classroom practices for an education methods class in reading and writing completed surveys answering questions about their writing and their health. Initial analysis of the data echoed the findings of previous studies: writing is healing. However, the more important observation became that on one of the health survey questions 92% of the subjects reported experiencing anxiety or stress. Consequently, the research evolved into a social action project to help college students cope with stress and anxiety; stress is a very common cause of a downward spiral to quality of life and overall health. By making a few positive changes in their lives, people can learn to deal with stress.

CURRICULUM INQUIRY USING RESEARCH NARRATIVES

Curricular change begins when researchers develop ideas with the purpose of implementing enduring effective change. It is one thing to notice a problem, another to solve it. Researchers can benefit from envisioning ideas from different perspectives and borrowing ideas from other fields. The field of city planning follows a research process that leads to implementation of detailed

DOI: 10.4018/978-1-7998-1931-8.ch007

plans; city planning shares similarities with the qualitative interpretive research fields of narrative inquiry and curriculum inquiry, since both rely on narratives to illuminate issues. Illuminating issues can lead to bringing purpose to life, whether a city planner looks at a piece of land and uses plans to create a new housing development or an educational researcher looks at data indicating college students experience stress and anxiety and uses plans to create a curriculum of healing.

Education endures multiple curricular incarnations throughout the decades, since the only constant in the curriculum of schools remains change. Marshall, Sears, and Schubert (2000) discuss the evolution of curriculum and provide the history that "more than any other philosopher, John Dewey influenced the thought of curriculum scholars throughout the twentieth century, and at the century's end curriculum questions remain easily related to his definition of education. The enduring curriculum question thus becomes "What adds meaning and direction or purpose to experience?" (p. 2). The question still remains today. What experiences bring purpose to life?

While researchers often study texts or programs from an existing curriculum, the stories of the people participating in a curriculum add another dimension to the inquiry process because looking at policies and procedures cannot take the place of witnessing the implementation of such policies and procedures when adding people to the process. Marshall, Sears, and Schubert (2000) believe, "through biography as curricular text we can see how individuals reconstructed themselves and their work, including the need to reread past decisions and changes" (p. 199). An idea may appear one way in theory on paper, but watching the idea unfold in practice may tell a different story. Educators want their stories to possess purpose; students may repeat the words of an excellent teacher years after that teacher's lifetime.

This curriculum inquiry research story alternates from the perspectives of the researchers being both participants and observers. Narrative inquiry is the qualitative interpretive discipline which encourages researchers to use first person when describing events and intertwine their own narratives with the narratives of the research participants. Clandinin and Connelly (2000) define narrative inquiry and explain, "it is a collaboration between researcher and participants, over time, in a place or series of places, and in social interaction with milieus. An inquirer enters this matrix in the midst and progresses in this same spirit, concluding the inquiry still in the midst of living and telling, reliving and retelling, the stories of the experiences that make up people's lives, both individual and social" (p. 20). Therefore, in narrative inquiries, researchers learn about a story, report on the story, and subsequently seek to offer their own contribution to the story already in progress. The sharing of stories serves as the methodology as Clandinin and Connelly elaborate, "in our work, we keep in the foreground of our writing a narrative view of experience, with the participants' and researchers' narratives of experience situated and lived out on storied landscapes as our theoretical methodological frame" (p. 128). Think of it as the researchers reading a poem and then adding their own verse at the end. The researchers are changed by the research setting and also change the setting by being part of it.

Curriculum inquiry uses narratives to study an existing curriculum and determine how the stories of the participants can lead to curricular change. Connelly and Clandinin (1988) discuss, "curriculum inquiry is a process in which teachers read and study curriculum materials in the same way that they would read and study potentially interesting texts" (p. 151). Simply studying curriculum materials, however, does not lead to change. According to city planner and former Florida Atlantic University president Catanese (1996), "for too many years we have not dealt with the most important lesson from the real world, which is that implementation is the most important part of planning" (p. 295). In order to implement lasting change as a result of research, researchers can learn from the process implemented by city planners. Harper (1996) explains, "when I was in graduate school I remember being surprised to learn that the planning process is almost identical to the scientific method of research I had already studied" (p. 194). Like narrative inquiry, city planning uses stories to frame problems and discover solutions. Learning stories and receiving feedback from the constituents impacted by the solutions becomes an essential part of the process because neither cities nor schools are empty places. Both contain people whose lives become transformed either positively or negatively by the implementation of change. Hoch (1995) elaborates, "we use elements of narrative and rhetoric to compose our stories. In planning tales, we usually combine logic and rhetoric, argument and poetics" (p. 295). The same description applies to any story told, whether a citizen writes a letter to a city planner or a student writes a journal entry in a classroom. Both writing processes involve the venting of feelings.

Change occurs not just with a process, but also with people. Change takes courage and requires a transformative leader to step up and lead the way. In order to use research to create curricular change, it helps the transformative leaders to participate in the change process instead of directing others to implement the change. Heifetz (1994) believes, "leadership is both active and reflective. One has to alternate between participating and observing" (p. 252). The extended metaphor of a dance is used to illustrate the concept.

To put it in other words, if you are chaperoning a school dance and are on the dance floor dancing the line dance The Electric Slide with the students, you know what it feels like to participate in the dance but can't see the entire picture. If the dance floor has a balcony where you can climb up to the top and look down, you see the entire picture of the dance but are detached from participating. Heifetz uses a ballroom dance example instead of The Electric Slide, but the philosophy remains the same since "to discern the larger patterns on the dance floor – to see who is dancing with whom, in what groups, in what location, and who is sitting out which kind of dance – we have to stop moving and get to the balcony" (p. 253). One of the researchers conducting the study discussed in this chapter needed to learn this lesson because the research took place in her classroom. She needed to alternate between living the subjective experience with her students and maintaining an objective distance. She also relied on the insights of her co-researcher, a medical consultant and physical therapist, because he could see the study from a different perspective and help her switch between the roles of researcher and professor.

HEALING VALUE OF WRITING

This research project began as a study to find connections between writing and healing. The authors of this research study previously conducted another research study and discovered that patients at a physical therapy clinic who used a strong positive writing voice on short answer survey questions demonstrated greater healing gains on existing objective physical therapy measures. The results illustrated writing can influence physical healing.

Other previous studies illustrated the link between writing and health. In a 1983 study, psychologist Pennebaker (1997) assigned college students at Southern Methodist University to one of four writing groups where they would vent about their emotions related to a trauma, write the facts of the trauma, write the facts of the trauma while venting about emotions, or write about superficial topics; he discovered that students in the writing group who both wrote the facts of the trauma while venting about emotions visited the student health center fewer times than students in the other three writing groups and concluded, "writing about their deepest thoughts and feelings about traumas resulted in improved moods, more positive outlook, and greater physical health" (p. 34). A follow up study where Pennebaker collaborated with doctors from the Ohio State University College of Medicine to draw blood samples from college students before and after they wrote revealed that "people who wrote about their deepest thoughts and feelings surrounding traumatic experiences evidenced heightened immune function compared with those who wrote about superficial topics" (p. 37).

Writing professor DeSalvo (1999) concurs with Pennebaker's research and elaborates, "the more people described positive emotions in their writing, the more likely they were to be healthier afterward. But describing negative emotions either excessively or very little or not at all correlated with poorer health. Describing negative emotions in moderation correlated with improved health" (p. 60). Social work researcher and professor Brown (2012) also corroborates Pennebaker's research and explains, "when people shared their stories and experiences, their physical health improved, their doctor's visits decreased, and they showed significant decreases in their stress hormones" (p. 82). Conner (2008) uses her experiences as viewing writing as a spiritual practice to discuss Pennebaker's research through the lens of improved academic performance for college students and reports, "successive research projects demonstrated that students who wrote in an open, meaningful way developed a more positive outlook on life, experienced reduced anxiety and depression, had an improved ability to fight infection with more active T-lymphocytes (the agents in the body that fight cancer), and had lower heart rates. They also - this is my favorite - received better grades" (p. 59). All of the analyses lead to the conclusion that writing leads to healing.

Writing also helps improve depression and anxiety. Helgoe, Wilhelm, and Kommor, (2005) discuss the implications of writing from the perspective of the medical community and elaborate, "'therapeutic journaling,' or writing down your feelings and concerns, has been associated with reductions in symptoms of depression and anxiety. In fact research by James Pennebaker found that immune function was enhanced for study subjects who wrote about their deepest feelings as compared to subjects instructed to write about trivial matters" (p. 260). Pennebaker's research illustrating writing leads to healing even resonates beyond the academic community. In the popular magazine *Oprah,* Kamenetz (2013) discusses Pennebaker "who had found that students who wrote about the worst thing that had ever happened to them felt sadder initially, but six months down the road were visiting doctors less frequently" (p. 140). She used the study as inspiration to discuss how writing helped her and stated that as a result of writing, "I felt no fear or hesitation, just deep gratitude – and an eagerness to write the next chapter" (p. 141). But can writing benefit writers who write about topics other than traumas?

Writing helps people process emotions so they can heal both physically and emotionally from difficult experiences. As DeSalvo (1999) explains, "the act of linking feelings with troubling events, then, makes our bodies display responses associated with yoga and meditation. This explains why writers who stop work soon feel out of sorts – why they become edgy, irritable, anxious, even depressed. This explains, too, why people who begin writing report feeling a greater sense of well-being – why they become calmer, more capable of coping with stress, more serene, even when facing life's challenges, than they'd been before" (p. 23). However, the writing questions on the survey the researchers used at the physical therapy clinic did not ask patients to write about traumatic experiences; instead, patients wrote about their perspectives and goals for healing. Furthermore, through personal experiences with their own writing as well as through informal observations and conversations with high school and college students in English classes, the researchers observed that students benefit from writing about topics other than traumatic ones. In fact, while the occasional student wants to explore a deep emotional issue in writing, most students write on less emotional topics and still report feeling more peaceful after writing. Gruwell (2007) writes of her students, the students known as *The Freedom Writers*, "writing became liberating, as each student discovered they had a story and found comfort in the computer. Although they couldn't change the cast of characters, the computer became their confidant, their therapist, and their outlet, and many of them hoped that they could rewrite their endings" (pp. 151-152). Could the act of completing the writing process have healing benefits for patients regardless of the topic discussed?

RESEARCH METHODS

For this research study, Florida Atlantic University students in the College of Education who chose to volunteer completed two surveys. One survey was a writing survey designed by the researchers, and the other survey was a health survey called the HRQOL (Health Related Quality of Life) survey, a general health survey in the public domain and able to be used by researchers without securing permission or paying copyright fees. The two surveys were stapled together to eliminate the need to match up surveys. Students completed the surveys anonymously, meaning specific responses could not be traced back to individual students. Students received a consent form explaining that completing and returning the survey indicated consent to participate in the research study. The consent form also contained phone numbers for the student health center and student counseling center in case students wanted to discuss a physical or emotional health issue with a professional after writing.

Survey administration took place on February 4, 2014 and February 5, 2014. The researcher informed her two classes that met on February 4 and her one class that met on February 5 that they would have the opportunity to volunteer to participate in a research study, with participation not being connected in any way to the class grade. The class then proceeded as normal with a writing workshop that takes place every semester as part of normal classroom practices. As part of the writing workshop, students were asked to write on post it notes how they felt both physically and emotionally before writing, with a score of 1 being excellent and a score of 5 being poor. At the conclusion of the writing workshop, students were asked to write on post it notes how they felt both physically and emotionally after writing. For example, when the professor completed this activity, her scores were as follows:

Before writing: Emotional = 1, Physical = 3
After writing: Emotional = 1, Physical = 2

Emotionally, she loves teaching and writing, so she felt great before writing, she enjoyed writing in her journal, and continued to feel great after writing. Physically, she had a headache at the beginning of writing, during writing didn't notice it as much, and felt better after writing. She shares her own examples to illustrate the process students experienced, even though students reported only the numbers ranking how they felt, not the reason why they assigned a specific number to their physical and emotional feelings.

Students chose a topic to write about for the first writing session and wrote for ten minutes about the topic. Students were then given the opportunity to read aloud all or part of their writing and share it with their classmates if they chose, but sharing was optional and students were not required to share if they didn't want to read their writing aloud. Several students in each class used the opportunity to share their writing. The process was repeated three more times. For each of the three following writing sessions, students could either continue to write about their first topic or choose a different topic. Each writing session lasted ten minutes, and at the end of each session students had the opportunity to share their writing. The professor participated in the writing workshop and read aloud her writing at the end of each session.

Between the second and third writing sessions, the class took a dance break to stand up and stretch. Some students chose to complete dance moves from the popular dances YMCA and The Electric Slide even though there was no music, while others used the two minute break to simply stretch their arms over their heads. Writing then resumed.

At the conclusion of the writing workshop, the professor distributed the surveys while reminding the students that participation was optional and responses would remain anonymous. The professor then left the room so she would not see who completed surveys and who didn't. A manila envelope was left on a desk in the classroom and students placed surveys in the envelope when finished. A volunteer student from each class retrieved the professor from the hallway after all students who chose to participate placed the surveys in the envelope and class proceeded with a discussion of additional writing strategies and stress management techniques.

SURVEY RESULTS AND ANALYSIS

On the writing survey, for each of the four writing sessions, each student who completed the survey was asked to list the writing topic chosen, describe in one word how he or she felt about the topic, and describe the topic as emotional or neutral. Each student was then asked to answer two yes/no questions, with one question asking if he or she chose to share his or her writing by reading it aloud and the other question asking if he or she completed journal writing outside of the writing time in class. The professor wrote about twelve topics instead of four because she completed the writing in all three of her classes. Her topics and how she described them were: love of photography (emotional), first year of teaching (emotional), describing chair arrangements in the classroom (neutral), love of teaching (emotional), required exams (emotional), graduation (emotional), her aunt and role model (emotional), finding her way as a teacher (emotional), required exams (emotional), deeper themes of Disney movies (neutral), required exams (emotional), her writing process (neutral).

On the health survey, students were asked to answer general questions about their health by circling numbers. An example of a question on the Health Related Quality of Life Survey (2011) was:

Would you say that in general your health is:

1. Excellent 1
2. Very good 2
3. Good 3
4. Fair 4
5. Poor 5 (http://www.cdc.gov/hrqol/hrqol14_measure.htm)

Other questions asked students about specific health issues, such as:

During the past 30 days, for about how many days have you felt worried, tense, or anxious?

- Number of days (space for number)
    - None
    - Don't know/Not sure
    - Refused (http://www.cdc.gov/hrqol/hrqol14_measure.htm)

While the HRQOL contained numerous other questions, the one about feeling worried, tense, or anxious is included here because that question provided the most significant information for the research study.

When scoring the surveys, each survey received a number from 1-64, because 64 subjects chose to participate in the research study. Results were then entered in a table under each survey number to easily keep track of the data. Results are listed in the following summary, and a detailed analysis follows the numbered list to illustrate how a study intended to illuminate connections between writing and healing led to the discovery of anxiety reported by college students and the design of a social action project to help students manage stress.

1. Correlations in SPSS showed no significant relationship between:
    a. Writing about emotional topics and overall health (HRQOL)
    b. Writing about neutral topics and overall health (HRQOL)
    c. Emotional topics and emotional change (pre/post writing)
    d. Emotional topics and physical change (pre/post writing)
    e. Neutral topics and emotional change (pre/post writing)
    f. Neutral topics and physical change (pre/post writing)
    g. Emotional change (pre/post writing) and physical change (pre/post writing)

2. One sample chi square showed equal probabilities of sharing vs. not sharing when compared to general health, as well as equal probabilities of writing at home vs. in class when compared to general health.

Observations: The act of writing is not influenced by topic, whether or not students share, or whether or not they write outside class. This could be a good thing because students receive equal benefits from writing regardless of other factors. The only thing all subjects have in common is they wrote in journals.

3. Physical change during writing: 43 subjects reported no change in the way they felt physically pre/post writing, 15 felt better and 6 felt worse.

Observations: Most students reported excellent or good health to begin with, meaning there was nothing to improve or change. The few who reported severe physical pain would not see it cured by writing; they need to see a doctor. Writing may have caused an increase or decrease in physical health if students relaxed during writing, causing their muscles to be less tense, but there may be other factors such as uncomfortable desks in the classroom. Interestingly, numbers of how students felt pre/post writing did not always correspond to the overall health score on HRQOL, meaning students could have good health overall but had a bad health day or vice versa.

4. Emotional change during writing: 28 subjects reported no change in the way they felt emotionally pre/post writing, 26 felt better and 10 felt worse.

Observations: Some students reported excellent or good health to begin with, meaning there was nothing to improve or change. The increase or decrease in emotional health can be explained by choice in topic; overall, the students who used optimistic words to describe their writing felt better and the students who used pessimistic words felt worse. Also, sometimes when writing about a difficult topic, the writer feels worse initially but better over time.

5. On the HRQOL question that asked during the last 30 days, how many days have you been worried, anxious, or tense, only 5 students responded 0 days, or none of the time. Some used words like all days, parts of every day, and 11 students responded 30 days, or all of the time. The

next most common number was 10 days (9 students) followed by 20 days (4 students) and the rest of the students gave varying responses.

6. Most common other health complaints were lack of sleep, low energy, and sadness/depression. Most students who reported a large number of days with lack of sleep also reported a large number of days with low energy. Exactly half, 32 students, reported no physical symptoms but the most common physical symptom reported by 13 students was back and neck pain, which can be a physical manifestation of emotional stress.

Observations: Students are experiencing anxiety and stress, and better methods of managing stress are needed.

7. A significant correlation in SPSS was found between the first word students used to describe their emotions about writing and the number of anxiety days reported on the HRQOL. The correlation was found using the following steps:

   a. Converted the number of anxiety days each student experienced each month into a scale with 20-30 days = high anxiety, 10-19 days = mid anxiety, and 0-9 days = low anxiety.
   b. Scored anxiety using a scale where 1=high anxiety, 3=mid anxiety, 5=low anxiety. The few students who left the question blank received the neutral response of 3.
   c. Looked at the first word students used to describe their feelings about their first writing topic.
   d. Scored the word using the same artistic writing scale rubric used for other writing surveys such as the survey used at the physical therapy clinic, with 1=negative, 3= neutral, 5=positive. The few students who left the question blank received the neutral response of 3.

The correlation between the numerical anxiety scale and the positive artistic writing is significant, meaning a trend exists where students who use more positive language have less anxiety.

Table 1 illustrates the significant correlation discussed above.

Observations: These results dovetail with the results of the previous study at the physical therapy clinic because students who used a positive writing voice demonstrated lower anxiety.

Table 1. Correlation between more positive language and less anxiety

		Positive Artistic First Word	Anxiety Numeric
Positive artistic first word	Pearson Correlation	1	.265*
	Sig. (2-tailed)		.035
	N	64	64
Anxiety numeric	Pearson Correlation	.265*	1
	Sig. (2-tailed)	.035	
	N	64	64

*. Correlation is significant at the 0.05 level (2-tailed).

8. Students with high anxiety typically chose to write about school issues before other topics.

Observations: Listing the topics each student chose to write about is a qualitative notation without quantitative statistical analysis in SPSS, but it was interesting to notice a trend that the first topic students who reported higher anxiety wished to explore in writing focused on school issues such as upcoming exams, current field experience internships, and plans after graduation, while students who reported lower anxiety chose a broader range of topics such as family, favorite books, current events, and other issues unrelated to school experiences.

THE SIGNIFICANCE OF FIRST IMPRESSIONS

Initial analysis of the data from the 64 subjects who completed the survey echoed the findings of previous studies: Writing is healing. Writing also seems to have benefits for people who take the time to put pen to paper regardless of the topic chosen. However, the more important observation existed in the fact on one of the health questions asked on the Health Related Quality of Life Survey (HRQOL), all but five subjects reported experiencing anxiety or stress. This research study did not begin with the intent of studying anxiety in college students, but consequently, the results caused the research to evolve into a social action project to help college students cope with stress and anxiety. Diagnosing a problem raises questions and the need for answers in the form of providing solutions.

As previously mentioned, the results of this research study dovetail with the previous research study the researchers conducted at the physical therapy clinic. College students who used a positive writing voice demonstrated lower anxiety and stronger emotional health, just like physical therapy patients who used a positive writing voice throughout their treatment interventions demonstrated higher recovery gains for objective measures on pre-existing physical therapy surveys. The results illustrate that a strong positive writing voice can help people heal both physically and emotionally.

Voice in writing was assessed using a writing rubric that incorporates both the technical and artistic dimensions of writing. The technical dimension of writing reflects specificity, while the artistic dimension reflects voice. Romano (2013) believes a successful rubric reflects both artistic (holistic) and technical (required) elements of writing and explains when examining writing, "the rubric helps me pay attention to its totality. The holistic portion allows me to open myself to what the paper is doing, to feel it, just as I want to feel other crafted writing I read. The required elements remind me to examine how well students executed specific skills, strategies, and genres I've taught" (p. 167). The artistic dimension of the writing rubric highlighting voice correlated with the amount of anxiety, as students who demonstrated a more positive writing voice showed lower anxiety.

Writing teachers and theorists believe that the first thoughts are the truest thoughts, because the more people write, the more they self-censor. As Goldberg (1986) argues, "first thoughts have tremendous energy. It is the way the mind first flashes on something" (p. 9). That is why the focus of the student writing on the survey became the first topic they chose to write about and the word they used to describe that topic. Most students wrote about multiple topics, but the first topic represents what is really on their minds and how they feel about it. Goldberg (1990) believes, "we need to learn to accept our minds. Believe me, for writing, it is all we have" (p. 53). First thought writing can illuminate a writer's true feelings. When beginning to write about a topic, frequently writers will have a flash of insight that causes them to be honest with themselves when writing. Some writers will continue to reflect on their honest feelings as they continue to write, but other writers will start to question their ideas, worry about what others may think even if no one else is reading the writing, or feel vulnerable and not remain as open to their thoughts when continuing writing. Goldberg (2013) explains, "these moments are a flash, an insight when we see through the confusion of our constant thinking to something clear" (p. 30). Writing captures the insightful moments that illuminate honest first impressions before the writer revises due to second thoughts.

As students participated in the writing workshop, they had time to think about their writing, listen to their classmates' read writing, and add to their original writing. Any of these factors could cause students to censor their own unique writing voices, even though the student writing was not collected for the survey and if students did not choose to share no one else saw or heard the writing. Sometimes writers reread their own words and want the story to be different from what actually happened, not to lie but to make the truth sound better, make more sense, or hurt less. DeSalvo (1999) believes, "we resist chaos narratives. We resist reading them. Sometimes we resist writing them, penning a neater, more hopeful though fraudulent version of events we've survived. We want narratives that demonstrate the resilience of the human spirit. We don't want to admit defeat" (p. 197). Mistakes happen in life, but since we are the authors of our own individual stories, we often chose to cast ourselves as the hero rather than admit sometimes our best thinking got us to a place we don't want to be. But before the doubt that leads a writer to second guess those first thoughts creeps in and tells a new story, the writer's true voice reveals itself. And as Graves (1994) writes, "it is a writer's voice that gives me the best sense of his or her potential" (p. 82). Just like with the physical therapy patients, the college students were using their writing voices to tell stories. We had to figure out what stories.

THE AGE OF ANXIETY

Because the majority of college students surveyed reported experiencing stress and anxiety, we as the researchers decided to help university administrators brainstorm potential strategies to help the students. In order to implement effective solutions to this situation that will improve health for college students, it helps to first understand the problem. Nurse practitioner Clark (2006) explains that, "Anxiety conditions appear as a result of cumulative stress over time" (p. 2). The terms anxiety and stress may be used interchangeably, but they are different. Helgoe, Wilhelm, and Kommor (2005) elaborate, "stress implies external pressure, whereas anxiety describes an internal experience" (p. 26). There is agreement among practitioners in the medical field that some anxiety can actually be helpful. Clark (2006) argues, "mild anxiety can be a good thing. Without it, you'd be constantly drifting off to sleep, probably couldn't hold a coherent discussion or achieve any of your goals. Mild anxiety is necessary for learning to take place" (p. 15). Helgoe, Wilhelm, and Kommor (2005) concur and add, "anxiety is considered healthy when it motivates us to take action in the name of accomplishment" (p. 22). However, anxiety frequently crosses the line and becomes unhealthy. Stress/anxiety over a long time is not healthy. This is called chronic stress. Chronic stress can cause physical symptoms such as headaches, potential weight gain, inability to concentrate, inability to sleep, increased risk for a stroke and/or heart attack, and depression (http://www.helpguide.org/mental/stress_signs.htm). There are different types of stressors which cause stress. External Stressors can be pain, weather, working conditions, abusive relationships. Internal Stressors can be physical or psychological such as infections, inflammation, worrying. (http://umm.edu/health/medical/reports/articles/stress)

In the field of education, the most common reference to anxiety is test anxiety. As English teacher Johnson (1998) advises teachers, "you don't have to make your exams easier in order to improve grades and student motivation in your classroom; you do need to reduce the stress and anxiety your students feel about taking exams" (p. 26). Unfortunately, numerous teachers get pulled into the vortex known as standardized testing and professional obligations eclipse personal wellness. Clark (2006) cautions, "as anxiety increases, your perception of what is going on around you decreases" (p. 16). Many people find themselves trapped in this cycle. Increased anxiety leads to decreased perception, which in turn leads to increased anxiety. College students can become especially vulnerable to anxiety as they struggle to make decisions about their future.

Another author named Johnson (2009) writes about anxiety from the perspective of a minister and observes, "contrasting the past to the present, the not knowing to the knowing, it creates a totally different point of focus. Before I was anxious; now I am free. Why? Because now I know the outcome. When we know the outcome, we're not nearly as constrained by the process of getting there. To be sure, we are free to rise above the moment and savor the intricacies of the journey" (p. 15). The fact that the next chapter in life remains unwritten can make the journey simultaneously exciting and anxiety provoking.

People may say they have fear of the future, but fear and anxiety are different. Clark (2006) elaborates, "although you may not know the difference between anxiety and fear, the two terms refer to entirely different feelings. Fear is usually directed at an external danger" (p. 11). Conversely, "anxiety has no such easily recognizable source and is often called an unexplained discomfort" (p. 11). However, Helgoe, Wilhelm, and Kommor (2005) highlight the similarities instead of the differences between anxiety and fear by stating, "anxiety is fear without a clear threat. Whereas fear is a natural reaction to an obvious, literal threat to your physical well-being, anxiety often feels abnormal and without use or function" (p. 4). It is also easy to discuss anxiety from the outside looking in at the issue instead of experiencing it. What may seem abnormal to people who haven't experienced anxiety is a normal part of the day for people who live with anxiety. Journalist Smith (2012) describes his personal experiences with anxiety and believes, "and yet to talk about anxiety as directionless and formless and fear as focused and specific only says how the two experiences are different, not how they're related. It also suggests in a backhanded way, that fear is normal, a hardwired Darwinian response, and that anxiety is abnormal, a sort of postindustrial, urban affliction. No experts say this outright, or even at all" (p. 124). Stossel (2013) also shares his personal experiences with anxiety as well as advice from his therapist and elaborates, "yet enough of us do suffer from anxiety that perhaps writing about my own ought not to be an occasion for shame but an opportunity to provide solace to some of the millions of others who share this affliction. And maybe, as Dr. W. often reminds me, the exercise will be therapeutic. 'You can write yourself to health,' he says." (pp. 28-29).

FBI profiler and security expert DeBecker (1997) describes a nonmedical perspective on fear and explains, "worry, wariness, anxiety, and concern all have a purpose, but they are not fear. So anytime your dreaded outcome cannot reasonably be linked to pain or death and it is isn't a signal in the presence of danger, than it really shouldn't be confused with fear" (p. 286). Echoing the sentiment that anxiety decreases when the outcome of a situation becomes more certain, DeBecker continues, "predictions in which you have high confidence free you to respond, adjust, feel sadness, accept, prepare, or to do whatever is needed. Accordingly, anxiety is reduced by improving your predictions, thus increasing your certainty. It's worth doing, because the word anxiety, like worry, stems from a root that means "to choke," and that is just what it does to us" (p. 292). To feel more certain about predictions encompassing the way people could potentially behave and the resulting outcomes, DeBecker reminds people to use intuition. Intuition represents the first flash of insight that DeBecker believes is often correct. The first mental insight, just like the first thought in writing, is more accurate because second thoughts do not have time to occur.

FOR THE GIRLS

Because more female students than male students completed this survey, it became enlightening to examine factors that may cause college women to experience stress and anxiety. Self-defense expert Baty (2003) references DeBecker's research and advises, "whatever your fears are, the goal is to become proactive" (p. 201). The context of that quote encourages women to take ownership of their own safety, but it nevertheless highlights another interesting observation about the college students who reported anxiety. Because the survey responses remained anonymous, there is no way of knowing if students who indicated high anxiety were male or female. However, the majority of students from the potential pool of respondents were female. This is due to the population composition of the College of Education. With a few exceptions, in most education classes women outnumber the men. Therefore, while the anonymity of the responses prevents this next observation from being stated as a clear fact, it is a safe bet to assume that more women than men completed surveys.

Twenty years ago, educators sounded the alarm that girls endured more stress and anxiety than boys did because antiquated notions of stereotypical gender roles from past generations refused to dissipate. Sadker and Sadker (1994) conducted extensive research in classrooms and made the disturbing observation, "as the snapshots continue, the underlying gender messages become clear. The classroom consists of two worlds: one of boys in action, the other of girls' inaction" (p. 42). The Sadkers painted a troubling portrait of girls sitting back in the classroom while boys volunteered to share their ideas. Sadly, twenty years later Sandberg paints the same troubling portrait of women sitting back in conference rooms while men volunteer to share their ideas. Sandberg (2013) urges women to lean in and make their voices heard without being afraid to speak up because "fear is at the root of so many of the barriers that women face. Fear of not being liked. Fear of making the wrong choice. Fear of drawing negative attention. Fear of overreaching. Fear of being judged. Fear of failure" (p. 24). Twenty years later, the same conversation still takes place.

Even though society should have evolved to the point where a woman can live any life she wants to live, women still experience the pressure of mixed messages. Popular magazines with a target audience of women reveal the messages portrayed on one page emphasize accomplishments while the messages portrayed on the next emphasize appearance. Cohen-Sandler (2005) discusses the effects stress can have on girls and reports that parents and teachers often do not recognize signs of distress because "many signs of stress are so common that they are accepted as the normal, even expected, cost of leading busy, productive lives" (p. 13). But consequences occur when being busy and productive transforms into being overscheduled and overwhelmed. Cohen-Sandler continues, "with a distinct lack of downtime, girls are less able to relax, sleep, read for pleasure, and exercise. This undermines their ability to combat both anxiety and depression. Similarly, without the benefit of solitary activities such as writing in journals, reading, and creating music or art, girls can't soothe themselves as well" (p. 17). Moreover, while Cohen-Sandler concluded through her research that all teens need strategies for coping with stress, girls need more help than boys since "what I discovered is that all girls, even highly functioning ones, can be toppled into crises by a constellation of circumstances: temperament, personality style, past history, school dynamics, and community cultures" (p. 23). Boys are not immune to sociocultural pressures, but Pipher (1994) states that with girls, "calmness is replaced by anxiety" (p. 23). She argues that girls become vulnerable to silencing their own voices because as they try to answer life's questions of their place in the world, "American culture has always smacked girls on the head in early adolescence" (p, 23). And the mixed messages linger for college women. If they have a career, will time run out to have children? And why when they win awards does someone always compliment their cute shoes before their intelligence?

Writing proved healing for girls to process conflicting feelings and mixed messages. The blank page of a journal also gives them space to find their voices. As Barbieri (1995) asks, "for isn't every girl's voice worth saving?" (p. 28). English teacher Barbieri devoted class time for writing so her students, all girls, could share their stories. Shandler (1999) read Pipher's research and developed her own project encouraging girls to share their stories, in the process discovering that "invited to speak honestly, girls told treasured and hidden stories. They wrote to communicate, to heal themselves, and to help other girls. With intelligence, they reflected on the most important experiences in their lives. Sometimes, their stories made me laugh. More often, they made me cry" (p. xv). Writing led to healing because it enabled the authors to identify their feelings, name their fears, and have an audience for their stories. It provided another method of becoming proactive by naming fears and processing them.

As a therapist, Pipher (1994) encouraged patients to express their pain through writing and other creative outlets as she describes, "I teach girls to sit with their pain, to listen to it for messages about their lives, to acknowledge and describe it rather than to run from it. They learn to write about pain, to talk about it, to express it through exercise, art dance or music" (p. 257). Writing highlights the source of the stress and while writing about a problem may not solve it, it may prevent the author from living in denial of the pain. And denial can lead to anxiety. As DeBecker (1997) explains, "denial is a save-now-pay later scheme, a contract written entirely in small print, for in the long run, the denying person knows the truth on some level, and it causes a constant low-grade anxiety" (p. 10). Through writing about issues and discussing them, perhaps both men and women can alleviate anxiety caused by outdated social pressures and crazy busy lives full of stress so that twenty years from now but preferably much sooner, a different conversation takes place.

ANXIETY AND HEALTH

Regardless of the factors which cause an individual to have anxiety, anxiety influences that person's health. It can help people to comprehend the impact anxiety and stress have on their bodies; it can also help people to know methods for managing anxiety and stress. Clark (2006) states, "anxiety has physical, emotional, mental, even spiritual effects" (p. 12). Emotional distress often leads to physical symptoms. Tindle (2013) discusses her medical research and concludes, "depression, anxiety, and chronic pain are classic examples of chronic "whole body" stressors. Based on the research and my clinical experience, I believe that certain attitudes can be chronic whole body stressors, too. Over time, learning to blunt our own tendencies toward negative automatic responses may reduce overall wear and tear on our bodily organs" (pp. 103-104). She provides the example that a thought about something that causes stress can lead to anxious feelings followed by physical queasiness. Rankin (2013) also discusses her medical research and shares the belief that stress can create illness, elaborating that, "intuitively, we know this, and when we're stressed out, we crave relaxation. But too often, we go about it the wrong way, seeking out unhealthy forms of stress relief like alcohol, tobacco, and illegal drugs, which only exacerbate the problem. There are, however, healthy ways to elicit the relaxation response – such as meditation – that are the best medicine we can take for the treatment of life's stresses" (p. 147). Exercise is also a great way to decrease stress levels. According to the Mayo Clinic (2011) it can decrease depression, increase dopamine, improve self-esteem, improve confidence, decrease risk of stroke, decrease risk of type 2 DM, help you fall asleep quicker, decreases risks of certain types of cancer, helps with arthritis (http://www.mayoclinic.com/health/exercise/HQ01676).

Sometimes when people crave relief from the stressors in life, they don't always make the best decisions. Despite the fact that an apple is a healthier nutritional choice than a cookie, in a moment of pain people may not see the value of making short term sacrifices for long term gains. It may seem fulfilling at the moment eating an unhealthy food item when stressed, yet there are many more long-term health factors you should consider first before making this a routine for coping. Unhealthy eating and physical inactivity can lead to four of the six leading causes of death along with other diseases including: heart disease, diabetes, obesity, hypertension, stroke, osteoporosis, and many cancers. The cancers include colon cancer, prostate cancer, mouth cancer, throat cancer, esophagus cancer, lung cancer, and stomach cancer (http://www.cspinet.org/nutritionpolicy/nutrition_policy.html#eat).

Other times, making life changes that may lead to less anxiety may seem like an insurmountable obstacle. Rankin (2013) continues, "can't quit your stressful job? Not ready to leave your unhappy marriage? Haven't found the love of your life yet? Not interested in going to church? That's okay. I'm not suggesting you have to do everything I've covered in this book in order to be optimally healthy. But I am suggesting that if you're exposed to stressors you either can't change or aren't ready to change, you must prioritize activities that include the relaxation response as a way to counterbalance the stresses in your life" (p. 153). In theory, it may be easy to think of following a stressful activity such as a long commute to work with a relaxing one such as reading a novel, but some people find it difficult to relax. Life coach Beck (2008) conducted her own experiment to see how her thoughts influenced her physical health and describes, "hooked up to that brain-mapping computer, I learned that just remembering times of great fear and then repeating my 'surrender mantras' brought my anxiety-related beta waves down, down, down. Gradually, this taught me how to calm myself. After all those hours of brain-training, hooked up to the mapmakers' computer, I'm less anxious overall" (p. 96). By being able to see how her calm thoughts she called surrender mantras influenced her neurological patterns, Beck learned the value of living in the moment, facing her fears, and letting go of things beyond her control.

Nevertheless, when parts of life feel beyond control, it can be difficult to let go. Numbing the pain through anything that provides a temporary high or just staying too crazy busy to reflect about life becomes easier than facing fears. Brown (2012) discusses the need for people to numb their pain and explains, "the most powerful need for numbing seems to come from combinations of all three – shame, anxiety, and disconnection" (p. 138). Often people feel embarrassed by their stories, especially when the story presents the storyteller in a less than perfect light. No one is alone in this world, but when you make a mistake, fail to reach a goal, or live with pain, it is easy to think no one else has ever felt what you feel. Brown adds, "shame enters for those of us who experience anxiety because not only are we feeling fearful, out of control, and incapable of managing our increasingly demanding lives, but eventually our anxiety is compounded and made unbearable by our belief that if we were just smarter, stronger, or better, we'd be able to handle everything" (p. 139). A lack of connection also contributes to feelings of isolation and loneliness.

With social media and modern technology, it should be easier for people to stay in touch with each other than ever before. Yet how many times do we send a text or an email instead of picking up the phone and calling someone? Social media sites often encourage an individual to share only events worth bragging about without showing the real person behind the screen. College students have more ways of connecting to others than ever, but sometimes feel more alone than their parents and grandparents who remember what it was like not to constantly have a phone in front of them. As Brown (2012) explains, "with disconnection it's a similar story. We may have a couple hundred friends on Facebook, plus a slew of colleagues, real-life friends, and neighbors, but we feel alone and unseen. Because we are hardwired for connection, disconnection always creates pain" (p. 139). Does this disconnection contribute to the anxiety the college students reported? Only future research will tell. But for now, we can use the information we have to implement practices that will lead to increased connection and decreased stress.

THE PROBLEM: IMPLEMENTING STRATEGIES FOR COLLEGE STUDENT SUCCESS

Highlighting an issue such as stress and anxiety raises awareness of it, but brainstorming potential success strategies will not lead to change unless people implement the strategies. While the following strategies focus on helping college students, like the students who were the subjects of this research study, anyone can use these strategies to create a curriculum of community. In discussing community, once again the city planning process mentioned previously can provide a template for implementing change.

As city planner Johnson (1997) believes, "planning for cities begins when we look around us and say, 'this could be different!'" (p. 1). The same applies to planning curriculum change for college students. We as transformative leaders need to believe that the way things are can be different. Johnson explains the planning process, the same process used to design the curriculum change solutions. He continues, "we could think of planning for a given geographic area as a cycle with three major stages. In the first stage, governmental and private planners set goals and criteria to guide the succeeding steps" (p. 10). Later, "in the second stage in the cycle, planners select actions that give the goals tangible form" (p. 10). And finally, "third, planning leads to implementation of the choices" (p. 10). And just as in planning a city, planning to help college students requires a community vision to implement a detailed plan. As Harper (1996) states, "the visioning process may also result in guidance for the comprehensive plan goals and objectives. If there is a community vision, the plan can become an implementation tool" (p. 196). The university community needs to build a vision and work together to meet the needs of its students. Faculty members and university leaders have struggled with the same problems as our students; perhaps we still struggle with the same problems our students do. Regardless of our own experiences, we need to take action.

Kinematics professor Kepler (1973) discusses a physics principle of motion and explains, "kinetics is the study of forces acting on rigid bodies in motion and the effect of such forces in changing the motion" (p. 1). The same physics principle applies to curriculum change: We need to be the force that changes the motion of people. We can use our expertise to share our knowledge and lead the way to create change. We can become the understanding role models students, especially students confronting anxiety, need. College students experiencing anxiety need resources to make healthy choices, a safe supportive community, and a space to share their stories.

THE SOLUTIONS: MAKING HEALTHY CHOICES

Each person's life represents a series of decisions. Behaviors, whether they include the amount of exercise, food choices, or writing about feelings, all influence health. If the choices do not lead to health and happiness, it's never too late to make new choices. On the topic of stress, Juhan (1998) states, "it is clear then that neither the extreme of altogether avoiding stress nor the extreme of altogether ignoring it are really very helpful to the individual who wants to live a long and productive life. The real point is to learn how to handle stress, how to sustain our efforts without burning out, how to keep the nose to the grindstone without grinding it off" (p. 302). However, in order to incorporate the consistently changing medical field while simultaneously dovetailing academic theory with practical advice for the readers of this chapter, websites respected by numerous medical professionals that reflect current practices intertwine with texts from the fields of writing and medicine to present an eclectic approach of using methods that promote healthy behaviors. Juhan (1998) elaborates on this theme of behavior choices enhancing health by sharing the example of a ballet dancer preparing for a recital because "the dancer, if she is to be a successful professional, has no choice but to confront each symptom and discover the way to work through it, not by ignoring nor avoiding its causes, but rather by learning to form a working relationship with the stresses of her activity. She trains herself to produce strength at every point where a weakness develops" (p. 302). Too often, people think of having anxiety as a weakness, but methods exist for coping with it and living a healthy life.

Solutions to the problems discussed in this research utilize a myriad of resources from the fields of writing and medicine to illustrate the benefits of choosing health and limiting stress. Consider identifying sources of stress and implementing the strategies discussed. After all, theories about healthy living must become a lifestyle in order to achieve elite and effective results. It is possible to take initiative and manage stress. Don't lose hope.

SOLUTION #1: MANAGE TECHNOLOGY

Technology enhances people's lives. Cameron (1998) describes that technology can enhance writing, "because it is instantaneous, email tricks people into evading their censor" (p. 33). While the use of email, like other technology, can enhance people's lives, too often people abuse the technology. Carter (2015) asks the questions, "Do you check your email, texts, voicemails, Facebook, Instagram account, or Twitter feed within an hour of waking up or going to sleep? While you're in line at the store? During dinner with your family? Would you check it at church while waiting for a funeral to start? If so, ya ain't alone" (p. 97). Carter explains that there is a reason for such behavior. She elaborates, "there is something gratifying about constantly checking our email and social-media feeds. The distraction is pleasurable because it gives us what researchers call 'variable ratio reinforcement.' In other words, we are drawn to our smartphones in the way we are drawn to slot machines. We never know when we'll get a satisfying message on Facebook or an email with good news, so we just keep checking" (p. 97). Even though people can rationalize their actions, it doesn't mean it is healthy behavior. Brickman (2015) observes, "so far, I haven't missed any career or life-changing moments by not facing the morning with a first-thing phone fling" (p. 20). He recommends easing into the morning before checking technology.

Brown (2012) discusses research on anxiety and elaborates, "when it comes to anxiety, we all struggle. Yes, there are different types of anxiety and certainly different intensities. Some anxiety is hardwired and best addressed with a combination of medication and therapy, and some of it is environmental – we're overextended and overstressed" (p. 143). Brown observed differences between two groups of people and discovered, "participants from both groups often used today's dominating technology as an example of an anxiety-producing source during the interviews" (p. 143). While both groups shared the experiences of anxiety from technology, one group found ways to manage the anxiety while the other changed behaviors that led to anxiety. Brown provided the example that the first group constantly checked emails and made sure they were all answered although sometimes at the expense of sleep, while the second group asked people not to send unnecessary emails and indicated it might take several days for a reply. Brown concluded, "when we asked that group about the process of setting boundaries and limits to lower the anxiety in their lives, they did not hesitate to connect worthiness with boundaries. We have to believe we are enough in order to say, 'Enough!'" (pp. 144-145). Because abuse of technology can cause anxiety, it helps to set boundaries for use.

Carter (2015) concurs that there is a connection between technology and anxiety with the explanation, "even though our brain tends to seek that variable ratio reinforcement, which suggests pleasure, usually we aren't consciously checking our email for fun or recreation. We check constantly to abate our anxiety that we are missing something" (p. 98). Carter offers suggestions such as disabling push features that provide instant alerts on phones and computers, designating spaces in which technology will be used, and deciding on times when not to use technology. She concludes, "what all this means is that unless we want to feel overwhelmed and exhausted, we need to unplug. A lot" (p.

99). Following this advice may not seem easy, but it becomes necessary for a life filled with less stress.

Enayati (2015) discusses the connections between technology and stress and explains, "the effects of stress are compounded by the fact that we are rarely turned off and are always connected. Stress in its various forms has access to us at all times. In the old days people got up and were able to go for a walk to get away. Now we are never far from all sorts of bad news. The solution: turn it off! Go on technology fasts" (pp. 158-159). Enayati concludes, "we can choose narratives that help us reframe stressors, thereby strengthening our ability to withstand (or avoid) the stress coming our way and to counter it with positive emotions" (p. 159). Choosing and reframing a narrative can change a person's perspective on stress and anxiety.

SOLUTION #2: FINDING A HEALTHY LIFESTYLE

One solution to help with stress and anxiety is to live a healthy lifestyle. Medical doctor Winner (2008) provides the reminder, "anxiety disorders and depression are medical conditions. It should not be viewed as weakness to take medication for these problems, any more than it is weakness to take medication for diabetes" (p. 214). The solutions discussed can provide relief from stress and feelings of anxiety. Nevertheless, they cannot take the place of advice from a supportive medical professional such as a physician, physical therapist, psychiatrist, or counselor. There is no shame in seeking medical help, talking to a medical professional, or taking medication to help with anxiety.

It remains essential to acknowledge the connection between stress and health. As Handler (2013) states, "stress can make you sick" (p. 175). Through her research of interviewing doctors, Handler learned, "looking back at a stressful situation tends to create stress in the present moment" (p. 175). It therefore becomes important to remember that recovery takes time, and people suffering from anxiety may notice slow progress and may not feel better immediately. Pennebaker (1997) learned from his writing study, "as it turned out, writing about horrible things made people feel horrible immediately after writing" (p. 34). Over time, however, feelings improved. College students often struggle to find themselves and may change their belief systems. This can lead to anxiety and depression because as Pennebaker discusses, "when beliefs about the world are threatened, traumatized individuals experience intense anxiety, depression, or denial because their worlds don't make sense. With time, individuals may reorient their lives in order to force new experiences into their existing belief systems. Alternatively, peoples' original belief systems may gradually return by their having positive experiences" (p. 76). For college students, they may define a trauma as being homesick, preparing for a test, or feeling uncertain about a career choice. That doesn't mean their problems are more trivial than their counterparts experiencing severe illness or a death in the family.

It also helps for people experiencing anxiety to get moving. Clark (2006) explains, "exercise is one of the most effective ways to reduce anxiety, and even panic attacks. Panic is simply the physical and emotional experience of an excessive surge of adrenaline" (p. 102). What's the recommended amount of exercise? The American College of Sports Medicine (2011) recommends the amount of time for each adult to put in for cardiorespiratory exercise is "at least 150 minutes of moderate-intensity exercise each week." The ACSM elaborates, "exercise recommendations can be met through 30-60 minutes of moderate-intensity exercise (five days per week) or 20-60 minutes of vigorous-intensity exercise (three days per week)." For resistance exercise it is recommended by the ACSM that "adults should train each major muscle group two to three days each week." How many repetitions for each exercise? The ACSM advises, "8-12 repetitions improve strength and power, 10-15 repetitions improve strength in middle-age and older persons starting exercise, and 15-20 repetitions improve muscular endurance." Including flexibility exercises and balance exercises can also be beneficial (http://www.acsm.org/about-acsm/media-room/news-releases/2011/08/01/acsm-issues-new-recommendations-on-quantity-and-quality-of-exercise). If you are unable to meet all of these minutes it does not mean that you are unhealthy. Gradually work up to it. Over time increase your amount of minutes, followed by increased intensity levels. Even taking a short break to take a walk around campus or play on the swings outside the residence halls enables a person to receive the benefits of exercise. Going to the dining hall for a salad can also have more health benefits than ordering pizza and drinking beer multiple times a week.

SOLUTION #3: CONNECTING THROUGH CREATING CLASS COMMUNITY

Another strategy to help with stress and anxiety is to feel part of a supportive community. While students are in the classroom it is important to make the classroom a home away from home. Heard (1995) writes, "we know where we feel most at home" (p. 5). Teachers want to believe that all students leave the classroom and go home to supportive families. Sadly, for some students, the place where they feel most at home is the classroom because once they leave, they confront difficulties at home. For college students, some may be living away from family for the first time in their lives. Nontraditional students frequently juggle families and jobs in addition to classes and the classroom may provide the only respite in a busy day. So teachers and professors need to create classroom communities where students feel safe and supported. Routman (2003) discusses the value of building a strong class community because "no one talks about bonding, and we need to. Curriculum and standards must first connect with the lives and spirits of our children if we're to have any lasting success. Unless we reach into our students' hearts, we have no entry into their minds" (p. 12). Building a community means encouraging students to trust each other and share their voices. The community can then provide a support network for students by providing strength when a community member struggles.

People only have a certain number of hours in a day, so why not make the time spent in the classroom as enjoyable as possible? Most people strive to find balance in their lives, and students in the College of Education who completed surveys for this research study not only have the stress of completing their own assignments for classes, but also the added pressure of designing inspiring lessons for the students who are in their classrooms during required field experiences and later, student teaching. Time management can be difficult for teachers because, even with constant multitasking, there never seem to be enough hours in the day to accomplish all of the learning goals. Routman (2003) encourages teachers to rethink their schedules and states, "the elusive balanced life remains a mirage. Your time is valuable. Spend it in the most meaningful, productive ways possible" (p. 202). She also encourages teachers to get a life outside of school and tells the story of a friend who almost gave up tickets to the ballet to grade papers. Routman told her friend to go to the ballet and be an interesting person because "you can't come to work each day enthusiastic about teaching if all you did the night before was grade papers. You want to be able to have dinner with a friend, go to a movie. Read a book, cook for fun, reflect about what's just happened. We are not only role models for learning but role models for living" (p. 202). Professors of future teachers need to become role models for students to live balanced lives.

This is easier said than done, because most teachers feel like Codell (1999) at the end of the school year who says "of course, I cried. There was so much I wanted to say. But the sands of the hourglass fell, and they left me, single file" (p. 185). There will always be one more lesson that could have been taught, one more comment that should have been said, and one more idea that would have fit fabulously into class if only there was more time. Gruwell (2007) describes this feeling as "I knew going in that my student teaching position was supposed to last only a semester, but as finals approached, I started getting anxious. There were still so many things I wanted to do, so many stories I wanted to read, and so many places I wanted to take them" (p. 35). College of Education students who prepare to student teach may share the sentiment of wanting to prove themselves as excellent student teachers while not having enough time with their students. But regardless of whether they are in kindergarten or college, once students leave the classroom for the last time, they will remember how they felt as part of a strong class community and that strength will sustain them as they begin the next chapter of their careers.

Furthermore, teachers feel responsible for all their students. Gruwell (2009) describes this feeling as, "as my students became more like a family, I was surprised by how difficult a balancing act being a teacher really is. At the end of each day it became more impossible to leave my students' problems in the classroom. Then there was the fact that my social life was beginning to implode, and I was spending way too much of my own money on school supplies" (p. xviii-xix). As teachers, we want to be role models for students to enjoy their time in the classroom without experiencing stress; yet, secretly, we may be about to collapse from the stress in our lives ourselves. English teacher Johnson (2005) advises teachers, "stress is a serious problem all by itself." (p. 132). She encourages teachers to take mental health breaks as needed and shares the reminder, "teaching is difficult work, but if you make up your mind that you truly want to teach, your determination and sincerity will lead you in the right direction" (p. 135).

But why go through experiences alone? Sandberg (2013) discusses her movement to create community support networks and encourage conversation. Her movement, called Lean In because she wants people to face their fears and lean in to life, begins with the idea "you can also create and join Lean In Circles, small peer groups that meet in person for ongoing encouragement and development" (p. 173). Descriptions of successful Lean In Circles appeared in recent issues of *Glamour* and *Cosmopolitan*, two publications more popular with college students than chapters like this one. Creating a Lean In Circle on a college campus can bring its students together.

Sandberg (2014) successfully implemented Lean In Circles on college campuses and encourages college students to start their own Lean In Circles because "when you need help – and we all do – please look for it. No one needs to navigate this world alone" (p. xvii). Whether participating in Lean In Circles or other forums of conversation such as a discussion between classes, college students need to know they are not alone.

SOLUTION #4: REFLECTING THROUGH WRITING

Another strategy to help with stress and anxiety is to express thoughts and feelings through writing. To create a strong community, people who belong to the community need to feel they are not alone. Barbieri (1995) discusses her method of using writing to build community at the school where she taught all girls and describes, "I had explained our curriculum for the year. We would write every day on topics of our own choosing, and yes, I would write with them" (p. 18). She discovered that her students used their writing practice time to discuss issues on their minds and asked the question, "should writing be used as therapy for the girls to work out their developmental issues?" (p. 21). After reflection, she concluded that she wanted to provide a safe community for students to write and discuss their writing with each other because, "their writing practice entries brought me back to earth, as I came to know again that the real magic of writing lies in what it can do for the writer. I should have remembered. How many times had I survived stress, crisis and grief by sitting up at night writing furiously? How many times had I written my way out of confusion, anger, or despair? I should have remembered" (p. 27). When there is no one around to listen, or when the author is not ready to share thoughts and feelings with others, writing can help the writer write right through the pain.

Writing cannot solve all the problems that create anxiety, but it can provide an effective coping mechanism. Murray (1985) argues, "writing is therapy. I tried to avoid that issue as a writing teacher, mostly because I had colleagues who accused some of us of using writing as therapy. I can no longer avoid the fact that writing is therapy – for me and for my students. We write because we need to write, and the act of writing rarely solves our problems, but it is a way of dealing with problems and achieving a momentary distance from them. The act of writing about the most painful subjects – in my case the death of a daughter – seems both necessary and therapeutic" (p. 217). Writing does not take the place of a conversation with a supportive emotional therapist, and sometimes talking to a therapist may be the best method to deal with a difficult issue. Pipher (2006) who is a therapist, believes in the power of writing and sharing stories, whether in written or conversational form as she states, "stories are the most basic tool for connecting us to one another" (p. 11). Sharing stories serves as another facet of community building and bringing people together to alleviate isolation and loneliness. Pipher (2006) adds, "healing stories give people hope, teach them empathy, and encourage action" (p. 12). In a community of writers, if one person hears another person's story of healing, that person may feel inspired to survive similar circumstances.

Writing can also provide an effective method to relieve anxiety. Helgoe, Wilhelm, and Kommor (2005) provide the medical perspective on writing and elaborate, "it may be that, by just putting the feelings on paper, we are able to back away from the intensity of the situation and better evaluate things. Often, we are able to sort out feelings and reach insight and clarity through writing. Also, writing slows us down, which is a real benefit to anxiety sufferers" (p. 260). Nurse practitioner Clark (2006) concurs and adds, "journaling, or journal writing, is a way to establish a permanent record of your thoughts, feelings, and situations that evoke anxiety" (p. 146). By rereading journal entries, it becomes possible for the author to discover the source of the anxiety. Or if the author lacks the distance or expertise to provide a self-diagnosis, a supportive audience such as a counselor can help. This is similar to completing a pain journal of physical pain and sharing it with a physician or physical therapist. Pipher (2006) continues the discussion of the healing benefits of writing by stating, "paradoxically, even though writing is anxiety provoking, it is also therapeutic. Once we are immersed in writing, we forget our anxiety. Focusing on clarity and beauty calms us down" (p. 79). Sometimes writing can illuminate issues and motivate the author to create change because, as Pipher believes, "stewing in our own stress is not a good way to handle difficulty. Action ameliorates anxiety" (p. 79). If a writer also belongs to a supportive community, the community members can encourage the writer to take steps toward achieving a goal.

And any step becomes progress. As Cameron (2002) believes, "most blocked creatives have an active addiction to anxiety. We prefer the low-grade pain and occasional heart stopping panic attack to the drudgery of small and simple daily steps in the right direction" (p. 143). Writing can raise awareness so the writer can determine the real issue and take steps to process any pain instead of turning to unhealthy choices to numb it. Cameron highlights the value of this process and continues, "as we become aware of our blocking devices – food, busyness, alcohol, sex, other drugs – we can feel our U-turns as we make them. The blocks will no longer work effectively. Over time, we will try – perhaps slowly at first and erratically – to ride out the anxiety and see where we emerge. Anxiety is fuel. We can use it to write with, paint with, work with" (pp. 165-166). And when anxiety becomes fuel, it can provide help instead of hurt for the individual experiencing it.

SOLUTION #5: CHOOSE TO SHARE STORIES

Whatever an individual's story may be, it influences health. Rankin (2013) discusses this issue from a doctor's perspective and elaborates, "when you work in a hospital, you often hear inspiring stories of optimism linked to disease remission and pessimism associated with disease progression" (p. 127). She also observes, "the body is the physical manifestation of the sum of your life experiences" (p. 173). Tindle (2013) shares this belief that outlook influences health and explains, "we – meaning people in general, but also the larger medical and scientific community – may understand that there is some relationship between outlook and physical health. What we may not fully realize, however, is just how intimately tied our outlook is to our own health and aging over the course of our lives, from our humblest beginnings as babies to the adults we are today, to the older people we'll become tomorrow" (p. 14). However, in her career as a doctor, Tindle discovered most patients don't change their behavior because short term incentives become more enticing than long term health. She adds, "given that humans are hardwired to overvalue rewards now and undervalue rewards later, this answer seems understandable and satisfying, until one thinks about that elusive 1 percent of people – those who achieve ideal cardiac health, or even the 19 percent who get a little more than halfway there, with predictably fantastic health results. How do they do it? What motivates them?" (p. 24). She continues, "I believe that a big part of the mystery of the 1 percent is in our outlook – whether we can envision a positive outcome and muster the confidence and drive to work toward it, taking stock in our own abilities, our friends, and family to help us through" (p. 24). So if outlook can lead to positive health benefits, why isn't it easy to change outlook?

If an individual stops to think about all the factors causing stress, it is possible to feel his or her body getting tense. People often have to deal with urgent tasks, such as emails, work deadlines, and phone calls that require immediate attention. Conversely, if that individual stops to think about beloved things, his or her body will start to relax. People know the things important to them, such as spending time with family, pursuing a favorite hobby, or following dreams. But too often the urgent eclipses the important. Pipher (2006) advises, "one of my rules as a therapist was: Don't let the urgent crowd out the important" (p. 91). She explains how people can apply her advice to their lives and elaborates, "writers too can guide readers toward the important rather than the urgent" (p. 91). People all have urgent tasks that demand attention, but the urgent should not cause neglect of the important. How often do people go out to dinner with their families and answer ringing cell phones even when they know the calls are not emergencies?

Sometimes the best way to delineate between the urgent and important in life is to write about choices. Cameron (1998) believes writing reminds people that "each day, each life, is a series of choices, and as we use the lens of writing to view our lives, we see our choices" (p. 94). A person can complete a variety of activities to identify what gives energy and what takes it away, such as a list of daily activities, a pie chart as a graphic organizer balance wheel of how time is spent, or writing about whatever is on his or her mind. Graves (2001) explains, "I know that you already have a sense of what takes energy, gives it, and is a waste of time. What you need now are the specifics from your own life in order to chart a different course from the one you know" (p. 11). Charting a new course can mean something as simple as minor adjustments to daily habits. If reading a favorite magazine brings energy but waiting in line takes away energy, read the favorite magazine while waiting in line. Other times, charting a new course means needing to make major life changes. That part of the journey can feel scary because it means rewriting a life story.

Rewriting a life story and starting on the path to a healthier lifestyle means people must meet themselves where they are. Individuals must forgive themselves if they aren't happy with their life choices and know the ending of that life story remains unwritten. Brown (2012) discusses her research on shame and vulnerability by explaining, "when we bury the story we forever stay the subject of the story. If we own the story we get to narrate the ending" (p. 80). This means celebrating past accomplishments and taking steps in the present to achieve future goals. Thinking about a goal already achieved can provide motivation when tackling a new goal. Brown (2010) provides the reminder, "owning our story can be hard but not nearly as difficult as spending our lives running from it" (p. 6). Many people do choose to run from their stories and numb physical and emotional pain with unhealthy results. This behavior causes Brown (2012) to observe, "Americans today are more debt-ridden, obese, medicated, and addicted than we ever have been" (p. 138). Individuals often worry about what other people think. Those individuals may feel the need to be perfect, when just being themselves is more than enough for the people who truly care about them. Each individual should know that the people who deserve to be in his or her life are the ones who will listen to a story while providing acceptance and support, no matter what the story may be. Often people who are perfectionists are harder on themselves than anyone else could ever be. Furthermore, Brown (2010) shares, "the stories of our struggles are difficult for everyone to own, and if we've worked hard to make sure everything looks 'just right' on the outside, the stakes are high when it comes to truth-telling. This is why shame loves perfectionists – it's so easy to keep us quiet" (p. 39). But keeping quiet and not sharing a story can lead to problems with physical and emotional health. It can lead to physical muscle tension, high blood pressure, headaches, potential weight gain, increased risk of a stroke, increased risk of a heart attack, decreased confidence, depression, reduction in productivity, inability to sleep, diarrhea or constipation, loss of sex drive, frequent colds, nervous habits, neck pain, using of alcohol, cigarettes, or drugs, as well as emotional isolation (http://www.helpguide.org/mental/stress_signs.htm). To find the courage to choose health and make some changes, find a supportive audience who will encourage success.

SOLUTION #6: CHOOSE EXERCISE

Obesity is at its all time high and continuing to grow. From the American Heart Association (2013) it shows that "23.9 million children ages 2 to 19 years are overweight or obese" and "among Americans 20 years of age and older, 157.4 million are overweight or obese" (http://www.heart.org/idc/groups/heart-public/@wcm/@sop/@smd/documents/downloadable/ucm_319588.pdf). There is a vast amount of co-morbidities associated with obesity and being overweight. Research by Guh, Zhang, Bansback, Amarsi, Birmingham, and Anis (2009) shows that "statistically significant associations with obesity were found with the incidence of type II diabetes, all cancers except esophageal (female), pancreatic, and prostate cancer, all cardiovascular diseases (except congestive heart failure), asthma, gallbladder disease, osteoarthritis and chronic back pain" (http://www.biomedcentral.com/1471-2458/9/88). These are just some of the reasons for the significant importance of living a healthy lifestyle.

Exercise provides numerous benefits. Exercise decreases obesity, decreases the chance of a heart attack, decreases the chance for diabetes, lowers blood pressure, lowers cholesterol, decreases depression, and allows a person to think clearer. Exercise helps control obesity since it burns off calories and helps raise one's metabolism. One study reported by Neporent (2011) shows that "fit men who completed a super-high intensity, 90-minute strength workout, performing 60 sets with little rest in between, experienced an 11 percent metabolism increase for about two hours after the workout. The next morning, 15 hours after the workout, their metabolism was still elevated by a substantial 9 percent, which translated into about 150 extra calories burned" (http://www.thatsfit.com/2011/03/23/does-exercise-really-boost-your-metabolism/). Although this is an extreme example, there is still an "afterburn effect" with normal exercise. With the average workout, Neporent reports, "during a more typical workout -- say, three sets of ten exercises -- researchers say a generous guesstimate for afterburn add up to no more than 50 to 75 calories total" (http://www.thatsfit.com/2011/03/23/does-exercise-really-boost-your-metabolism/).

Exercise can decrease the chance of a heart attack and helps with cholesterol as well. The Mayo Clinic (2011) shows that "being active boosts high-density lipoprotein (HDL), or "good," cholesterol and decreases unhealthy triglycerides. This one-two punch keeps your blood flowing smoothly, which decreases your risk of cardiovascular diseases" (http://www.mayoclinic.com/health/exercise/HQ01676). Not enough reasons to be motivated for starting exercise? It also helps elevate one's mood. The Mayo Clinic shows that "physical activity stimulates various brain chemicals that may leave you feeling happier and more relaxed. You may also feel better about your appearance and yourself when you exercise regularly, which can boost your confidence and improve your self-esteem" (http://www.mayoclinic.com/health/exercise/HQ01676).

What if a person feels he or she does not have enough time in a busy schedule to exercise? Exercise will actually allow people to be more productive and think clearer. This by itself proves that it is even more important for very busy people. Blaylock (2013) talks about this and states that "exercise improves blood flow to the brain and increases protective antioxidant enzymes. People with minimal cognitive impairment, thought by some to be an early stage of dementia, can reverse memory problems with regular exercise combined with a proper diet" (http://www.newsmaxhealth.com/Dr-Blaylock/exercise-benefits-brain-repair-neurotrophins-Alzheimers/2013/06/26/id/511942?s=al&promo_code=13FC0-1). These are all just some of the benefits of exercise.

What if a person has never exercised, doesn't know how long to exercise, or what intensity to start with? Start with light exercise and slowly progress with the amount and time of exercise. Schmidt (2012) recommends that "at the beginning of the program, the frequency and duration of the activity is more important than the intensity. Aim for exercising four or five days a week for 30 to 60 minutes. If you were previously sedentary, these sessions can be broken up into three 10-minute sessions, with gradual increases in duration" (http://www.acsm.org/access-public-information/articles/2012/01/19/obesity-and-exercise). Another option is to complete simple tasks such as taking the stairs, going to a park, playing games rather than watching television, or parking further from the destination to lose weight. The American College of Sports Medicine (2011) recommends for cardiorespiratory exercise that "adults should get at least 150 minutes of moderate-intensity exercise each week." Furthermore, the ACSM elaborates, "exercise recommendations can be met through 30-60 minutes of moderate-intensity exercise (five days per week) or 20-60 minutes of vigorous-intensity exercise (three days per week)." And finally, for resistance exercise it is recommended by the ACSM that "adults should train each major muscle group two to three days each week." Specifically, the ACSM advises, "8-12 repetitions improve strength and power, 10-15 repetitions improve strength in middle-age and older persons starting exercise, and 15-20 repetitions improve muscular endurance." It is also beneficial to include flexibility exercises and balance exercises (http://www.acsm.org/about-acsm/media-room/news-releases/2011/08/01/acsm-issues-new-recommendations-on-quantity-and-quality-of-exercise).

Remember that all of this can be a goal to progress to achieving. Doing even less than just half of the recommended amount of exercise is significantly better than nothing at all. Exercise also decreases risks for falling as a person ages and therefore it is beneficial to add in exercises that challenge the neuromotor system. If a person is having joint pain, it is beneficial to do specialized exercises that appropriately build muscle strength around the key structures to take the stress off of the joints and/or spine. It is always beneficial to first talk to a physical therapist, exercise physiologist, or physician prior to starting an exercise program.

SOLUTION #7: CHOOSE NUTRITION

Nutrition can have more of an impact on image and overall health than exercise alone. Nutrition is something that most Americans do not know enough about or choose not to learn more about. It is always very easy to choose an unhealthy dish at the dinner table than demonstrate discipline and choose the healthy option. Although having a good diet requires a lot of discipline, it is worth it for the feelings of being more energetic, stronger, more confident, more alert, and healthier overall. If that doesn't provide motivation, four out of the six leading causes of death are attributed to poor diet and physical inactivity. These are heart disease, cancer, stroke, and diabetes. Each person is at increased risk for these complications with a poor diet and sedentary lifestyle. Many cancers such as colon, prostate, mouth, throat, esophagus, lung, and stomach are related to this as well. The estimated costs of diseases associated with poor diet and physical inactivity are cancer ($180 billion), coronary heart disease ($112 billion), obesity ($117 billion), diabetes ($98 billion), stroke ($49 billion), high blood pressure ($47 billion), osteoporosis ($14 billion) per year (http://www.cspinet.org/nutritionpolicy/nutrition_policy.html). To put into perspective the interests of Americans for marketing at this time, "the federal government's largest nutrition education program for the general public (the 5 A Day program) has an annual communications budget of about $3.6 million. Mars spends 68 times that to promote M&Ms candies ($68 million). McDonald's spends 1000 times more than 5 A Day on advertising and promotions ($1 billion)" (http://www.cspinet.org/nutritionpolicy/nutrition_policy.html). This should be a huge eye opener just to see where money is being spent and what is being promoted for the general population. Clearly everyone has a significant amount to learn, but motivation and awareness provide a place to begin.

So what is the recommended amount of food to eat and also the type of food to eat? Before answering these questions it is of ample importance to talk about caloric intake versus caloric expenditure. Caloric intake is the amount of calories a person consumes in a day while caloric expenditure is the amount of calories a person expends (or burns off in a day). If a person consumes more than he or she actually burns off, (regardless of the type of food) that person will gain weight. However if a person consumes less than he or she expends, he or she will lose weight. A few things need to be understood prior to basing nutritional information from the previously stated information. A person can consume too little and the basal metabolic rate (BMR) will decrease. The basal metabolic rate is the amount of calories one's body burns off for an individual to stay alive (for vital organs) without including any physical activity at all in a day. BMR should always be accounted for when trying to figure out how many calories are burned off in a day. Most people seem to burn off more calories from their BMR than they do with their daily activities along with exercise. The BMR can be accurately determined in a laboratory with an exercise physiologist or cardiologist, or a basic calculation can be used which seems to be fairly accurate overall. The calculation which determines the BMR factors in sex, weight, height, and age. The equation for BMR for women is: 655 + (4.35 x weight in pounds) + (4.7 x height in inches) – (4.7 x age in years). BMR for men is: 66 + (6.23 x weight in pounds) + (12.7 x height in inches) – (6.8 x age in years) (http://www.bmi-calculator.net/bmr-calculator/bmr-formula.php). After you determine this, it is good to calculate the amount of calories that are expended with exercise as well. This final equation will provide an accurate amount of calories that are expended throughout the day. People can compare this to their calorie intake to see whether or not they are on track for losing or gaining weight.

If caloric intake seems to be higher than the calculations and one is trying to lose weight, then it is time to cut back on some food. If someone is trying to lose weight it is important to do it more gradually than very quickly. It is recommended by the Mayo Clinic (2010) to try to set a goal losing one to two pounds per week. They state that in order "to lose 1 to 2 pounds per week, you need to burn 500 to 1000 calories more than you consume each day, through a lower calorie diet and regular exercise" (http://www.mayoclinic.com/health/weight-loss/HQ01625). Losing weight at that rate is important in order to maintain muscle mass, have a better chance at maintaining weight loss goals, and to not impact health in a negative way. Before trying to figure out what that would require, an individual can do a few different things. One option is to determine the amount of calories currently consumed (this includes salad dressings, liquid calories, and butter) and decrease that amount overall in a week to meet these goals. Adding in exercise to a daily routine will burn off the calories that way. Or, an individual can decrease the amount of overall calories consumed in a week and add in more exercise. The last option is actually the best option since it'll be easier to maintain muscle mass while losing weight. If an individual strictly loses weight by diet alone, muscle mass might be lost at the same time.

So what are the recommended types of foods to eat? It is good to realize that the main goal for all of these is healthy food including proper protein, good carbohydrates, fruits, and vegetables, as well as staying properly hydrated, and consuming good fats. Nutrition seems to change each year for the recommended percentages of carbohydrates, protein, fats, and dairy, but below are the current recommendations. They are broken down into different categories since each person should have a different diet. For example, an athlete should eat significantly different than a person who is sedentary. Also someone that is lactose intolerant or has diabetes should eat different than the "average" person. According to the Harvard Medical School Family Health

Guide (2006), the average male measurement that is used for nutritional guidelines is a 175 lbs. male that is moderately active and requires about 2,800 calories per day. The average female they refer to is 125 lbs. and is moderately active consuming 2,000 calories a day (http://www.health.harvard.edu/fhg/updates/update0906b.shtml).

One food pyramid (for the "average" American) (2005) states that based off of a 2,000 calorie diet in one day a person should have 6 ounces of grains (half of them should be whole grain), 2.5 cups of vegetables (different types), 2 cups of fruit (variety and easy on juices), 3 cups of milk (low-fat or fat-free), and 5.5 ounces of meat and beans (lean cuts, seafood, and beans, avoid frying) (http://www.washingtonpost.com/wp-srv/nation/daily/graphics/diet_042005.html). Again, that is for a 2,000 calorie diet. This amount of food might be good, but don't forget to find out how many calories are actually burned off in a day first. The Harvard School of Public Health (2008) designed a healthy eating plate. This plate states that a majority of food intake should be in the following order: vegetables, whole grains, protein, and fruits. They state that healthy oils (like olive and canola oil) should be used for cooking, on salad, and at the table while avoiding trans fat. Milk and dairy should be limited to 1-2 servings and juice to one small glass per day. They recommend while drinking water, tea, and coffee have very limited sugar added. They say to eat plenty of fruits and of multiple colors to get in all of the proper vitamins. For vegetables it is recommended to have a variety not including potatoes or French fries. For whole grains choose a variety (whole-wheat bread or pasta, brown rice) and limit refined grains (white rice and white bread). For protein choose fish, poultry, beans, nuts, while limiting red meat and cheese, cold cuts, and processed meats (http://www.hsph.harvard.edu/nutritionsource/what-should-you-eat/pyramid/). The Dietary Guidelines (2011) have a few tips for nutrition as well saying very similar advice as recommended from above. They recommend that people "consume more of certain foods and nutrients such as fruits, vegetables, whole grains, fat-free and low-fat dairy products, and seafood. Consume fewer foods with sodium, saturated fats, trans fats, cholesterol, added sugars, and refined grains" (http://www.health.gov/dietaryguidelines/2010.asp#overview).

As stated previously, athletes must eat differently than the "average" human. It does depend on what type of athlete as well. Some athletes need more carbohydrates to provide fuel for their muscles for a longer period of time, while other athletes might not need as much. Some athletes need to maintain a very low body weight (wrestlers, gymnasts) while others might want to try to strictly build muscle mass (football players, weight lifters). Rodriguez,

DiMarco, and Langley (2009) break down a few different types of athletes and list the American College of Sports Medicine recommendations for each. Keep in mind this does vary with age, sex, and type of sport. For endurance athletes the ACSM recommends the amount of protein consumption to be "1.2 to 1.4 grams per kilograms per day" (p. 715). Additionally, "ultra-endurance athletes who engage in continuous activity for several hours or consecutive days of intermittent exercise should consume that same amount of protein or even slightly higher" (p. 715). Strength athletes actually need more protein for their muscle recovery due to the type of training they need to be able to endure. This is necessary since "additional protein, essential amino acids in particular, is needed along with sufficient energy to support muscle growth" (p. 715). Therefore, "recommended protein intakes for strength-trained athletes range from 1.2 to 1.7 grams per kilograms per day" (p. 715). Athletes also should have more carbohydrates overall than most people. The ASCM states that "approximately 50-60% of energy during one to four hours of continuous exercise at 70% of maximal oxygen capacity is derived from carbohydrates and the rest from free fatty acid oxidation" (p. 712). Furthermore, "a trained individual uses a greater percentage of fat than an untrained person does at the same workload" (p. 712). Consequently, "carbohydrate recommendations for athletes range from 6 to 10 grams per kilograms of their body weight per day" (p. 710). These are just a few changes in diet that athletes should consider, but there are many more categories as well.

The main thing to get out of all of this is to realize that nutrition is very important and improves health. Having and maintaining a great nutrition can save people's lives. Nutrition needs to not only be making the right choices, but should become a lifestyle. Don't forget that these recommendations stated above will change if a person has other co-morbidities such as diabetes, thyroid problems, or any heart problems. It would be wise to first see a nutritionist for further details about getting on a proper diet.

SOLUTION #8: CHOOSE JOURNALING

People all have moments in life where they feel lost, alone, and uncertain. Whether these feelings exist because of an emotional trauma, ongoing stress, or simply the feeling of having too many things to do and not enough hours to do them, life can feel overwhelming sometimes. Too often, people don't cope with such feelings in a healthy manner. They head to the local bar or the mall and add a hangover or credit card debt to their list of problems. Everyone has a favorite coping mechanism, so why not use writing as a method for processing thoughts and feelings?

Goldberg (2007) discusses the value of writing and says, "you have to speak. That's why you put the pen in your hand to begin with: in order to not blank out or turn your back" (p. 33). Writing provides a method of saying what needs to be said to a blank piece of paper. A notebook won't judge or talk back, thus giving the author the freedom to write anything and everything that may cause stress. Journal writing is not a formal assignment for a class; it becomes whatever the author wants and needs it to be. Journal writing can be a schedule of a day to see if the majority of time is spent on activities that do not provide happiness. Journal writing can be a letter to someone who has died or a letter to someone who is alive that will never be sent. Journal writing can be a list of gratitude declaring everything appreciated in life. Journal writing can be a prayer for what is needed. Journal writing can be a list of past accomplishments or future goals. It then becomes the decision of the author whether or not to share the writing with an audience.

Goldberg (2000) advises writers to put pen to paper and see where the writing leads since, "you keep your hand moving, you stay in there, you move closer and closer to the edge of what scares you" (p. 86). That's the most important thing about writing. A writer can always write, "I don't know what to write about" until inspiration occurs. People all have things that scare them and things they are afraid to feel. An individual may be afraid to admit he or she doesn't like something about life because then change is required, and this takes courage. Writing, however, can provide a sense of control to life. Romano (2004) believes, "there is so much in our lives we cannot control. We can, however, control our writing" (p. 218). Admitting feelings is better than locking emotions inside. That creates stress, which can lead to health problems.

Writing experts have differing opinions about whether or not writing is a form of therapy. Goldberg (1990) believes, "it's not therapy: it's the root of literature, direct connection with your mind" (p. 69). Conversely, Cameron (1998) counters, "without my writing, I would not have seen this dynamic. If this sounds as if I am saying writing is therapy, let me be clear that I feel writing is something therapy often is not; writing is therapeutic" (p. 94). Regardless, when writing about a difficult issue, it may help to share that writing with someone. Medical professionals can interpret physical symptoms or emotional issues and provide advice for how to help heal.

When sharing writing, it helps to find a trusting audience. Lamott (1994) believes the right audience is essential for writers to feel comfortable sharing their writing and suggests, "if you look around, I think you will find the person you need" (p. 171). Finding a person to trust with thoughts and feelings makes sharing easier and helps the confidant provide help after learning the story. A supportive audience can also help see patterns in one's life that the author cannot because either the author lacks information or feels too close to the situation to see clearly and achieve clarity. Heard (1995) believes larger patterns emerge when studying seemingly small events because, "by looking at the small, everyday circumstances and happenings, we find ideas to fill volumes" (p. 12). Sometimes small circumstances, whether they result in notes in a journal discussing pain symptoms or observations about behavior patterns, can fit into a larger picture that symbolizes a life story. Cameron (1998) shares the perspective, "what writing brings to a life is clarity and tenderness" (p. 83). Writing can illuminate events and make sense of them. However, when making sense of a life story, people need to forgive themselves for their mistakes. Everyone makes them, and writing illuminates behavior patterns. To make life changes, people have to take control and trust their own voices. Goldberg (1986) reminds people to believe they have something valuable to say because, "we have trouble connecting with our own confident writing voice that is inside all of us, and even when we do connect and write well, we don't claim it" (p. 154). It is never too late to claim that confident writing voice and make different decisions if existing behavior patterns don't lead to improved health. Articulating goals will provide strength to achieve them.

SOLUTION #9: CHOOSE TO CONSULT A MEDICAL PROFESSIONAL

Writing about thoughts and feelings can relieve stress because of the act of putting emotions on paper instead of holding them inside. As Pennebaker (1997) discusses, "although not a panacea, writing can be an inexpensive, simple, and sometimes painful way to help maintain our health" (p. 197). While writing can heal, at times it may feel painful to explore certain topics. People may find themselves writing about an emotional issue that is traumatic, or a physical issue where the symptoms seem confusing. Individuals who have those feelings should share them with someone who can provide help. Nothing a person can read or write will take the place of a conversation with a supportive medical professional.

As the editor-in-chief of *The Merck Manual of Medical Information*, medical doctor Berkow (1997) cautions, "no book can replace the expertise and advice of health care practitioners who have direct contact with a patient" (p. v). Sometimes people may attempt to provide self-diagnosis by reaching for a book or a computer, but that can lead to incorrect information or unnecessarily scary information. The best way to alleviate any concerns is to share them with a doctor, physical therapist, or other medical professional. As medical doctor Rankin (2013) discusses, "patients get well, at least in part, because they believe in the power of modern medicine and expect to feel relief when they see doctors and other health care specialists they trust" (p. 40). It becomes essential for patients to trust their medical professionals. Don't be embarrassed by what a doctor might think. Medical professionals want to help their patients heal, but they can't help if they don't know all the symptoms.

When a person writes about how he or she feels both physically and emotionally, the writing can illustrate patterns in life and in health. As Sharp (2000) says of writing thoughts and feelings, "this writing does not need to be interesting, or funny, for anybody. Think of it as a record book of your life, day by day. Assume that no one will ever see them. This will open you up and help the truth to appear on the page" (p. 18). While it is true that writing for an audience of only oneself provides the writer with the chance to vent about feelings, if that writer keeps a pain journal but lacks the medical knowledge to know what the symptoms mean, it becomes time to trust medical professionals and share. Pipher (2006) discusses the value of connection and explains, "writing to connect is 'change writing,' which, like good therapy, creates the conditions that allow people to be transformed" (p. 8). If an individual completes a pain journal of the intensity of pain felt, when it is felt, and what actions were taken when the pain was felt, it keeps that individual from forgetting what to tell a doctor, physical therapist, emotional therapist, or other medical specialist.

This type of connection between patient who writes and medical professional who reads and diagnoses can lead to health transformations. DeSalvo (1999) states, "for when we deal with unassimilated events, when we tell our stories and describe our feelings and integrate them into our sense of self, we no longer must actively work at inhibition. This alleviates the stress of holding back our stories and repressing or hiding our emotions, and so our health improves" (pp. 24-25). She discusses the value of sharing writing and elaborates, "when we share our writing, someone else knows what we've been through. Someone else cares. Someone else has heard our voice. Someone else understands. We learn that we are no longer alone and that we no longer need be alone" (p. 213). When faced with pain or illness, an individual may feel scared and alone. A caring person who knows the story and also has the medical expertise to provide help and healing provides a reminder that no one is alone and everyone has someone on his or her team to provide support during the healing journey.

Everyone has a story. Brown (2010) believes, "if we can find someone who has earned the right to hear our story, we need to tell it." (p. 40). Supportive medical professionals earn the right to hear their patients' stories by providing valuable advice; similarly, patients trust their medical professionals to listen to their stories and put the pieces of health puzzles together. Brown (2012) encourages sharing with a supportive audience "because sharing appropriately, with boundaries, means sharing with people with whom we've developed relationships that can bear the weight of our story" (p. 46). If people develop a strong collaborative professional relationship with doctors and other medical specialists in their lives, those medical professionals can take any detail of the stories shared with them to provide support and information for their patients to feel happier and healthier. As Graves (2001) states, "it is in the giving of energy that energy returns to us" (p. 175). Energy given with a record of symptoms for a doctor leads to energy returned in the form of improved health.

SOLUTION #10: CHOOSE SPIRITUALITY

To preface this section, it does not advocate the following of specific spiritual beliefs. Instead, it illustrates how spirituality can enhance health. As Cameron (2002) explains, "life is what we make of it. Whether we conceive of an inner god force or an other, outer God, doesn't matter. Relying on that force does" (p. 64). Sometimes when people go through a difficult time, it helps them to know they are not alone in the world. Rankin (2013) discusses the health benefits of spirituality and describes, "in addition to the relaxation responses induced by supportive community, faith in a higher power may also induce positive emotions, which counteract stress and contribute to the state of physiological rest necessary for the body to repair itself" (p. 89). Of course, people don't have to go to church in order to stop and reflect on life experiences. Tindle (2013) calls this practice contemplation and elaborates, "note that contemplative practice, just like the other techniques we're discussing, does not necessarily mean that you instantly feel better. Rather it means that you remain 'sober' enough to see your way to the next step, which may be to exercise or to ask for spiritual help, or identify another way to safely metabolize your tension" (p. 110). Becoming emotionally sober means being aware of thoughts and feelings and most importantly, asking for help when needed. That help may be prayer or a hug from a friend, or the knowledge that life's path does not need to be a solitary journey.

Regardless of an individual's beliefs, the science of healthy living and spirituality can coexist. Alexander (2012) discusses how he reconciled the science of his medical training with his spirituality after he spent time in a coma and believes, "certain members of the scientific community, who are pledged to the materialist worldview, have insisted again and again that science and spirituality cannot coexist. They are mistaken" (p. 73). Similarly, Neal (2012) discusses the connection between spirituality and healing after she reconciled her spiritual experiences with her scientific orthopedic surgery training and elaborates, "although the medical profession has recently, and somewhat tentatively, recognized the spiritual component of healing and of dying, patients have experienced this connection throughout the ages" (p. 25). She continues, "I encountered many patients during my training who wanted to tell me about their spiritual experiences. It was usually done apologetically and with a tone of embarrassment, as they did not want to offend me and did not think 'medical people' would listen or believe. Science and spirituality were presumed to be incompatible" (p. 25). Spirituality can lead to individuals feeling more confident, which can lead to increased health.

Often people feel stress when searching for the answers to life's questions. Cameron (2002) feels, "there is a path for each of us. When we are on our right path, we have a surefootedness. We know the next right action – although not necessarily what is just around the bend" (p. 194). Uncertainty about life can lead people to look for signs along the way in the form of coincidences as the puzzle pieces of life fall into place. Rushnell (2012) believes that coincidences aren't really coincidences and states, "additional signposts for you, providing you allow yourself to see them, will be godwinks, the messages from above that pop up like little coincidences all along your way" (pp. 149-150). Again, regardless of personal beliefs, the most important thing is to have faith in something. Believing in something provides hope for endeavors endured in life. It provides help through the hard times and allows people to set morals to follow. With good morals come good things. Good morals allow people to live the lifestyle they have always wanted to live or become the even better person they have wanted to become, which in turn will decrease stress levels. Decisions about which morals to set are different for each religion and personal to each individual. However, living a life demonstrating kindness to others and kindness to oneself can provide happiness and create less stress than carrying around feelings of anger and sadness.

SUSTAINING HEALTHY CHOICES

Each person controls the series of decisions that comprises a life story. The choices made will determine that individual's health story. As Lamott (2005) states, "your problem is how you are going to spend this one odd and precious life you have been issued" (p. 303). Often people feel overwhelmed by life and their choices, which can cause stress. Therefore, the key to healthy choices remains taking initiative by identifying and managing stress. Each individual possesses the power to write the next chapter in his or her story; the commitment to choosing health can lead to more peace and less stress as that unwritten chapter unfolds. As Beck (2008) explains, "in the gym – and in life – the point of endeavor is not sustaining the apex of achievement. The point is falling from that apex and finding our way back, over and over" (p. 217). Engaging in healthy habits represents a journey. Some days will always seem more difficult than others, but the goal becomes to be healthy and learn what triggers unhealthy behavior. Or as Beck (2012) believes, value exists in learning from experiences and making changes because "great artists embrace the full catastrophe of our condition and find beyond it an even deeper truth of peace, healing, and redemption" (p. 243). And know that tomorrow can begin a new chapter.

CONTRIBUTE A VERSE

This research study began with the goal of adding insights to the conversation of writing as healing and led in the unexpected direction of helping college students cope with anxiety and ongoing stresses in life. Psychologist Clark (2018) provides hope for people experiencing anxiety with the explanation, "whether anxiety is experienced loudly as fear, quietly as worry, or physically as stress, it is an undeniable presence and force in all our lives. Getting a handle on what it is, what it feels like for us, and what we call it is fundamental to harnessing it" (p. 38).

Since one of the researchers was also the professor of the students who participated as subjects in the study, even though the student survey responses were anonymous, a strong level of trust existed in the classroom for students to feel comfortable sharing their thoughts in writing on the surveys even though the researchers would never know who wrote what. Perhaps the students can relate to Zimmermann (2002) who shares, "fear of the future paralyzes us with anxiety" (p. 34). Her advice for coping? She suggests, "take several deep, centering breaths. Now write for at least fifteen minutes" (p. 35). The journal writing will continue during class sessions after the conclusion of this research project, with the hope writing will help the writers discover the answers they need. Both researchers also plan to provide additional help to students by sharing stress management strategies.

Every semester, the writing professor/researcher strives to establish a safe community in her classroom. As DeSalvo (1999) writes, "by sharing our stories under the safest conditions, we learn from one another that we need not engage in shame and self-hatred. They are the result of what happened to us, of what we survived. In time, we can learn to transform those feelings; we can learn to value ourselves and love ourselves" (p. 169). Because students found the courage to share, the responsibility now becomes that of the university community to use the information to increase student retention and decrease student stress. Heifetz (1994) writes of transformative leaders, "their lives would be less stressful if they did not care" (p. 252). But we have to care and make a difference. We as leaders also need to manage our own stress so we can help students manage theirs. Heifetz cautions, "to lead and yet sustain the personal stresses that come with leading requires inner discipline" (p. 252). University leaders can also benefit from the stress management techniques discussed in this chapter and can simultaneously take care of themselves while taking care of students. Let's build a community vision for change, where everyone works together with the purpose of helping college students succeed. Through this method, research can become the catalyst for additional conversations.

That's the long term goal. The short term goal echoes the sentiment of Gruwell (1999), who writes, "I encouraged the Freedom Writers to use a pen as a means of revolution. Through their writing, they discovered they shared a common identity, which united them into a community that connected them, not separated them from the world" (p. 276). The wish is for every student to have the opportunity to write in a journal and belong to a class community. Doing so will help them find their purpose in life. This chapter ends with the same question in which it began. The question still remains today. What experiences bring purpose to life?

Walt Whitman (1855) gives us the answer in his poem *O Me! O Life!* "That you are here – that life exists and identity, that the powerful play goes on and you may contribute a verse" (p. 341).

Make your verse a good one.

ACKNOWLEDGMENT

The preceding chapter contains excerpts from the following previous IGI publications:

Bird, J.L. (2018). Constantly connected: Managing stress in today's technological times. In V.C. Bryan, A. Musgrove, & J. Powers (Eds.), *Handbook of research on human development in the digital age* (pp. 385-402). Hershey, PA: Information Science Reference.

Bird, J.L., & Wanner, E.T. (2015). Research as curriculum inquiry: Helping college students with anxiety. In V.C.X. Wang (Ed.), *Handbook of research on scholarly publishing and research methods* (pp. 273-295). Hershey, PA: Information Science Reference.

Wanner, E.T., & Bird, J.L. (2014). Choose health: Tools for a healthy lifestyle. In V.C.X. Wang (Ed.), *Adult and community health education: Tools, trends and methodologies* (pp. 183-197). Hershey, PA: Information Science Reference.

REFERENCES

Alexander, E. (2012). *Proof of Heaven*. New York, NY: Simon and Schuster.

ASCM Staff. (2011). ACSM issues new recommendations on quantity and quality of exercise. *American College of Sports Medicine*. Retrieved from http://www.acsm.org/about-acsm/media-room/news-releases/2011/08/01/acsm-issues-new-recommendations-on-quantity-and-quality-of-exercise

Barbieri, M. (1995). *Sounds from the heart*. Portsmouth, NH: Heinemann.

Baty, K. (2003). *A girl's gotta do what a girl's gotta do*. New York, NY: Rodale.

Beck, M. (2008). *Steering by starlight*. New York, NY: Rodale.

Beck, M. (2012). *Finding your way in a wild new world*. New York, NY: Free Press.

Berkow, R. (Ed.). (1997). *The Merck manual of medical information*. Whitehouse Station, NJ: Merck & Co.

Blaylock, R. (2013). Exercise repairs the brain. *Newsmax Health*. Retrieved from http://www.newsmaxhealth.com/

BMR Calculator. (2013). *BMI Calculator*. Retrieved from http://www.bmi-calculator.net/bmr-calculator/bmr-formula.php

Brickman, J. (2015). *Soothe*. New York, NY: Rodale.

Brown, B. (2010). *The gifts of imperfection*. Center City, MN: Hazelden.

Brown, B. (2012). *Daring greatly*. New York, NY: Gotham Books.

Cameron, J. (1998). *The right to write*. New York, NY: Tarcher/Putnam.

Cameron, J. (2002). *The artist's way* (2nd ed.). New York, NY: Tarcher/Putnam.

Carter, C. (2015). *The sweet spot*. New York, NY: Ballantine.

Catanese, A. J. (1996). Lessons learned. In B. W. McClendon & A. J. Catanese (Eds.), *Planners on planning* (pp. 287–295). San Francisco, CA: Jossey-Bass.

Centers for Disease Control and Prevention. (2011). Health Related Quality of Life. *Health Related Quality of Life Surveillance Program*. Retrieved from http://www.cdc.gov/hrqol/hrqol14_measure.htm

Clandinin, D. J., & Connelly, F. M. (2000). *Narrative inquiry*. San Francisco, CA: Jossey-Bass.

Clark, A. H. (2018). *Hack your anxiety*. Naperville, IL: Sourcebooks, Inc.

Clark, C. C. (2006). *Living well with anxiety*. New York, NY: HarperCollins.

Codell, E. R. (1999). *Educating Esme*. Chapel Hill, NC: Algonquin Books.

Cohen-Sandler, R. (2005). *Stressed-out girls*. New York, NY: Viking.

Connelly, F. M., & Clandinin, D. J. (1988). *Teachers as curriculum planners*. New York, NY: Teachers College Press.

Conner, J. (2008). *Writing down your soul*. San Francisco, CA: Conari.

DeBecker, G. (1997). *The gift of fear*. Boston, MA: Little, Brown and Company.

DeSalvo, L. (1999). *Writing as a way of healing*. Boston, MA: Beacon Press.

Enayati, A. (2015). *Seeking serenity*. New York, NY: New American Library.

Go, A. S., Mozaffarian, D., Roger, V. L., Benjamin, E. J., Berry, J. D., Borden, W. B., ... Turner, M. B.American Heart Association Statistics Committee and Stroke Statistics Subcommittee. (2013). Heart disease and stroke statistics—2013 update: A report from the American Heart Association. *Circulation*, *127*, e6–e245. Retrieved from http://www.heart.org/idc/groups/heart-public/@wcm/@sop/@smd/documents/downloadable/ucm_319588.pdf PMID:23239837

Goldberg, N. (1986). *Writing down the bones*. Boston, MA: Shambhala.

Goldberg, N. (1990). *Wild mind*. New York, NY: Bantam.

Goldberg, N. (2000). *Thunder and lightning*. New York, NY: Bantam.

Goldberg, N. (2007). *Old friend from far away*. New York, NY: Free Press.

Goldberg, N. (2013). *The true secret of writing*. New York, NY: Atria.

Graves, D. (1994). *A fresh look at writing*. Portsmouth, NH: Heinemann.

Graves, D. (2001). *The energy to teach*. Portsmouth, NH: Heinemann.

Gruwell, E. (2007). Teach with your heart. New York, NY: Broadway.

Gruwell, E. (2009). Teaching hope. New York, NY: Broadway.

Gruwell, E., & the The Freedom Writers. (1999). The Freedom Writers diary. New York, NY: Broadway.

Guh, D. P., Zhang, W., Bansback, N., Amarsi, Z., Birmingham, C. L., & Anis, A. H. (2009). The incidence of co-morbidities related to obesity and overweight: a systematic review and meta-analysis. *BMC Public Health*. Retrieved from http://www.biomedcentral.com/1471-2458/9/88

Handler, J. (2013). *Braving the fire*. New York, NY: St. Martin's Griffin.

Harper, A. N. (1996). Tooling up for effective planning. In B. W. McClendon & A. J. Catanese (Eds.), *Planners on planning* (pp. 190–198). San Francisco, CA: Jossey-Bass.

Harvard Medical School Family Health Guide. (2006). *Good nutrition: should guidelines differ for men and women?* Harvard Health Publications. Retrieved from http://www.health.harvard.edu/fhg/updates/update0906b.shtml

Heard, G. (1995). *Writing toward home*. Portsmouth, NH: Heinemann.

Heifetz, R. A. (1994). *Leadership without easy answers*. Cambridge, MA: The Belnap Press of Harvard University Press.

Helgoe, L. A., Wilhelm, L. R., & Kommor, M. J. (2005). *The anxiety answer book*. Naperville, IL: Sourcebooks, Inc.

Helpguide. (2013). Stress symptoms, signs, causes. *Helpguide.org*. Retrieved from http://www.helpguide.org/mental/stress_signs.htm

Hoch, C. (1995). Teaching ethics and planning theory. In S. Hendler (Ed.), Planning ethics (pp. 281-300). New Brunswick, NJ: Rutgers.

Johnson, B. (2009). *But now! Awakening faith in an age of anxiety*. Belleville, Canada: Essence Publishing.

Johnson, L. (1998). *Two parts textbook, one part love*. New York, NY: Hyperion.

Johnson, L. (2005). *Teaching outside the box*. San Francisco, CA: Jossey-Bass.

Johnson, W. C. (1997). *Urban planning and politics*. Chicago, IL: American Planning Association.

Juhan, D. (1998). *Job's body*. Barrytown, NY: Station Hill.

Kamenetz, A. (2013). Power of the pen. *Oprah, 14*(12), 140–141.

Kepler, H. B. (1973). *Basic graphical kinematics* (2nd ed.). New York, NY: McGraw Hill.

Lamott, A. (1994). *Bird by bird*. New York, NY: Anchor Books.

Lamott, A. (2005). *Plan B: further thoughts on faith*. New York, NY: Riverhead.

Marshall, J. D., Sears, J. T., & Schubert, W. H. (2000). *Turning points in curriculum*. Upper Saddle River, NJ: Merrill/Prentice Hall.

Mayo Clinic Staff. (2010). Weight loss: 6 strategies for success. *Mayo Clinic*. Retrieved from http://www.mayoclinic.com/health/weight-loss/HQ01625

Mayo Clinic Staff. (2011). 7 benefits of regular physical activity. *Mayo Clinic*. Retrieved from http://www.mayoclinic.com/health/exercise/HQ01676

Murray, D. M. (1985). *A writer teaches writing* (2nd ed.). Boston, MA: Houghton Mifflin.

Neal, M. C. (2012). *To Heaven and back*. Colorado Springs, CO: WaterBrook Press.

Neporent, L. (2011). Does exercise really boost your metabolism? *That's Fit*. Retrieved from http://www.thatsfit.com/2011/03/23/does-exercise-really-boost-your-metabolism/

Nutrition Policy Staff. (2013). Why good nutrition is important. *Center for Science in the Public Interest*. Retrieved from http://www.cspinet.org/nutritionpolicy/nutrition_policy.html

Nutrition Source. (2008). Healthy eating plate and healthy eating pyramid. *Harvard School of Public Health*. Retrieved from http://www.hsph.harvard.edu/nutritionsource/what-should-you-eat/pyramid/

Pennebaker, J. W. (1997). *Opening up: the healing power of expressing emotions*. New York, NY: The Guilford Press.

Pipher, M. (1994). *Reviving Ophelia*. New York, NY: Grosset/Putnam.

Pipher, M. (2006). *Writing to change the world*. New York, NY: Riverhead.

Rankin, L. (2013). *Mind over medicine*. Carlsbad, CA: Hay House.

Rodriguez, N. R., DiMarco, N. M., & Langley, S. (2009). American College of Sports Medicine position stand. Nutrition and athletic performance. *Medicine and Science in Sports and Exercise*, *41*(3), 709–731. PMID:19225360

Romano, T. (2004). *Crafting authentic voice*. Portsmouth, NH: Heinemann.

Romano, T. (2013). *Fearless writing*. Portsmouth, NH: Heinemann.

Routman, R. (2003). *Reading essentials*. Portsmouth, NH: Heinemann.

Rushnell, S. (2012). *Divine alignment*. New York, NY: Howard Books.

Sadker, M., & Sadker, D. (1994). *Failing at fairness*. New York, NY: Charles Scribner's Sons.

Sandberg, S. (2013). *Lean in*. New York, NY: Alfred A. Knopf.

Sandberg, S. (2014). *Lean in for graduates*. New York, NY: Alfred A. Knopf.

Schmidt, S. (2012). Obesity and exercise. *American College of Sports Medicine*. Retrieved from http://www.acsm.org/access-public-information/articles/2012/01/19/obesity-and-exercise

Shandler, S. (1999). *Ophelia speaks*. New York, NY: HarperCollins.

Sharp, C. (2000). *A writer's workbook*. New York, NY: St. Martin's Press.

Smith, D. (2012). *Monkey mind: A memoir of anxiety*. New York, NY: Simon & Schuster.

Stossel, S. (2013). *My age of anxiety*. New York, NY: Alfred A. Knopf.

Tindle, H. (2013). *UP: How positive outlook can transform our health and aging*. New York, NY: Hudson Street Press.

University of Maryland Medical Center. (2014). *Stress*. Retrieved from http://umm.edu/health/medical/reports/articles/stress

U.S. Department of Agriculture. (2005). The new food pyramid. *The Washington Post*. Retrieved from http://www.washingtonpost.com/wp-srv/nation/daily/graphics/diet_042005.html

U.S. Department of Health and Human Services. (2011). Dietary guidelines for Americans, 2010. *Office of Disease Prevention and Health Promotion*. Retrieved from http://www.health.gov/dietaryguidelines/2010.asp#overview

Whitman, W. (1993). O Me! O Life! In *Leaves of grass* (p. 341). New York, NY: Random House. (Original work published 1855)

Winner, J. (2008). *Take the stress out of your life*. Philadelphia, PA: Da Capo.

Zimmermann, S. (2002). *Writing to heal the soul*. New York, NY: Three Rivers Press.

KEY TERMS AND DEFINITIONS

Anxiety: Different clinicians have different definitions of anxiety, and someone who lives with anxiety will describe it from a different point of view than a clinical definition in a textbook, but the general consensus is that anxiety is chronic fear or stress that can result in panic attacks and a person feeling an inability to cope with life's stressors.

Artistic and Technical Writing: English teachers design rubrics which incorporate both artistic and technical writing when evaluating student essays. Artistic writing is the writer's tone of word choice, also known as voice, while technical writing is the writer's specificity of word choice.

Community Development: Designing a place where people feel welcomed and supported, whether it is a neighborhood, a classroom, or a network of colleagues who provide support for an individual.

Curriculum Inquiry: A form of narrative inquiry made popular in the field of research by F. Michael Connelly and D. Jean Clandinin, curriculum inquiry is a qualitative interpretative form of research that focuses on the telling, retelling, and sharing of stories through the lens of curriculum to implement program changes.

HRQOL (Health Related Quality of Life) Survey: A general health survey in the public domain and able to be used by researchers without securing permission or paying copyright fees.

Lean in Circles: Sheryl Sandberg's movement to encourage community support and discussion groups that motivate participants to face their fears and lean in to life.

Planning Process: Used in the fields of city planning as well as curricular change, this process encompasses the following steps: survey, analysis, plan, implementation, and feedback.

Writing as Healing: Although numerous studies have been conducted investigating the influence of writing on physical and emotional health, James Pennebaker is considered to be the pioneer in this field that discusses the health benefits of writing.

Writing Voice: Voice in writing highlights a writer's word choice and tone to compose a journal entry or other written composition that reflects the writer's personality. Every writer has a unique writing voice, just like each person has a unique speaking voice.

Chapter 8
Narratives of Teaching Methods

Jennifer Lynne Bird
Oxbridge Academy, USA

ABSTRACT

While technology leads to innovative teaching strategies, technology also leads to disconnection as people seek coping strategies to deal with stress and the constant flood of information. This narrative addresses the health consequences of stress and the need for authentic connections instead of focusing on images portrayed in social media. Methods such as RICE (reflection, innovation, collaboration, evaluation) and MICE (motivation, importance, confidence, expression) illustrate techniques for managing stress, managing technology, setting goals, and creating change.

RICE

My writing, teaching, and research reflects my philosophy of RICE (Reflection, Innovation, Collaboration, Evaluation). All of us will be patients at some point in our lives, and I want these innovative methods to inspire you to be an educated patient and collaborate with the medical experts who want to help heal you. Educators, whether they are a teacher in a classroom or a medical practitioner in a clinic, need to reflect on their practice. They also need to use innovation to develop a lesson plan or a treatment plan. Collaboration, whether teachers collaborate with their students or medical practitioners

DOI: 10.4018/978-1-7998-1931-8.ch008

collaborate with their patients, becomes essential for learning to take place. And finally, educators need to evaluate the needs of their students or patients.

For teachers, the process is RICE, because like all teachers I need to reflect on each class I teach before planning the next one. However, physical therapists and other clinicians need to complete the evaluation step first with patients so their process is ERIC. When we first started working together, my physical therapist colleague, Dr. Eric Wanner, found it interesting that his work was the same as his name. We discovered English professors and physical therapists can learn from each other's fields of expertise. My research professor colleague, Dr. Claudia Jayne Brahler, reminded me to bring my own area of expertise as an English teacher to the medical field. In addition to teaching writing, my life as an English teacher involves motivating students, discussing literature, demonstrating leadership, managing stress, and using technology. In this chapter, I invite you to travel with me into the world of teaching and apply educational strategies to your life.

MICE

When people align their goals with their vision and values, they become more likely to enact change in their lives. Change begins with four components: motivation, importance, confidence, and expression. I use the acronym MICE to refer to these components. By using both conversational methods such as motivational interviewing and writing strategies such as expressive writing, health coaches can help patients identify the stories they are telling themselves. Rankin (2015a) argues, "it's not life's stressors per se that make us sick and miserable. It's the stories we make up about these events, which translate into negative beliefs that activate chronic repetitive stress responses, shorten our life expectancy, and lead us into despair" (pp. 37-38). Conversely, Rankin (2015b) believes, "when the mind heals from loneliness, anxiety, fear, depression, resentment, anger, and negative beliefs about health and life, at least a percentage of the time, the health of the body follows suit" (p. 204). As far as implications for your life, you do not have to be a patient to practice the components of MICE which will help you the next time you set a goal that requires sustained behavior change.

PART I: MOTIVATION

Motivation manifests as two types, extrinsic and intrinsic. In other words, what inspires you to do something? External or internal factors? Does a student write a research paper to earn a specific grade or for the love of the topic? Does a patient complete exercises to earn a compliment from a physical therapist or for a personal desire to heal? One of the foundations of health coaching is the field of motivational interviewing. Caldwell, Gray, and Wolever (2013) explain, "while some professionals are actually using the terms health coaching and MI synonymously, this analysis suggests there are overlapping but also distinct elements to health coaching" (p. 55). Despite the slight delineation, the essence of both motivational interviewing and health coaching is in the conversation. Miller and Rollnick (2013) clarify, "motivational interviewing is a collaborative conversation style for strengthening a person's own motivation and commitment to change" (p. 12). While strengthening motivation and commitment to change is important in all areas of a person's life, it especially enhances the health care field. As Rollnick, Miller, and Butler (2008) explain, "MI works by activating patients' own motivation for change and adherence to treatment" (p. 5). From this perspective of collaboration, a patient sees the health care provider as a partner, not an authority figure giving orders. Miller and Rollnick (2002) elaborate, "we define motivational interviewing as a client-centered, directive method for enhancing intrinsic motivation to change by exploring and resolving ambivalence" (p. 25). Or as Tindle (2013) addresses patients, "You know what you want to do. The big question is, how do you get there? MI helps answer that question. It's a tool that helps the road open up before you. MI shows you how to see the path and gives you a starting push in the right direction" (pp. 117-118). As they begin a treatment plan, this question is on the minds of numerous patients. They want to feel better, but how do they get there? Sometimes the road ahead can seem long and overwhelming. The key is following the road in small, manageable, yet productive steps.

Motivation is frequently connected to the sense of purpose a person has in life. Pink (2009) asks the question, "as you contemplate your purpose, begin with the big question: What's your sentence?" (p. 155). In other words, at the end of your life, if you could only have one sentence on your memorial stating what you accomplished in life, what would that sentence be? It may seem unsettling to contemplate mortality, but we don't always have as much time as we think. Looking backwards from a future point in time can help us figure out how we want to live in the present. My sentence would be: Helped others find their voices and use writing to heal both physically and emotionally while simultaneously living a strong life filled with family and faith.

Other researchers argue that moving beyond extrinsic motivation to intrinsic motivation can make people happier. Enayati (2015) believes, "this reason to be happy – this essential "why" – is why we must be resolute in our quest to move beyond extrinsic motivations" (p. 135). Since extrinsic motivation involves doing something to either please someone else (getting a compliment from a doctor when complying with a medical treatment plan) or avoiding pain from someone else (getting a lecture from that same doctor when not complying with that medical treatment plan) we can experience stress. Enayati explains, "we volley emotions back and forth all the time, as part of every interaction – however brief or extended – that we have with one another. We can "catch" other people's stress, all with amazing speed" (p. 154). Visit a college campus around the time of midterms or finals, and witness students collectively getting stressed because while they are sharing the same community experience; that community experience is one of stress. Carter (2015) believes, "we also need intrinsic motivation, or passion – and the space to pursue our passions" (p. 183). This intrinsic motivation means finding the things that bring joy in life and provide both passion and purpose, such as signing up for a dance class for the pure joy of it or following a medical treatment plan for the desire to lead a healthier life regardless of what the doctor thinks.

Pursuing passions can lead to improved health. As Carter (2015) explains, "when we are happy, we are more creative and motivated, more productive and skilled socially because blood flows freely to our pre-frontal cortex, allowing us to make better decisions than we would if we relied on the more primitive, instinctive regions of our brain that are activated when we are under stress" (p. 20). So while there are times in life where we may need extrinsic motivation from others to help us get through a situation, it also becomes essential to find the internal motivation that drives us to succeed and makes us happy.

Finding purpose and self-motivation can lead to growth. Dweck (2006) describes students with the growth mindset as "even if they thought the textbook was boring or the instructor was a stiff, they didn't let their motivation evaporate. That just made it all the more important to motivate themselves" (p. 61). The goal of learning eclipsed the potential barriers of a boring textbook or a passionless instructor. Of course, in an ideal education world, students

we want to act in the present, even if we can't explain the feeling. Or maybe we notice something out of the corner of the eye that we know is significant information before the brain has the opportunity to process it. Dimitrius advises, "since your intuition depends on the quality and quantity of your information, your first step is clear: Improve the database" (p. 218). The more experiences people have, the more they are able to synthesize the experiences and file the information away in the database to help in the future. Starratt (1993) states, "professionals develop intuitions of what works over years of experience" (p. 39). What seems like magic or everything falling into a place is a result of a person collecting experiences and calling up those experiences when they are most needed to appear in a moment of intuitive insight.

As an FBI security expert, DeBecker (1997) tells people that intuition helps keep them safe and always provides helpful information. He explains, "intuition is always learning, and though it may occasionally send a signal that turns out to be less than urgent, everything it communicates to you is meaningful" (p. 70). So if something catches our attention, it is important to pay attention to it, because our intuition is trying to communicate something to us. DeBecker provides the valuable advice, "listen to your intuition" (p. 74).

Deep inside, we know the answers for what we truly feel is important in our lives. The key is to stop and listen. Baty (2003) concurs, "you hear it time and time again: Listen to your gut instinct, or intuition. Fact is, it works" (p. 3). Why does it work? Baty answers, "intuition just means acknowledging what you already know inside" (p. 4). If we ask ourselves the questions and trust our intuitive insights, we frequently get the answers right. DeBecker (1997) emphasizes the importance of listening without judgement because, "when free of judgment, we inherently respect the intuition of others" (p. 25). In medicine, it's always best to consult a medical professional if you have an intuitive sense something is wrong with your health. But if in your personal life, if you sense someone sinister behind you, listen to your intuition and keep yourself safe.

While security experts focus on the value of intuition to keep you safe, intuition can also help you assess what is important to achieve your goals in life. Beck (2001) believes, "your intuition has a more refined understanding of your right life than any other part of your consciousness" (p. 221). By listening to our intuition, we become aware of what we find important and what we value. If we are asked to do something we don't find important, intuition helps delineate whether we need to do that thing anyway to reach a goal or achieve a dream, or whether we think that thing is unimportant because it has no benefit. Beck describes this feeling as, "the more you listen to your intuition, the more it will change your life; and the more bravely you set forth into the territory of change, the more you'll come to rely on it" (p. 239). You are more likely to achieve success if you listen to your intuition and follow the path that makes you happy instead of listening to anyone who doubts your insight. You know yourself better than anyone else.

How does intuition relate to the field of medicine? Groopman (2007) explains, "clinical intuition is a complex sense that becomes refined over years and years of practice, of listening to literally thousands of patients' stories, examining thousands of people, and most important, remembering when you were wrong" (p. 20). So for medical professionals, their clinical intuition becomes refined by learning from experiences and listening to patients. Groopman cautions against relying too heavily on intuition, because in the medical world, feelings about a diagnosis must often be supported with factual data.

However, medical professionals place value on both their own and patients' intuition. Rankin (2015a) explains that people often feel fear in life and "although false fear can illuminate areas in your life that need your attention, healthy decisions that guide appropriate behavior never arise from false fear; they arise from intuition and integrity" (p. 51). Inherently, people know what they need to do to make healthy decisions and take care of themselves. And that sense of purpose helps them feel the importance of their actions. Rankin discovered, "the people I interviewed who had cultivated and learned to trust their intuition felt like they were always being guided, and they were supported by this guidance more than they were controlled by their fears" (pp. 142-143). She admits that the busy pace of a doctor's schedule doesn't allow as much time with patients as doctors would like, but she learned that if she partnered with her patients and took the time to listen to their stories, it helped her make a diagnosis and adjust her treatment plan. Rankin (2015b) learned, "my new patient intake form was 12 pages long, and what these questions revealed about my patients' lives shocked me. When combined with the intuitive information I sometimes received from patients, I started to get a sense of the link between their physical health and their emotional health" (p. 120). Her story illustrates how a medical professional trusting her own clinical intuition and the intuition of her patients in the stories they shared with her helped patients heal.

PART III: CONFIDENCE

Do we feel we have the ability to change? The answer to that question is how confident a person feels about making a change. Miller and Rollnick (2002) explain, "sometimes a person feels willing but not able to change" (p. 11). We may feel that making a change is important, but we don't have the confidence we can make the change.

Connected to confidence is another word that starts with C, compassion. Connected to confidence is compassion, specifically the self-compassion we must have with ourselves when things don't go as planned. Often people can be their own worst critics, and when something doesn't happen the way we want it to happen, it becomes easy to give up and focus on self-blame instead of searching for methods to overcome the obstacles and other pathways to achieve the goal. Germer (2009) defines, "self-compassion is simply giving the same kindness to ourselves that we would give to others" (pp. 33-34). Since we cannot change the past, all we can do is move forward and show ourselves the same kindness that we demonstrate for others. Neff (2011) believes something meaningful can happen from a less than perfect experience and states, "by giving ourselves unconditional kindness and comfort while embracing the human experience, difficult as it is, we avoid destructive patterns of fear, negativity, and isolation. At the same time, self-compassion fosters positive mind-states such as happiness and optimism" (pp. 12-13). No one is immune from negative events, both the minor annoyances of daily life as well as the major life changing catastrophes, but keeping a positive attitude and demonstrating the kindness to ourselves that we would demonstrate to others can diminish the severity of an event's impact.

If a person practices self-compassion and sees that the hard times in life can be obstacles to overcome rather than insurmountable barriers, he or she can get creative in problem solving and build confidence in the process as each problem is solved. Germer (2009) explains the value of practicing self-compassion because, "research on self-compassion is demonstrating that it softens the impact of negative events in our lives. Self-compassionate people are more likely to recognize when their efforts turn out badly and to take responsibility for their part" (p. 98). Neff (2011) adds, "by giving ourselves unconditional kindness and comfort while embracing the human experience, difficult as it is, we avoid destructive patterns of fear, negativity, and isolation. At the same time, self-compassion fosters positive mind-states such as happiness and optimism. The nurturing quality of self-compassion allows us to flourish, to appreciate the beauty and richness of life, even in hard times. When we soothe our agitated minds with self-compassion, we're better able to notice what's right as well as what's wrong, so that we can orient ourselves toward that which gives us joy" (pp. 12-13). Self-compassion is not the same thing as self-confidence, but self-compassion can contribute to self-confidence. Once someone achieves or overcomes something, it becomes possible to draw on that memory of confidence to know something similar that was achieved in the past can be achieved in the future.

It can be easy to be faced with fear and lack of confidence when encountering a new situation. Cameron (2002) calls these moments creative U-turns; just like a car may need to make a U-turn when going the wrong direction on the road, people may have to make U-turns when going the wrong direction in life. Cameron encourages, "have compassion. Creative U-turns are always born from fear – fear of success or fear of failure. It doesn't really matter which. The net result is the same" (p. 157). Whatever caused the U-turn, it led to the discovery of a new way to overcome an obstacle along with the confidence of finding a solution to a problem.

When we demonstrate compassion for others and ourselves, we find a support system of people to walk with us on our journey. Brown (2012) believes, "self-compassion is key because when we're able to be gentle with ourselves in the midst of shame, we're more likely to reach out, connect, and experience empathy" (p. 75). When people accept us and our stories, we experience the confidence that we are okay as we are and that we do not need to be anyone other than ourselves. Our confidence decreases when we feel shame at what we have done or how we have acted. By finding the courage to share our stories and be compassionate with ourselves, we own our story and while we cannot rewrite what has already happened, we can find the confidence to pick up a pen and write a new ending. Brown (2012) describes this story sharing process as, "whether we're on the purging end or the receiving end of this experience, self-compassion is critical. We have to give ourselves a break when we share too much too soon, and we have to practice self-kindness when we feel like we weren't able to hold space for someone who hit us with the floodlight" (p. 161). When we find the right person with whom to share our story, we have the confidence that we will not be judged and that our words will be heard.

By demonstrating compassion, people earn the right to hear our stories. Goldberg (2013) advises writers, "always have tremendous kindness for yourself. You'll get a lot more writing done" (p. 21). The same advice applies to all parts of life; demonstrating self-compassion means a lot less time thinking about regrets and a lot more time getting things accomplished.

How does compassion relate to the field of medicine? Tindle (2013) reports that self-compassion "has been linked to better self-care and healthier behaviors" (p. 77). How does this happen? Carter (2015) argues, "self-compassion – being warm and supportive toward ourselves, and actively soothing ourselves – has many benefits over self-criticism. It leads to less anxiety and depression, and greater piece of mind" (p. 219). And since emotional health is linked to physical health, if emotionally we are more compassionate to ourselves, physically we feel less tense from anxiety and stress. Self-compassion can provide the insight that a one day divergence need not derail an entire nutrition or exercise plan. Tindle (2013) reminds us, "self-compassion and the deep sense of self-worth that it fosters are at the very foundation of our physical and mental health" (p. 182). Because when people believe they have value, that confidence is reflected in their health.

PART IV: EXPRESSION

Are we ready to change? The answer to that question is the expression of where change falls on a person's priority list. Miller and Rollnick (2002) explain, "One can be willing and able to change, but not ready to do so" (p. 11). We may feel making a change is important and we may have the confidence to make the change, but we are not ready to take action.

Expression is articulating a plan for what is needed to be done in order to enact change. It means stating one's goals and making a commitment to the accountability of achieving them. This is often difficult for people, because it is one thing to say you will do something, but another thing to actually do it. Expression, however, allows for the exploration of possibilities. It puts experiences into words. This is often best done in writing. Goldberg (2016) believes, "you don't have to change a thing. Writing doesn't ask you to be any different from who you are right now" (p. 161). When writing, you are who you are. Looking at a piece of paper and seeing a plan for achieving goals in writing is a method of making the plan seem like a series of concrete steps to focus on and be accountable for instead of a series of ideas swirling around in one's head. Like a camera lens focusing on a subject, everything suddenly zooms into possibility. Seeing the words on the page allows an issue to become present and eliminate the maybe someday attitude people have when thinking of specific steps needed to transform a dream into reality.

People can experience success when speaking their goals or drawing pictures of them; however, expressive writing possesses power. Romano (2000) provides a description of expressive writing as, "we use expressive writing when we are trying to explain or render something for the first time, when we're seeking to recover information, make connections, generate ideas. Expressive writing is exploratory and new and focused on meaning" (p. 137). As all writers know, rarely is a first draft perfect. Elaborating on ideas is when the process of revision happens. Nevertheless, by capturing our words on paper, we not only share our story of what happened to us, but also explore what we want to happen next. Pennebaker and Evans (2014) explain, "expressive writing (EW) – can positively affect people's sleeping habits, work efficiency, and their connection to others. Indeed, when we put traumatic experiences into words, we tend to be less concerned with the emotional events that have been weighing us down" (pp. 3-4). Brown (2015) concurs that Pennebaker's work with writing as healing is "some of the most important and fascinating research I've seen on the power of expressive writing in the healing process" (p. 87). While Pennebaker and Evans have studied the positive effects of people writing about traumatic experiences, writing does not always have to be negative and people always have the power to rewrite their narratives. Gruwell (1999) named the students in her English class The Freedom Writers and helped them use writing to "create a sense of community and an outlet for expression" (p. 275). That outlet for expression enabled them to share their past experiences as well as future dreams and built a strong class community where they shared their stories with both themselves and each other to enact change in their lives and the lives of their community.

Indeed, while certain practitioners have always used the sharing of stories in the medical field, it is only recently becoming more of a mainstream practice. Therefore, the most interesting discussion of the value of expression comes from the field of writing. With healing, just as in writing, it becomes essential to trust the process. According to Goldberg (1986) "we must continue to open and trust in our own voice and process" (p. 12). She provides the encouragement, "understanding this process cultivates patience and produces less anxiety" (p. 15). Writers know that revision is always possible; the first few pages of a draft might not end up being used, but may provide an idea that can later be implemented.

Similar strategies apply when designing a plan for achieving a goal. The initial plan may not end up being used, but may provide an idea that can later be implemented. Sharp (2000) describes this writing process when telling the story of an author who "one day after rereading the first four hundred pages, she decided that the novel really began on page 401. She threw out the first four hundred pages, and the novel hit its stride. The author realized that she had to have written those first four hundred pages in order to have reached page 401" (p. 19). Similarly, a physical therapy patient may develop an initial plan of completing exercises at home in the evening before falling asleep. However, the competing priority of the need for sleep at the end of the day wins and that plan doesn't work. The patient uses the idea that it makes sense to complete exercises during an uninterrupted time instead of trying to fit exercises in during the day and adjusts the plan to complete exercises first thing in the morning. The initial draft didn't work, but in the revision, the essence of the idea remains to enable the enactment of change. Lamott (1994) agrees, "there may be something in the very last line of the very last paragraph on page six that you just love, that is so beautiful or wild that you now know what you're supposed to be writing about, more or less, or in what direction you might go – but there was no way to get to this without getting through the first five and a half pages" (p. 23). Capturing the first draft leads to the beginning of idea exploration.

Exploration of the initial draft may lead the writer to discover that he or she is believes a version of the story that is not entirely true. A simple example of this are physical therapy patients who tell themselves the story that they have no time to complete their at home exercise plans. Using expressive writing and capturing this idea on paper may reveal that while the no time argument may be believed to be true, there may in reality be moments of time when the exercises can be completed. Brown (2015) advises that when writing, "don't hold back. There is no rising strong without a true accounting of the stories we're making up" (p. 92). And when we hold ourselves accountable for the stories we're making up that we may emotionally believe to be true but that factually may not be true, we do become emotionally strong so we can become physically strong in our health as well.

Writing also allows the writer to turn negative emotions into positive ones. As Cameron (1998) observes, "we are so skilled in the art of negative imagination, we are so adroit at the art of writing out of anxiety, what might our writing and our world look like if we allowed ourselves to inhabit our positive imagination?" (pp. 125-126). And what might our world look like if we reframed a negative attitude into a positive one and realized there is more than one road that can lead to our destination?

TEACHING AND TECHNOLOGY

I began my high school English teaching career in a school with a tremendous amount of caring for teachers and students, but not a significant amount of resources. The classroom contained a chalkboard, an old television and VCR, and an overhead projector. I made the best of it. When the overhead projector, named Elmo for the company that manufactured it, broke, I placed Hawaiian leis on it with the note "Elmo is on vacation." For presentations, I used video clips from old VHS tapes. I wrote notes on transparencies (once Elmo started functioning again) and washed them in the restroom sink to reuse. I waited (sometimes patiently, sometimes not) for one of the four computers in the faculty workroom when I needed to send emails to parents. I returned to the same restroom sink and filled a bucket with water to scrub the chalkboard. But the lack of technology did not interfere with learning. Students loved taking out their journals and putting pen to paper to record their thoughts. When did all this take place? This was only about ten years ago. While technology enhances teaching presentations, sometimes students still prefer taking out their journals and putting pen to paper.

WRITING WITH TECHNOLOGY

Writing prompts enable students to explore their thoughts and feelings. When several students in my classes last semester said they could not remember the last time they received a handwritten letter, I designed a class activity where everyone took out a sheet of paper and wrote a note to a friend or family member. But when I compose my own writing for chapters such as this one, I rarely handwrite anything first. Instead, I love the feeling of my fingers flying across the keyboard and seeing words appear on the screen. As Goldberg (1986) observes, "sometimes, instead of writing in a notebook, you might want to directly type out your thoughts. Writing is physical and is affected by the equipment you use" (p. 6). And a flash drive with writing is easier to carry than a pile of notebooks. Goldberg continues, there is a time and place for both because "I have found that when I am writing something emotional, I must write it the first time directly with hand on paper. Handwriting is more connected to the movement of the heart. Yet, when I tell stories, I go straight to the typewriter" (pp. 6-7). Regardless of whether students use pen and paper or their laptop computers, I want them to write.

I value my role as a writing role model for students. Johnson (2005) advises teachers, "here's your chance to provide that role model" (p. 26). I illustrate the writing process by projecting one of my computer typed drafts onto the large screen in the room so students can offer feedback while observing me adding, deleting, and revising phrases. If I want to be a writing role model, I need to provide my students with the same writing opportunities. Kearns (1997) describes, "word-processing programs can help our students be better writers by encouraging students to write before they compose – to brainstorm, plan, select, focus, draft, revise, and publish." (p. 114). She elaborates, "computers can also reduce writing apprehension. For some students, writing becomes easier to manipulate and motivation becomes higher" (p. 114). Some students see a finished handwritten draft as a work of art not to be disturbed; conversely, technology enables them to save multiple drafts of an essay with a quick click of a computer mouse. Revision also becomes easier with a typed draft, since deleting a word makes it disappear without any of the crossed out words or erasing required of handwritten drafts. Heard (1995) writes, "there are times when revision isn't necessary. These are the rare moments when what I write the first time is exactly what I want" (pp. 121-122). Like Heard, when I write a piece right with the first draft it is a special occasion. In fact, the words you are reading represent the fourth draft of this sentence. My computer made the magic of revision possible within a few seconds. While I will never lose my admiration for a powerful handwritten composition, technology provides methods of making writing easier and more fun for students.

MULTIGENRE WRITING

Students do not always need to respond to a text using writing. Artwork and song lyrics provide additional outlets for creative expression. Rief (1999) observes, "by watching my students and collecting their work over the years, I've learned how vision and voice matter to them. Their reader's-writer's journals are filled with sketches, drawings, and photographs; they are filled with poems and song lyrics" (p. 32). Students can effectively demonstrate their comprehension of a text using multiple genres including original paintings and drawings as well as song lyrics and musical performances.

One of my favorite projects is the multi-genre project, where students view a text through multiple genres and multiple lenses. As Tompkins (2011) explains, "children generally use three or more genres in a multi-genre project and include both textual and visual genres. What matters most is that the genres would not have to deal with such obstacles. Every classroom would be like the one Johnson (1998) describes for teachers as, "you can harness the power of words to motivate and inspire your students by displaying inspirational quotations in your classroom where students will see them every day. Some teachers ask their students to discuss the quotations or write responses to them in their journals. Others let them speak for themselves. Whether you discuss them or not, your students will read them and think about them – although they may never admit that they do" (p. 141). The power of words is not limited to classrooms with desks. The power of words can be used with patients, clients, students, friends, family, colleagues, and anyone else we encounter in the classroom of life.

By sharing words and stories, we support each other. We rely on our own intrinsic motivation but know where to find positive extrinsic motivation when needed. Sandberg (2013) states, "sharing emotions builds deeper relationships. Motivation comes from working on things we care about. It also comes from working with people we care about" (p. 88). There is a place for both extrinsic motivation and intrinsic motivation to coexist beautifully in supportive environments where people care about each other and encourage each other to achieve positive change.

PART II: IMPORTANCE

Are we willing to change? The answer to that question is how important change is to a person. Miller and Rollnick (2002) explain, "one factor is the extent to which the person wants, desires, or wills change. We tend to talk about this dimension as the perceived importance of a particular change" (p. 10). We all know there are things we probably should do. But the importance of each thing to us determines if we make a change.

Connected to importance is another word that starts with I, intuition. People often have an intuitive sense of what is truly important to them. Individuals who have a strong sense of intuition can appear to others as having a psychic sixth sense of what to do and when to do it. While intuition is unique to each person and highly individualized, a significant amount of theory exists to explain the practice of intuition. Dimitrius (1998) provides the description, "what we call intuition is nearly always the surfacing of a submerged memory, a barely noticed event, or some combination of the two" (p. 216). Perhaps we have experienced something similar in the past, so we have a feeling of how amplify and extend the repetend" (p. 333). A repetend can also be referred to as a narrative thread that connects the genres of a project and focuses on a central theme. For example, if a student completes a multi-genre project about a novel, the narrative thread is that each project illuminates a different aspect of the text. Romano (2013) elaborates, "instead of producing expository papers, students are writing in many genres. Although each piece is self-contained, making a point of its own, taken together, all the writing creates a unified whole" (p. 2). Technology adds a new dimension to multi-genre projects, as students now design digital collages, blogs from a character's perspective, and movies starring their friends and family to recreate scenes from the novel. Students then include a short section of end notes to explain why they designed the projects they did. Clandinin and Connelly (2000) remind me that "the teacher is part of the curriculum and therefore part of the establishment of the goals in the first place and part of the ensuing achievement" (p. 29). In my classroom, I observed students learning more if they can have fun in the process, so my goals which lead to student achievement incorporate both creativity and critical thinking.

TEACHERS AS REFLECTIVE LEADERS

Most importantly, teachers need to meet the needs of students, regardless of the format in which strategies are implemented. As Romano (1987) observes, "in a classroom full of opinionated teenagers, the last thing a teacher wants to feel is more vulnerable. The job is tough enough" (p. 39). But when teachers share their stories, students experience the practice of learning instead of only the theory.

One powerful strategy for reflecting happens when a person opens a journal and begins writing in a notebook. The page will not argue, which frees the author to write a list of goals, vent about frustrations, celebrate successes, or process thoughts and feelings. Goldberg (2007) believes, "writing is the act of reaching across the abyss of isolation to share and reflect" (p. xxi). Writing provides not only a place to reflect, but also a space to develop new ideas to share with others. Moreover, new ideas lead to finding a way to implement the goals of an organization. Beck (2012) explains, "Wayfinders, by definition, create paths where there are none and find destinations no one knew were there" (p. 280). Journal writing enables leaders, such as classroom teachers, to envision an idea and then make that vision reality. When rereading my journal from my first year of teaching, I observed my use of writing to wrestle with questions such as: What worked about this lesson? What didn't work? What would I do differently the next time? Writing helped me gain confidence in my leadership skills, something a new teacher of teenagers definitely needed!

Using writing as a method of reflection helps leaders rewrite their stories. Enayati (2015) reminds people to pay attention to the stories they tell themselves because, "there are stories that serve us. And stories that don't. What are the stories that you repeat to yourself over and over again? How mindful are you of your unspoken mantras? What are the threads that run through your everyday and eventually, your entire life?" (p. 8). Writing can make people aware of their narratives to know which stories need rewriting. Ideally, writing should become about the journey, not the destination. But ideas help no one if they stay in the pages of a journal. Eventually the leader must stop reflecting and return to action to implement a new strategy. Heifetz (1994) argues, "leadership is both active and reflective. One has to alternate between participating and observing" (p. 252). By alternating reflection with action, leaders develop a dream and share that dream with others to make it become reality.

Transformative leaders leave an organization better than when they found it. Starratt (1993) states, "transformational leaders enable subordinates to find fulfillment from striving for and achieving the high goals and purposes the leaders set for them" (p. 9). Transformative leaders enable everyone to invest in the community's shared vision and values, while simultaneously establishing goals and a sense of purpose. One example of this is when Sandberg (2013) writes of the Harvard Business School, "they laid out a new, communal definition of leadership: 'leadership is about making others better as a result of your presence and making sure that impact lasts in your absence.' They held students responsible for the impact their behavior had on others" (p. 157). And the ripple effect continues.

TECHNOLOGY AND STRESS

It is not yet five in the morning. My alarm goes off, and as I reach over to shut it off, I grab my iPhone from my bedside table. I check the texts I received since I went to sleep, then check my email. I haven't even been awake for two minutes, but already I am typing a reply to a coworker that can certainly wait until I've had breakfast. My mind is racing thinking of my endless to do list before my feet even hit the floor. The tone has been set for the day, and I'm not sure it's a good one.

Technology makes the world a better place by connecting people. My out of state relatives are only a text message away, and we can send each other pictures on our phones to bridge the distance between us. It makes my life as a writer and researcher easier to know a wealth of information awaits only a mouse click away when I type key words into a search engine. The flip side of the advantages of technology, however, is that we as a society are constantly connected. This constant connection can bring a feeling of stress.

When my parents were my age, they had a landline to call people. Before the invention of answering machines, if someone wasn't home, a call was missed. Even with an answering machine, my parents had to wait until they got home to know who called them. Their dinners at restaurants and trips to the movies were not disturbed by phone calls. Granted, they were difficult to reach if there was ever an emergency, but true emergencies are few and far between. My parents could actually look into each other's eyes at dinner. How many times have my friends and I been at a restaurant and everyone is looking at their cell phones instead of each other?

When my parents were my age, if they were gone when a favorite television show was on, they missed it. Thanks to the invention of the VCR, they could record their favorite shows, but only one show at a time. Members of my generation tend to get overwhelmed by the volume of television shows and all the recording options.

When my parents were my age, it may be difficult to fathom they lived in a world without social media or email. My mom wrote handwritten letters to her family and friends. My dad left work at the office and the only inbox he ever had to check was the paper one on his desk. Email brings people together while simultaneously making it difficult to disconnect. How many times have I been distracted by the ping of an email? Pipher (2006), advises, "don't let the urgent crowd out the important" (p. 91). Too often, the urgent email eclipsed the important activity that required more of my attention. The reality is that most people do not have the time to pick up a pen and write a handwritten letter, but they do have time to type a few lines from their phone or computer keyboard. Information can be transmitted quickly, and an entire conversation can take place in a matter of minutes if both people are checking their email. Technology itself is not stressful; it's the reaction by people to the technology that often creates stress.

DISCONNECTED

It is the middle of the week, and I am finished with work for the day. My family members have other plans on this weekday evening, and I am too tired from a busy day to call friends and go out for the evening. So I send some emails and text a few friends. Even though I have communicated with them, I feel restless and disconnected. Texting someone is not the same as looking a person in the eyes or sharing a hug. I open the YouTube app on my iPhone and discover that old television shows from my childhood are only a few clicks away. I watch a few clips, but don't feel the same happiness I did when I originally watched the shows years ago in the living room of my childhood home with my family. I talk to my cats, Lucy and Andy, just to be able to hear the sound of my own voice and know someone is listening even if they can't reply with anything other than a meow. I have difficulty sleeping and wake up the next morning tired, completely defeating the purpose of a quiet evening at home.

STRESS RELIEF STRATEGY #1: SELF-COMPASSION AND CONNECTION

Whether caused by technology or another source, stress can feel overwhelming. Perhaps from the tone of my writing voice in the last passage, you could infer that I wasn't being too kind to myself. It would have helped if I practiced self-compassion and did not mentally beat myself up for what I thought was a wasted evening of my life watching YouTube videos. Neff (2011) describes self-compassion as, "if we can compassionately remind ourselves in moments of falling down that failure is part of the shared human experience, then that moment becomes one of togetherness rather than isolation" (p. 65). I am certainly not the first person to use technology to waste time, and I will certainly not be the last. Therefore, the fact that I am willing to share my story in this chapter will perhaps cause you as the reader to smile, relate to it, and know that you are not alone either. Germer (2009) concurs, "self-compassion is the foundation for kindness toward others. When we're accepting of our own idiosyncrasies, we become more accepting of others" (p. 87). And kindness and connection with others can lead to less stress.

Even though I attempted to connect with friends through text messages, I didn't feel as happy as when I see them in person. I needed more connection than a text could provide. Rankin (2013) discusses the value of community and explains, "chronic social isolation can lead to loneliness, and multiple studies demonstrate that loneliness can trigger stress responses in the body, the same kind of fight-or-flight responses fear of bodily harm can elicit" (p. 93). Being part of a strong community can help reduce loneliness and consequently reduce stress. Used well, technology can bring people together. A text message can remind a person that a loved one is thinking about him or her. Skype enables people across the country and even around the world to see each other. But there is a time for technology and a time to get out of the house and get together with people in person.

Some people find strength in spirituality and their community in churches. Spirituality can provide comfort in times of need. Hale (2013) believes, "just like a puzzle, it takes time for all of the pieces in your life to come together" (p. 142). It can be disappointing when a story doesn't have the ending you want, but that means it becomes time to write another story and have faith in the new narrative. Arterburn (2011) concurs, "You lack a unifying understanding of why all these unrelated pieces are hanging together in your life. If so, the choice to serve may be the choice that puts it all together for you" (p. 370). Often people who have experienced physical or emotional pain in their own lives find careers in healing professions because they want to help others through similar experiences. Once we write new chapters in our own stories, we can turn around and help others on their healing journeys.

Furthermore, while some people find their community in a church, a church is not the only place to go for community connection. It is possible to find community in a gym, in a classroom, or around a table in a restaurant. No one needs to experience social isolation and there are numerous opportunities to reach out and connect with others. Germer (2009) believes, "connecting with others is another form of self-care – to stop isolating" (p. 108). He explains that this is important because "a sense of isolation can turn even ordinary unhappiness into despair or minor anxiety into dread" (p. 108). Technology can bring people together in the form of a community of practice, where a group uses technology as a platform to share their ideas and collaborate on projects.

Whether it is directed toward self or others, compassion becomes essential for increased health and happiness. Neff (2011) shares, "one of the most robust and consistent findings in the research literature is that people who are more self-compassionate tend to be less anxious and depressed" (p. 110).

She discovered that self-compassionate people had lower levels of the stress hormone cortisol and concluded, "self-compassion gives us the calm courage needed to face our unwanted emotions head-on" (p. 124). Remaining calm lowers stress while helping people assess a situation and take ownership of their emotions. The next time you make a mistake or feel isolated and lonely, try to be kind to yourself and rely on your community where others will demonstrate kindness toward you.

STRESS RELIEF STRATEGY #2: FOCUS ON YOUR HEALTH

Concerned about something you looked up on an internet search engine or worried about a friend's post on social media? It can influence your health. Tindle (2013) reports, "anxiety, self-doubt, and related thoughts and feelings are associated with increases in blood pressure, heart rate, and stress hormones such as adrenaline and cortisol, all of which pound our organs like waves on the beach" (p. 100). Tindle discusses that a positive outlook can lead to better health, and one way to change outlook is through exercise because "physical activity can temporarily catapult you out of the territories of depression, relapse, and other unsavory outlook addresses long enough to get your bearings and steer yourself in a different direction" (p. 138). For specifics about the right exercise plan for you, consult a physician or physical therapist.

Research has shown that stress can make people sick. Rankin (2015a) explains, "when exposed to stress, the body tends to whisper before it yells. Stress often manifests through less immediately life-threatening physical symptoms, such as backache, headache, eye strain, insomnia, fatigue, dizziness, appetite disturbances, and gastrointestinal distress" (p. 35). If you find yourself experiencing any strange health symptoms, check the stress level in your life and call your doctor, since emotional stress can manifest physically in your body.

If you are experiencing stress, meditation and letting everything go can help. Beck (2008) provides the reminder, "remember, you can't force this kind of calm; pressuring yourself to feel no anxiety merely creates more anxiety" (p. 101). It becomes very easy to focus on what you don't have, but stopping for a moment to think about gratitude and what you do have is an effective method of relaxing and relieving stress. Beck (2001) advocates facing fears and addressing anything that may be creating stress, and she describes an experience where writing down her anger at a situation helped with her back pain because "as soon as I wrote it down, I felt a tingle along my own spine, and the pain in my back relaxed significantly" (p. 195). As you will read in the next section, writing serves as a valuable resource for stress management; however, before you continue reading take a deep breath and give yourself permission to let go of any stress you may be feeling today.

STRESS RELIEF STRATEGY #3: WRITE YOUR STORY

Stressed? Pick up a pen and put it to paper or let your fingers roam over the keyboard of your computer. Writing, whether handwritten or typed, enables expression because a piece of paper or the computer screen won't criticize the writer, thus allowing for the emergence of writing voice. Pipher (2006) discusses the value of blogs because "writing a blog is instant self-publication, which is its own special kind of creativity" (p. 200). While technology allows blogs to be shared with a large audience, writing does not have to be shared if the writer does not wish it to be.

While there can be value in sharing written words, writing can have healing benefits even if no one sees it except the writer. Brickman (2015) believes journaling is a great method of self-exploration because, "it is a wonderful way to explore your life and figure out what's working and what's not. You'll also find reviewing your journal at the end of the year a great way to explore your accomplishments and figure out what you want to do over again" (p. 104). Writing helps reveal the stories we are telling ourselves. We can then choose the path our writing can take. Goldberg (1990) states, "think of something now that you sincerely want to tell and go ahead and tell it" (p. 7). We can share our writing with a trusted medical professional who can see patterns to our pain. We can publish our writing in a blog and share it with readers we may not even know. Or we can keep the writing private in a journal, letting the page worry about an issue so we can experience a little less stress and perhaps a little more sleep. Heard (1995) believes, "the task of every writer is to dig beneath the surface and find complexity in each situation" (p. 45). Life can be complex. Stories can be complex. Your story is your story. Sharing it, even with only yourself, can help you heal physically, heal emotionally, and relieve stress.

WELLNESS RESOURCES

To help you put the theories in this chapter into practice, here are some additional wellness resources. Sandberg (2013) writes, "we cannot change what we are unaware of, and once we are aware, we cannot help but change" (p. 156). Feel free to take these ideas and incorporate them into your life in whatever ways work best for you.

Heart Maps

Jen has become too involved in trying to think of a brilliant idea that she can no longer see the larger picture of how her research team's current goals relate to their vision and values. It's time to reflect and remember the things which really matters to her. She remembers she won't be able to help her team write a new research story if she can't help herself, so she needs to practice self-care and find her way back to her creative self by drawing a heart map.

When you look at heart pictures, you might think of love, Valentine's Day, and happiness. Or you might think of health or a trip to the doctor. Too often in life we worry about things, which can lead to stress on our bodies. Ever feel your heart race when you are nervous about something? One way to stress less and smile more is to spend time with people and things you love by creating a heart map.

During the routine of a busy schedule, one method people can use to remind themselves of people and things they value is to create a heart map. Heart maps help people remember not to make work their lives. Heart maps originally started as a writing strategy; teachers use them in classrooms when students can't think of a writing topic. What is important to you? Look in your heart map!

Writing teachers such as Georgia Heard discuss the value of falling in love with life and the sense of peace it can bring. Heard (2016) describes heart maps as, "heart mapping is a metaphor for what all writers know: to write is to delve into what matters to us, to keep our feelings alive, to be vulnerable, to tell the truth, to question, and to speak what many people only keep inside" (p. 1). I love drawing heart maps and creating artistic representations of my thoughts, feelings, ideas, hopes, and dreams; I also love seeing my journal writing and my formal writing that you now read as a written representation of my heart.

Heart maps can be a simple sketch or an intricate work of art. Heard (1999) instructs her students, "Today, I'd like you to make a map of all the important things that are in your heart, all the things that really matter to you. You can put: people and places that you care about; moments and memories that have stayed with you; things you love to do, anything that has stayed in your heart because you care a lot about it" (pp. 108-109). To create a heart map, draw a heart on a sheet of paper. In the heart, write the names of beloved people, places, and things. The important thing is to make the items in the heart map as much a part of life as possible. Heard (1999) instructs, "if it's something that you really care about then it belongs in your heart map. Only you can decide what should be in your heart map" (p. 109). In heart maps, the common thread is that the designer loves each item in it. Heard (1995) writes, "the seemingly random observations I make or the subjects I choose to write about are like the branches of a tree whose roots reach down to the depths of myself and reveal my obsessions" (pp. 69-70). Heart maps provide a vision of what the designer values.

Here's how to create your own heart map:

- Draw a heart on a sheet of paper. The artistic quality doesn't matter. What is important is that you leave enough blank space to write words inside the heart.
- Inside the heart, write down the names of people, places, and things you love. No one has to see this except you. Remember it's not always the big things in life but the small things that can cause you to smile. A walk in the park when it is sunny outside. Spending time with my family. A great book. That's part of my list. What makes you happy?
- Look at your list. How much of your day is spent with the people, places, and things in your heart map? If you are not spending part of your day with people, places, and things you love, how can you arrange your schedule so you can do this?
- No one has to see this heart map except for you, but you may want to use your heart map as a reality check. You may love things that are not healthy for you, and it's also fine to enjoy some things in moderation or occasionally, such as spending a Saturday watching reruns of a favorite television show or eating your favorite dessert. The key is balance.
- Don't have enough hours in the day for things you love? Try to rearrange your schedule to spend more time with the people and things in your heart map.
- Below is an example of a heart map I created.

Figure 1. Heart map designed by the author

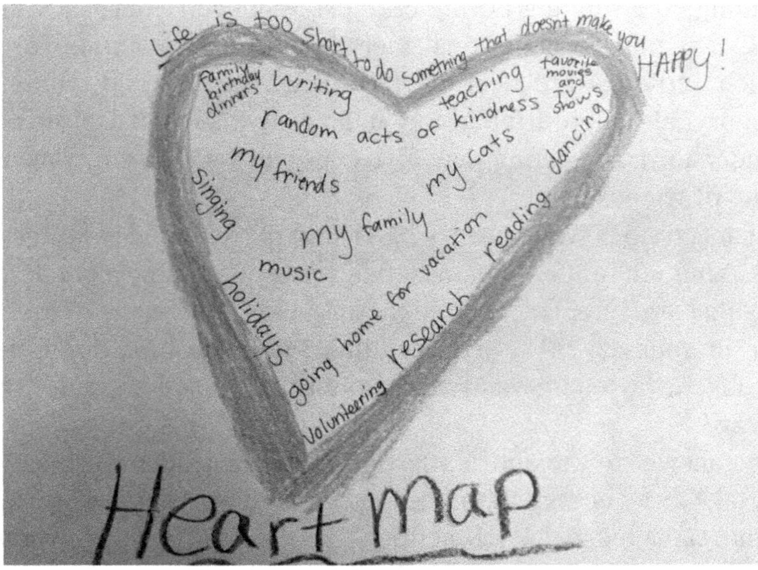

525,600 Minutes of What Brings You Energy

In the song *Seasons of Love*, a year is measured in 525,600 minutes. Everyone has an equal amount of time in a year. How do you use it? Teacher Donald Graves discusses four types of activities. Graves (2001) states, "I know that you already have a sense of what takes energy, gives it, and is a waste of time. What you need now are the specifics from your own life in order to chart a different course from the one you know. Awareness that grows out of the specifics of your own situation produces energy" (p. 11). What do you do that gives you energy? What do you do that takes away energy? What do you do that is neutral? What do you do that wastes energy? Time to take a look at how you spend your time.

- Write out your schedule, or choose a computer program or the calendar feature on your phone that will do it for you.
- Hour by hour, list how you spend your time during a day. Be honest with yourself. No one has to see this except for you. Now look at how your energy level feels with each activity.
- Which activities give you energy? For me, I love spending time with loved ones, teaching, and making a difference in the world. List yours.

- Which activities take away energy? For me, I hate waiting in long lines, cleaning, and running boring errands. Some activities, such as a long walk, may take away physical energy but bring you emotional energy.
- Which activities are neutral? I consider driving and eating in this category, although driving may take away energy if I'm driving in a thunderstorm and eating may give energy if I am having a meal with a group of friends.
- Which activities waste energy? I have to play computer solitaire until I win. After ten or eleven games, this wastes both time and energy.
- Now that you have categorized the activities, how many of each do you have in your day? Are you spending too much time doing activities that take away energy and not enough time doing activities that give energy?
- If the answer to the above question is yes, consider pairing activities that take away energy with ones that bring you energy. For example, I might read a magazine (something that gives me energy) while sitting in the waiting room during a car oil change (something that takes away energy).
- Can you eliminate activities that take away energy or waste energy from your schedule? In other words, if you said no to someone or something, how bad would the consequences be? If you can't make the dessert for the party, the odds are someone else will do it. Probably not a big deal.
- You should notice some connections between the activities that bring you energy and the ones in your heart map. More energy = the feeling of more hours in a day.

10-10-10

Suzy Welch designed a strategy called 10-10-10. Welch (2009) explains that to reclaim her life, she needed "to start making my decisions differently – proactively – by deliberately considering their consequences in the immediate present, near term, and distant future. In ten minutes….ten months….and ten years" (p. 9). What will be important to you ten minutes from now, ten months from now, and ten years from now? Dooley (2019) shares how she uses the process as, "make sure the big and small decisions you make are good for both Present You and Future You" (p. 158). Answer these questions in your own life. Sometimes what seems like a big deal now may not be a big deal later.

Here's an example of how I used this recently:

Issue: I have numerous emails to answer but also want to meet my family for dinner. I picture how the results of my decision might look in the short term, midterm, and long term future.

Life 10 minutes from now: I really need to answer these emails so I can start work tomorrow without having to worry about them, but I also don't want to disappoint my family.

Life 10 months from now: I won't remember the content of those emails, but I will remember dinner with my family and smile when I look at the pictures of that event.

Life 10 years from now: I love my job, but I love my family more. I don't want to be a person who was so distracted by work at the expense of family relationships. So I'm going to put aside the emails and focus on being in the moment with people I love.

So if an issue is bothering you…. How will you feel about it in the immediate, distant, and really distant future?

Important/Urgent

Stephen Covey designed a matrix of urgent vs. important. Covey, Merrill, and Merrill (1994) explain, "clearly, we deal with both factors – urgency and importance – in our lives. But in our day-to-day decision making, one of these factors tends to dominate. The problem comes when we operate primarily from a paradigm of urgency rather than a paradigm of importance" (p. 39). If something is both urgent and important (the bills need to be paid), people usually do it. If something is not urgent and not important (reading junk mail), people rarely do it. The middle categories can get confusing. Some things that seem urgent aren't that important. For example, the phone rings during a family dinner, you grab it, and it is a telemarketer. Don't take time away from family dinner (not urgent but important) to deal with the telemarketer (urgent but not important).

Here's an example of how I used this recently:

I'm working on lesson plans for class (urgent, important). Emails appear in my inbox (urgent, not important). I also want to have dinner with my family (not urgent, important). I wonder if I will have time to watch my favorite television show (not urgent, not important). I make my decisions based on my values and priorities of what is important. I finish the lesson plans and remind myself they do not have to be perfect, enjoy dinner with my family, save the emails for later, and will watch the television show if I have time.

Don't let urgent demands eclipse what is truly important in life.

LIVING A WELLNESS NARRATIVE

As a teacher, curriculum design enables me to think of the larger goals, themes, and objectives for my lesson plans. Connelly and Clandinin (1988) believe, "administering the curriculum meant the narrative living out of a personal philosophy of education" (p. 196). My personal philosophy consists of acronyms such as RICE and MICE, as well as providing both the students in my classroom and readers of this text with teachable moments.

ACKNOWLEDGMENT

The preceding chapter contains excerpts from the following previous IGI publications:

Bird, J.L. (2018). Constantly connected: Managing stress in today's technological times. In V.C. Bryan, A. Musgrove, & J. Powers (Eds.), *Handbook of research on human development in the digital age* (pp. 385-402). Hershey, PA: Information Science Reference.

Bird, J.L. (2017). Writing healing narratives. In V.C. Bryan & J.L. Bird (Eds.), *Healthcare community synergism between patients, practitioners, and researchers*. Hershey, PA: Information Science Reference.

Brown, S., Bird, J.L., Musgrove, A., & Powers, J. (2017). Leading learning communities with creative practice. In V.C.X. Wang (Ed.), *Encyclopedia of strategic leadership and management*. Hershey, PA: Information Science Reference.

Brown, S., Bird, J.L., Musgrove, A., & Powers, J. (2016). The digital journey: integrating technology into teaching and learning. In V.C.X. Wang (Ed.), *Handbook of research on learning outcomes and opportunities in the digital age* (pp. 612-643). Hershey, PA: Information Science Reference.

Bird, J.L. (2015). Preface. In J.L. Bird (Ed.), *Innovative collaborative practice and reflection in patient education* (pp. xiv-xxi). Hershey, PA: Information Science Reference.

REFERENCES

Arterburn, S. (2011). *Healing is a choice*. Nashville, TN: Thomas Nelson.

Baty, K. (2003). *A girl's gotta do what a girl's gotta do*. New York, NY: Rodale.

Beck, M. (2001). *Finding your own North Star*. New York, NY: Three Rivers Press.

Beck, M. (2008). *Steering by starlight*. New York, NY: Rodale.

Beck, M. (2012). *Finding your way in a wild new world*. New York, NY: Free Press.

Brickman, J. (2015). *Soothe*. New York, NY: Rodale.

Brown, B. (2012). *Daring greatly*. New York, NY: Gotham Books.

Brown, B. (2015). *Rising strong*. New York, NY: Spiegel & Grau.

Caldwell, K., Gray, J., & Wolever, R. Q. (2013). The process of patient empowerment in integrative health coaching: How does it happen? *Global Advances in Health and Medicine: Improving Healthcare Outcomes Worldwide*, *2*(3), 48–57. doi:10.7453/gahmj.2013.026 PMID:24416672

Cameron, J. (1998). *The right to write*. New York: Tarcher/Putnam.

Cameron, J. (2002). *The artist's way* (2nd ed.). New York, NY: Tarcher/Putnam.

Carter, C. (2015). *The sweet spot*. New York, NY: Ballantine.

Clandinin, D. J., & Connelly, F. M. (2000). *Narrative inquiry*. San Francisco, CA: Jossey-Bass.

Connelly, F. M., & Clandinin, D. J. (1988). *Teachers as curriculum planners*. New York, NY: Teachers College.

Covey, S. R., Merrill, A. R., & Merrill, R. R. (1994). *First things first*. New York, NY: Free Press.

DeBecker, G. (1997). *The gift of fear*. Boston, MA: Little, Brown and Company.

Dimitrius, J. (1998). *Reading people*. New York, NY: Ballantine.

Dooley, J. L. (2019). *Own your everyday*. New York, NY: Waterbrook.

Dweck, C. (2006). *Mindset*. New York, NY: Ballantine.

Enayati, A. (2015). *Seeking serenity.* New York, NY: New American Library.

Germer, C. K. (2009). *The Mindful path to self-compassion.* New York, NY: The Guilford Press.

Goldberg, N. (1986). *Writing down the bones.* Boston, MA: Shambhala.

Goldberg, N. (1990). *Wild mind.* New York, NY: Bantam.

Goldberg, N. (2007). *Old friend from far away.* New York, NY: Free Press.

Goldberg, N. (2013). *The true secret of writing.* New York, NY: Atria.

Goldberg, N. (2016). *The great spring.* Boulder, CO: Shambhala.

Graves, D. H. (2001). *The energy to teach.* Portsmouth, NH: Heinemann.

Groopman, J. (2007). *How doctors think.* New York, NY: Mariner Books.

Gruwell, E., & the The Freedom Writers. (1999). The Freedom Writers diary. New York, NY: Broadway.

Gruwell, E., & the The Freedom Writers. (2009). The Freedom Writers diary (2nd ed.). New York, NY: Broadway.

Hale, M. (2013). *The single woman.* Nashville, TN: Thomas Nelson.

Heard, G. (1995). *Writing toward home.* Portsmouth, NH: Heinemann.

Heard, G. (1999). *Awakening the heart.* Portsmouth, NH: Heinemann.

Heard, G. (2016). *Heart maps.* Portsmouth, NH: Heinemann.

Heifetz, R. A. (1994). *Leadership without easy answers.* Cambridge, MA: The Belnap Press of Harvard University Press.

Johnson, L. (1998). *Two parts textbook, one part love.* New York, NY: Hyperion.

Johnson, L. (2005). *Teaching outside the box.* San Francisco, CA: Jossey-Bass.

Kearns, J. (1997). *Where to begin: a guide to teaching secondary English.* Portsmouth, NH: Heinemann.

Lamott, A. (1994). *Bird by bird.* New York: Anchor Books.

Larson, J. (2005). Seasons of love [Recorded by the cast of Rent]. On Rent: Original motion picture soundtrack [CD]. Burbank, CA: Warner Brothers Records.

Miller, W. R., & Rollnick, S. (2002). *Motivational interviewing* (2nd ed.). New York, NY: The Guilford Press.

Miller, W. R., & Rollnick, S. (2013). *Motivational interviewing* (3rd ed.). New York, NY: The Guilford Press.

Neff, K. (2011). *Self compassion: the proven power of being kind to yourself.* New York, NY: HarperCollins.

Pennebaker, J. W., & Evans, J. F. (2014). *Expressive writing: words that heal.* Enumclaw, WA: Idyll Arbor.

Pink, D. (2009). *Drive*. New York, NY: Riverhead Books.

Pipher, M. (2006). *Writing to change the world.* New York, NY: Riverhead.

Rankin, L. (2013). *Mind over medicine*. Carlsbad, CA: Hay House.

Rankin, L. (2015a). *The fear cure*. Carlsbad, CA: Hay House.

Rankin, L. (2015b). *The anatomy of a calling*. New York, NY: Rodale.

Rief, L. (1999). *Vision and voice*. Portsmouth, NH: Heinemann.

Rollnick, S., Miller, W. R., & Butler, C. C. (2008). *Motivational interviewing in health care: helping patients change behavior*. New York, NY: The Guilford Press.

Romano, T. (1987). *Clearing the way*. Portsmouth, NH: Heinemann.

Romano, T. (2000). *Blending genre, altering style*. Portsmouth, NH: Heinemann.

Romano, T. (2013). *Fearless writing*. Portsmouth, NH: Heinemann.

Sandberg, S. (2013). *Lean in*. New York, NY: Alfred A. Knopf.

Sharp, C. (2000). *A writer's workbook*. New York, NY: St. Martin's Press.

Starratt, R. J. (1993). *The drama of leadership*. London, England: The Falmer Press.

Tindle, H. (2013). *Up: How positive outlook can transform our health and aging*. New York, NY: Hudson Street Press.

Tompkins, G. E. (2011). *Literacy in the early grades* (3rd ed.). Boston, MA: Pearson.

Welch, S. (2009). 10-10-10. New York, NY: Scribner.

KEY TERMS AND DEFINITIONS

Heart Maps: Writing teacher Georgia Heard believes in the value of heart maps, which ask writers to draw a heart and inside the heart write things that the writer loves.

Journal Writing: The process of a person responding to prompts and writing about his or her thoughts and feelings. While journal writing is typically associated with writing classrooms, writing teachers including Julia Cameron and Natalie Goldberg advocate that journal writing can be done by anyone, anywhere.

Motivational Interviewing: A method of using reflective statements and open-ended questions to enhance intrinsic motivation for change.

Multi-Genre Writing: Introduced to the field of education by Tom Romano, multigenre writing consists of creative writing in multiple genres and the writer's analysis of the genres.

Narrative Inquiry: Described in depth by F. Michael Connelly and D. Jean Clandinin, narrative inquiry is a qualitative interpretative form of research that focuses on the telling, retelling, and sharing of stories.

Self-Compassion: The act of demonstrating the same kindness toward oneself that one would demonstrate for others.

Story Sharing: By sharing a story with a supportive audience, either in conversation or in writing, it frees the storyteller of unneeded physical and emotional stress caused by holding the story inside and worrying about it. Brene Brown explains that it helps people to share stories instead of numbing pain with unhealthy choices.

Urgent vs. Important: Mary Pipher, Don Graves, and Stephen Covey all discuss the type of choices people make of how they spend their time and the resulting increased or decreased energy experienced.

Writing as Healing: James Pennebaker is a leader in the field which explores the health benefits of writing. Numerous studies have been conducted by researchers investigating the influence of writing on physical and emotional health.

Writing Voice: Voice in writing describes how a writer uses word choice and tone to reflect the unique personality of the writer. Just like each person has a unique speaking voice, each writer has a unique writing voice.

Chapter 9
Narratives of Journal Writing

Jennifer Lynne Bird
Oxbridge Academy, USA

ABSTRACT

How can writing help people heal? While writing cannot take the place of an evaluation by a trained medical expert, it can help the healing process. The process of writing serves as a valuable resource whether a patient writes about symptoms in a journal to share with a medical professional, a high school student writes about the day's events in a journal to deal with emotions, or an adult writes a prayer in a journal to cope with uncertainty. Regardless of the circumstances which motivated the writer to pick up a notebook and pen or type at a computer, writing releases thoughts and emotions from the mind to the page. When people transfer ideas to paper, stressful emotional events in the mind and physical tension in the body often improve. Therefore, writing can become a catalyst for healing.

I JUST WANT YOU TO KNOW WHO I AM

How can writing help people heal? This question served as the motivation for research and also led to discoveries in my roles as a high school English teacher, Stephen Minister at my church, and health coach. While writing cannot take the place of an evaluation by a trained medical expert, it can help the healing process. When a patient writes about symptoms in a journal to share with a medical professional, a high school student writes about the day's events in a journal to deal with emotions, or an adult writes a prayer in

DOI: 10.4018/978-1-7998-1931-8.ch009

a journal to cope with uncertainty, the process of writing serves as a valuable resource. Regardless of the circumstances which motivated the writer to pick up a notebook and pen or type at a computer, writing releases thoughts and emotions from the mind to the page. When people transfer ideas to paper, stressful emotional events in the mind and physical tension in the body often improve. Writing can therefore become a catalyst for healing.

This chapter uses first person and the method of narrative inquiry to share stories and apply artistic methods, such as writing in journals, to the practice of healing. The theory of narrative inquiry invites writers to own their writing voices and make stories accessible. Clandinin and Connelly (2000) explain, "questions of form for a narrative inquirer are with us from the outset of an inquiry. Even as we tell our own research stories prior to entering into the midst of the field stories, there is a tentative sense of plot. As we engage with research participants and live and tell stories with them, the plotlines under composition are restoried, that is, they are relived and retold. All of these tellings and livings prefigure the narrative forms of our research texts" (p. 165). Narrative inquiry, as a qualitative interpretive form of research, focuses on stories and the finding of narrative threads, or themes, in the stories. Narrative inquiries may include objective data, such as a tally of the number of times events occurred; however, a narrative inquiry also includes subjective data, such as the stories of participants. Consequently, the researcher in the field of narrative inquiry can choose to participate as a participant observer instead of only observing other people. If the researcher chooses the role of a participant observer, attention must be paid to the dual roles. Heifetz (1994) describes the dual roles by using the extended metaphor, "consider the experience of dancing on a dance floor in contrast with standing on a balcony and watching other people dance" (pp. 252-253). Narrative inquirers alternate between the balcony perspective of observation and the dance floor perspective of interacting with participants.

My research into writing as healing began with studying the stories of others during my doctoral dissertation, but expanded when the death of my mom caused me to unexpectedly find myself in the same position as the research subjects I interviewed. My research transformed from just another topic to study to having a larger purpose. My own experiences of how I used writing as healing mean as much to me as the stories of others. The research for this chapter exists as observational research and reflections of previous research projects. It serves as a qualitative interpretive analysis as well as an introduction to writing as healing for anyone looking to explore the concept in their lives.

In this narrative, the practice of writing meets the practice of medicine. This section's title, *I Just Want You to Know Who I Am*, is a line from the song *Iris* by the Goo Goo Dolls. It also describes how patients feel when seeking help: They want someone to know their stories. When seeking medical treatment, a patient wants to feel like his or her story is being heard and the medical provider sees a person and not just a name on a chart. Rankin (2015b) advises that despite demands from a sometimes frustrating medical system, those practicing medicine need to take the time to look their patients in the eyes and not stand with a hand on the door to the exam room because, "just as healers must stand up and reclaim the lineage of their professions, patients must reclaim their own power, standing up with their autonomy, their intuition, their willingness to question and participate in changing the system from within, and their vote. It all starts with change at the level of the healer-patient relationship" (p. 238). This narrative will explore the value of writing and how writing can be applied to the field of medicine to help people heal. Whether a patient talks to a health coach, receives prayers from a Stephen Minister, or writes in a journal, the important thing is that the patient feels the story is heard.

While a story can be spoken, writing enables the author to capture additional details of a narrative. Pennebaker (1997) theorized from his research as a psychologist, "if my experience was any indication, writing about upsetting issues must work in ways similar to talking about them" (p. 30). Any patient who has ever walked out of a doctor's office with the realization of forgetting an important question can benefit from writing notes to remember experiences. Brown (2015) summarizes, "Pennebaker's research, combined with what I've learned in my own work, has convinced me that even brief engagements with writing can lead to significant results" (p. 88). Patients therefore do not have to write a long narrative for their medical practitioners or themselves; a short series of notes or freewriting of a few sentences can be enough to share the story.

Journal writing may be relatively new to the medical field, but for years English teachers have used journal writing in their classrooms. Anderson and MacCurdy (2000) advise English teachers, "we are, however, arguing what we know to be true – stories about painful, traumatic events in the lives of students do appear in our classrooms, they have always appeared, and they will continue to appear, not because we want or don't want them to, but because writing is quite simply the medium in which, for many people, the deepest, most effective, and most profound healing can take place" (pp. 8-9). Writing in journals gives students a space to explore their thoughts and feelings. While some students do choose to write about painful events, students can also choose to write in their journals about other topics, such as their feelings about an inspirational quote. By writing, students transfer emotions out of their heads and onto the page. Gruwell (2007), whose students became known as the Freedom Writers, states, "I, like my students, realized that it would take more than just writing to feel better – but at least it was a start" (p. 148). The purpose of journal writing is for students to trust themselves and their first impressions while they write narratives. Students have a short amount of time, such as five or ten minutes, to write their first impression on a topic. The time limit is to capture the writer's first impression about an idea before self-criticism can create any doubt or second guessing.

Journal writing helps students find their writing voice. Lamott (1994) discusses her own experiences and shares, "so I sit for a moment and then say a small prayer – please help me get out of the way so I can write what needs to be written" (p. 117). Writing what needs to be written serves as a form of self-expression that leads to the discovery of writing voice. English teachers know that no matter what the story is now, students always have the power to rewrite their narratives. As Cameron (1998) states, "when we just let ourselves write, we get it 'right'" (p. 8). If we find the courage to write our stories and trust our writing voices, we write a new narrative.

BACKGROUND OF WRITING AS HEALING

Writing helped me through difficult situations by bringing clarity to my life. As a National Board Certified Health Coach, I advocate a holistic approach to healing. Writing helps me manage my stress most of the time, but it does not exist as the only option or a magic cure. A couple times in my life, losses such as the death of my mom caused my stress to transform into anxiety; I needed therapy and medication, and no shame exists in either option or in asking for help. Consequently, none of my words can become a good alternative for a conversation with your doctor if you experience anxiety or any other health issue. When everyday stress does not cross the line into anxiety, however, writing can help.

Research exists to support the theory of writing helping people heal, beginning with the work of psychologist James Pennebaker. Pennebaker and Smyth (2016) discuss Pennebaker's original study, which led to the discovery, "people who wrote about their deepest thoughts and feelings surrounding traumatic experiences evidenced enhanced immune function compared with those who wrote about superficial topics" (p. 21). They continue with the observation that improved health continued after the writing experience and elaborate, "people who wrote about their deepest thoughts and feelings related to stressful or traumatic experiences had reliable improvements in health in the two to three months after writing" (p. 25). Additional studies on wellness and writing followed. Evans (2010) summarizes the literature and reports, "wellness and writing are connected in ways yet to be fully researched and exploited, but the literature of several disciplines declares that for many people wellness and writing are connected in ways useful for emotional, physical, and spiritual health" (p. 3). In the years since Evans reported that the connections had yet to be fully researched, Sandberg and Grant (2017) report, "more than a hundred experiments have documented the therapeutic effects of journaling. It has helped medical students, patients with chronic pain, crime victims, maximum-security prisoners, and women after childbirth" (pp. 62-63). They continue, "writing about traumatic events can decrease anxiety and anger, boost grades, reduce absences from work, and lessen the emotional impact of job loss. Health benefits include higher T-cell counts, better liver function, and stronger antibody responses. Even journaling for a few minutes a few times can make a difference" (p. 63). Furthermore, people do not have to write about traumatic events to receive the benefits of writing. Brown (2015) described the participants in her research as, "many of them worked through their emotions in letters they knew they would never send but needed to write" (p. 87). The writing process can help anyone who feels willing to explore self-discovery.

Mindfulness expert Cameron (2018) explains, "whether you write for five minutes or 60 minutes a day, journaling helps you gain perspective and deepen self-awareness – revealing your thoughts, habits, strengths, and ways of interpreting the world" (p. 45). She continues, "although journaling is an excellent practice for self-awareness, insight, and clarity, it has also proven to be a tremendous tool for navigating times of change, uncertainty, and dealing with difficult emotions" (p.45). She encourages anyone interested in practicing journaling to use either prompts to explore ideas, or to open a notebook and put pen to paper as an act of mindfulness.

As a high school English teacher, I witness my students report that writing helps them calm their minds and organize their thoughts. Life as a high school student can be difficult. The words English teacher Johnson (1998) wrote twenty years ago remain true today when she gives teachers the advice, "don't belittle your student's concerns. Acknowledge their feelings, accept their right to have a bad day or a worry, just as adults do" (p. 174). Students appreciate when teachers treat them with respect. Journal writing can provide an outlet for describing feelings when students may not want to discuss something. I tell students that if they write something which concerns them to discuss it with me, their parents, or the school counselor. If you want to begin a writing practice, you do not need a medical credential to pick up a pen or open a blank document on your computer to receive the benefits of writing. Journal writing changed my life numerous times. I share my story while encouraging you to write the next chapter in your own story.

WRITING AND TEACHING

As soon as the bell rings, my students and I have a ritual: We reach for our journals. At the beginning of most of the high school English classes I teach, I allow about five minutes for journal writing time. I give students three options: Write about the quote I have on the board, write about the current work of literature we are reading, or write about whatever happens to be on their minds that day. At the end of each quarter, I hold individual conferences with each student where I flip through the journals to make sure they are writing, but I do not read their writing unless they request it. While I look through the journals, I ask students how they felt about writing. The majority of students tell me it helps them process thoughts and feelings. Several students tell me it helps manage stress. Students also describe that journal writing serves as practice, or warm-ups for formal essays. According to Carter (2015), "shoot for a perfect first draft and you are screwed, though; most people are paralyzed by the impossibility of that task" (pp. 204-205). I don't believe there is such a thing as a perfect first draft, but the imperfect first drafts that may not meet the requirements for a formal essay work perfectly for expressive writing in journals.

Journal writing encourages the writer to complete expressive writing. Writing teacher Romano (2013) describes, "expressive writing is where we start when we pour forth first words, seeking to make meaning from fragmented, chaotic inner speech. Expressive writing is writing closest to our speaking voice, the seedbed from which all other writing grows" (p. 189). Expressive writing focuses on the first thoughts before the voice of the internal censor starts questioning the words on the page. I want my students to feel like Lamott (1994) when she describes her process as, "so I'd start writing without reigning myself in. It was almost just typing, just making my fingers move" (p. 24). Some students prefer to type their journals, and they receive just as much as benefit as they process day to day issues in their writing. Sandberg and Grant (2017) believe, "turning feelings into words can help us process and overcome adversity" (p. 62). When adversity appears in the lives of my students, it becomes essential for me to honor their stories.

Student stories can lead to transformation. I love the work of teacher Erin Gruwell and her students, The Freedom Writers. My classes read *The Freedom Writers Diary* and discuss the philosophy of Erin Gruwell (1999), who describes of her students, "the students continued to write and began to forge stronger identities and to create a sense of community and an outlet for expression" (p. 275). My classes develop into strong communities when students care about each other and support each other. While I do not require them to share their writing during group discussions, when students do choose to share their writing with their classmates or me, they learn that others in the class share their feelings and they are not alone in their experiences.

While I choose not to share the writing of my students in this narrative to maintain the confidentiality I promised them, to give you an example of student writing I include a journal entry I wrote as a junior in high school. I keep my old journals and occasionally revisit them to reflect on my experiences.

Okay, I'm a junior. Let me see…what does that mean….more cafeteria food for one thing. Just kidding. For one thing, I'm not afraid of the school now, I know my way around (for the most part). I don't have to worry about graduation for another year. I guess I'm somewhere in the middle. I'll probably take ACTs and SATs this year, but I'm good at standardized tests so I'm not too worried. I do worry a lot though.

While it seems that my sixteen year old self wrote about surface things, at the end of the entry I started to process my thoughts and emotions about worrying. That insight comes from the writer years later after research and experience; my teenage self just enjoyed writing!

My students tell me writing in their journals at the beginning of class helps reduce the anxiety they feel during the school day. Medical doctor Rankin (2015a) describes, "anxiety is an emotional feeling of nervousness, unease, dread, or apprehension" (p. 11). As someone who has experienced anxiety, I can relate to the students and feel grateful that writing helps me sort out the stress in my life. Writing becomes part of a balanced wellness plan including exercise, nutrition, and perspective. Unlike the novel *The Scarlet Letter* students read, anxiety should never feel like a scarlet letter worn by anyone who experiences it. Szabo and Hall (2007) offer the encouragement, "it's time we all learned that each of us has a right – and a responsibility – to face our issues, be honest about our needs and emotions, and most importantly, to ask for help when we need it" (p. 221). Each day the bell rings and my students pick up their journals, I know the writing process helps them.

THE PROCESS

If you are a teacher or other educator and want to use journals in your classroom:

- Give students a choice of whether to write in a notebook or type their journals.
- Allow time for writing. A minimum of five minutes works well. Less than five minutes means students may not have the time to process their ideas.
- Maintain silence in the classroom so students can be alone with their thoughts and not distracted by classmates.
- It is your choice whether or not to read the writing, but make sure students know in advance if you will be reading their writing. Students do not want to be surprised if you tell them later you will be reading their personal writing.
- I recommend either not grading the writing or taking a participation grade. Students write differently when they know the content will be graded.
- You may have administrative tasks to complete, but take the time to write in your own journal when students are writing so they can see you as a writing role model.

WRITING AND EMOTIONAL PAIN

I first studied the field of writing as healing for my doctoral dissertation at Miami University in Oxford, Ohio. The topic of writing helping people heal emotionally became my purpose in life due to unexpected circumstances. In addition to helping other people, I also helped myself. My mom died in the middle of my graduate program, transforming me into not only an observer in my research study, but also a participant. Whenever my thoughts started racing or I missed my mom with an intensity which made me want to curl up on the floor and not get up again, I reached for my journal or my computer. My personal experiences with the transformative power of writing redefined my career and my life. I would trade all I have learned about writing as healing to be able to pick up the phone and call my mom again, but since I can't I choose to use my own experiences to help others.

While interviewing teachers about how they used writing to process their experiences, I also used writing to help me through the grieving process. Zimmermann (2002) believes, "writing allows you to access your wider mind, a wiser, more encompassing place deep within. Your story will unfold and through the writing of it, you will honor and embrace your sorrows, grow from them, and arrive at a place where life is more full and more joyful than you ever thought possible" (p. 19). Some days it became hard to feel when the emotional pain became too intense, but writing became my coping mechanism. Looking back at the writing, I can see my anger, devastation, and even moments of hope. This is an excerpt from my journal six months after my mom died when I traveled from Ohio to Delaware and Florida to visit my aunts, uncles, and cousins.

If the life you want isn't possible because of various circumstances, how do you piece together another life that may not be what you want but can still provide you with a little happiness? I think of all my dreams and my future plans that involved my mom. As I return from two weeks of visiting different cities and flying across the country on planes, I can't help but think that she would have been the first person I would have told of my adventures. I told her anyway; I know she was still part of my trip even though not in the way I wanted her to be.

After graduation, I decided to move from Ohio to Florida to make a new start and live closer to my family. Conner (2008) explains, "writing works amazingly well. If you want to engage in a vibrant conversation with the wisdom that dwells just a hair below your conscious awareness, write" (p. 57). In addition to helping me process my grief, writing helped me set new goals and dreams. By getting everything from my mind to the page, I gained clarity about my experiences. Sometimes when thoughts swirl around in a person's mind, the truth of the narrative becomes distorted. Social worker Brown (2017) elaborates, "the brain's self-protection mode often ramps up the stories we tell ourselves about what's happening, creating stories that are often not true or exaggerate our worst fears and insecurities" (p. 55). For days after my mom's death, I existed in survival mode and my subjective perspective of my life didn't always match my objective reality. My mind attempted to protect itself by processing pieces of the traumatic event at a time and when my thoughts couldn't focus, writing became a lifeline. Writer Heard (1995) believes, "a first memory is the first story embedded on the soul" (p. 72). Through a combination of writing and therapy, I refocused the first memory of the trauma and remembered the happy memories of my mom. I do not want to give the impression that writing solved everything for me during this difficult time; I also saw a therapist once a week to talk about my experiences and took an antidepressant at the advice of my doctor. Nevertheless, writing helped me on the days between therapist visits and especially the nights when I couldn't sleep and had already woken up my friends with phone calls. My journal and computer became reliable and constant companions who never gave advice and let me vent my emotions.

I could have stopped there; I did enough work on myself to not only survive but thrive. Still, perhaps because of my role as a teacher, I wanted to do more. Handler (2013) writes, "the passage of time between the event that caused grief and when the writer feels ready to pick up a pen or open the laptop is one place where your story is found. The person you were then, and the person you are now, create the voices that combine to tell the story" (p. 165). Immediately after the experience, my main focus was of course helping myself, but as time passed, I realized I wanted to share my story to help others. Along my journey I met people who cared about the topic as much as I did and we wrote together. I have to believe my words make a difference. That is my mom's legacy, and my legacy too.

THE PROCESS

If you are going through a difficult time emotionally and want to write about it:

- Remember no one has to see your writing except you.
- Stop writing if it is too difficult.
- Your writing and computer won't judge you, so don't judge yourself for anything you write.
- If you would be upset if someone else read your writing, keep your journal in a locked file cabinet or other safe place.

- If you find yourself writing about something that disturbs you, it's time to share with a trusted friend or professional therapist.
- It is not a sign of weakness if you need therapy or medication. Don't be afraid to ask for help if you need it.

WRITING AND PHYSICAL PAIN

While I knew writing could help people heal emotionally, another serendipitous moment on my journey led me to research how writing helps people heal physically. I found myself in physical therapy for neck pain and kept a journal to try to make sense of why I felt little pain one minute and intense pain the next. I couldn't make any sense of it, but fortunately for me my physical therapist used expert knowledge to interpret my writing, make a diagnosis, and help me heal. I felt grateful for his compassion and creative thinking, since not all medical practitioners would feel enthusiastic about a new idea. After my treatment ended, we continued to work together and research how writing helps patients heal. An enjoyable interdisciplinary collaboration led to research results that made a difference in the lives of patients.

When we asked patients to respond to short answer survey questions, we asked for their first impressions. Writing teacher Goldberg (2013) shares, "practice is not for something else. Practice is the practice of being here with your life and pen now. Go, across the page – or your computer screen – what are you thinking of? Put your life on the line" (p. 22). The process of trusting first impressions in writing not only works for high school English students in a classroom, but also physical therapy patients in a clinic. When I designed my pain journal, I needed to share my first impressions in order to have the most accurate information to share with my physical therapist. When patients responded using their first impressions, they shared the most accurate impression of what they felt before the self-censor could take over their thoughts. As Bernstein (2010) writes, "let your pen flow across the page and allow your mind to release its thoughts" (p. 23). When I shared my journal, I needed to trust my physical therapist to keep my information confidential and also use it to help me. I'm sure at times my writing entertained him while he read my thoughts about my neck pain!

Most of us will be patients sometime in our lives. While writing cannot heal physical pain on its own, it can contribute to healing. When people write and release their emotions, the decrease in emotional stress can lead to a decrease in muscle tension. Enayati (2015) argues, "in a way, extreme stress is self-fulfilling. The key is to switch the focus of both our perceptions and stories to post-traumatic growth" (p. 72). Even if the patient has no control over the physical pain, the patient does have control of how he or she feels about the pain. Writing can bring clarity and perception to the pain narrative and switch the mental focus from helplessness to achieving growth about this experience. Duckworth (2016) defines, "it was this combination of passion and perseverance that made high achievers special. In a word, they had grit" (p. 8). While this definition of grit applies to a variety of situations, passion and perseverance become important during the recovery process from physical pain. Pain can lead to frustration, but a positive attitude makes a difference. Beck (2008) explains, "in other words, the negative reaction cluster – the stress reactions, the emotional pain, and the physical weakness that are wired together in your brain and body – can be rewired. The associative learning that makes us feel depressed, anxious, and old can be unlearned" (p. 11). Writing holds us accountable by revealing our thought patterns. Once we illuminate our thought patterns, we can change them. Dalebout (2016) observes, "journaling allows you to stop identifying with your negative beliefs or thought patterns and instead see yourself as separate from them. You start to move from judging yourself to simply witnessing your thoughts, cozying up with them, learning from them, and ultimately letting them out" (p. 12). Letting out thoughts in the form of journal writing allows the page to worry about an issue while simultaneously serving as a stress release.

Another way writing can help with physical pain is by creating a journal to show medical professionals. How many times does the best question get thought of as soon as the doctor leaves the room? A pain journal or symptom journal ensures that all questions are asked and all information is conveyed to the person in charge of the patient's care. The most important quality of a pain or symptom journal is honesty. A doctor can best help a patient when he or she has all the information. Brown (2015) believes, "we can't get to our brave new ending if we start from an inauthentic place. So give yourself permission to wade through the sometimes-murky waters of whatever you're thinking and feeling" (p. 88). At times it may feel difficult to act vulnerable and authentic in front of someone in the medical field. Remember, most clinicians are compassionate professionals who will walk with you on your health journey. Medical doctor Rankin (2013) explains, "being unapologetically who we are – not just at work, but at home, in the schoolyard, at church, wherever – soothes the mind, halts the stress response, induces the relaxation response, and heals the body. Authenticity, in work and in life, can be medicine for the body" (p. 117). Not only can authenticity have health benefits by causing relaxation, when a person demonstrates a willingness to show vulnerability and articulate needs, clinicians appreciate knowing all the information so an accurate diagnosis can be made.

Despite my love of television medical dramas, I have no desire to observe a surgery. I did, however, have a desire to learn more about the health care field, so I earned my health coach certification from Duke University Integrative Medicine. According to Caldwell, Gray, and Wolever (2013), "health coaching entails a specific structure and provider relationship that reinforce each other. The coach-patient relationship is specifically centered on the patient's health goals and supporting the patient in those goals" (p. 55). Health coaches partner with the patient's medical team to align the patient's personal goals with the treatment goals and help the patient achieve the goals. Beck (2001) advocates, "today, take one turtle step toward your goal. Just one" (p. 323). A turtle step is a little step that, taken with numerous other little steps, leads to success. Health coaches help patients stay motivated to reach their goals. Writing does not eliminate pain, but can become part of the health plan. Writing about moments of success or moments of challenge can help determine the next best steps, as well as illustrate progress. Whether writing down goals, keeping a pain journal, or processing feelings about pain, writing exists as a resource for the healing process.

THE PROCESS

If you are sick or in pain and want to write about it:

- Obviously, if you have severe pain or illness, don't write. Seek medical help immediately.
- Be honest in your writing. Your medical team can best help you if you tell the truth about your symptoms and feelings.
- Members of your medical team want to help you. Don't fear that they will judge you for writing the truth.
- Try to keep a positive attitude. Healing is a journey, and small steps still equal progress. A great lesson my physical therapist, Dr. Eric Wanner, told me when I wanted my neck pain to heal immediately is to "think like a turtle" and make slow and steady progress. Turtles travel at a slow pace, but eventually reach their destination.
- An excerpt of my pain journal is below; feel free to use it as a model for your own pain journal.

Table 1. The author's neck pain journal

Fri 3/30	Right Side Pain Low = 2, High = 4, Average = 3	Best right after leaving physical therapy. Worst when looking down at notes and stressing about summer teaching schedule. Spend time with family today which leads to laughter.
Sat 3/31	Right Side Pain Low = 2, High = 4, Average = 3	Best when doing exercises. Going for a mellow experience and listening to Taylor Swift this time.
Sun 4/1	Right Side Pain Low = 3, High = 5, Average = 4 Was going to play an April Fool's joke on you and make the numbers really high so laughed thinking about that.	Best when out to lunch with cousins and laughing. Worst when trying to hold Grandma back and prevent wheelchair escape. Epiphany of day: This is a journey. Keep thinking like a turtle. You'll get there!

WRITING AND SPIRITUALITY

On a beautiful Florida winter afternoon, my students and I sit outside by the lake on the high school's campus. We discuss the poetry of Walt Whitman. Whitman (1855) writes in his poem *O Me! O Life!* "That you are here – that life exists and identity, that the powerful play goes on and you may contribute a verse" (p. 341). This leads to a conversation about the difference between spirituality and religion. My students give insightful answers. In their words, religion is what people practice while spirituality is how people feel. I explain that everyone has a right to his or her own religious beliefs, yet together as a class we have a spiritual moment sitting by the water in silence as we write in our journals and read poetry.

Religious institutions may choose to use writing with members of their congregations. Also, anyone may choose to use writing as a reflection and form of prayer. Niequist (2016) believes, "whatever it is that you clutch onto with angry fists, that you grab like a lifeline, when you release that thing, when you let it go, that's when you'll hear the notes between the music" (p. 97). Reflection and prayer allow for silence so the noise of a busy life becomes silent. Sometimes when life seems uncertain, people turn to destructive habits; writing serves as a healthy alternative to coping with a situation and provides a reminder that a lifeline to internal strength provides more power than external distractions Enayati (2015) explains, "adversity may or may not be out of our control, but we do have control over our stories: what we tell ourselves and others about our circumstances, and how we choose to respond to them" (p. 51). When we can't control the outcome of a situation, we can still control how we react.

Whatever your religious or spiritual practices may be, writing becomes accessible to all who choose to pick up a notebook and pen or reach for a computer. Does the story you tell yourself about your life and current situation reflect your reality? Is an obstacle a roadblock or an opportunity to learn? Brown (2015) explains, "the most dangerous stories we make up are the narratives that diminish our inherent worthiness" (p. 82). Putting thoughts on paper in the form of journal writing can clarify the difference between the actual truth of a situation compared to our interpretation of it. We remind ourselves of people and things we have for which we can show gratitude and determine what needs to change. Detours taken on the road of life can lead to new goals and opportunities.

In addition to my roles as high school English teacher and health coach, I serve as a Stephen Minister at my church. Haugk (2000) defines, "Stephen Ministers are lay Christians carefully recruited, selected, trained, commissioned, and supervised for lay caring ministry" (p. 17). With my role as a Stephen Minister, I use the same skills of reflective listening and partnering with people on their healing journeys as I do as a health coach. The difference with Stephen Ministry is that people may be experiencing a spiritual crisis instead of a health crisis, and I also have prayer as a resource. While I write about Stephen Ministry from the perspective of my experiences, the writing practices I describe are not meant to be seen only from the perspective of Christian faith.

Regardless of a person's views on religion and spirituality, the practice of self-compassion can lead to reflection and kindness toward oneself. Often people criticize themselves more harshly than other people ever could. While self-compassion can take place by thinking kind thoughts, writing can serve as an affirmation of thoughts of kindness. Neff (2011) suggests, "try keeping a daily self-compassion journal for one week (or as long as you like). Journaling is an effective way to express emotions and has been found to enhance both mental and physical well being" (p. 103). A daily self-compassion journal can remind the author to practice kindness and self-forgiveness. Whenever life seems challenging, we can enjoy the journey more by showing ourselves and others kindness and compassion. Mistakes happen as part of life, but since we cannot recapture the past like the main character in *The Great Gatsby* longs to do, writing can help us move forward. Germer (2009) shares, "keeping a journal is itself a contemplative practice and a self-compassion exercise" (p. 242). Contemplation shares characteristics with the practice of mindfulness, which promotes self-awareness and living in the present moment. Tindle (2013) explains, "the main difference between mindfulness and contemplation is that at its core, contemplation is a practice in which the contemplator seeks to come closer to a higher spiritual power" (p. 108). Some people may choose to practice mindfulness and remind themselves to refocus their attention to the present moment, while others may choose to pray as a form of contemplation.

While prayer exists mainly through spoken words, they may also appear in the forms of thoughts or written ideas. Cameron (1998) states, "it is my belief that all of us are naturally intuitive and that writing opens an inner spiritual doorway that gives us access to information both personally and professionally that serves us well" (pp. 206-207). Often, when a decision needs to be made, writing can provide guidance to the solution which makes the writer feel most at peace. Clarity appears on the page and offers valuable insight. Matousek (2017) believes, "like all forms of awakening practice, writing requires mindfulness. Just as we bring our attention back to the breath during meditation, you learn to observe the wandering mind without excessive control, and gently return your focus to the question at hand" (p. 5). Whatever question may bring the writer to the page, writing about it may provide the answer.

As a Stephen Minister, I often give short prayers. When I visit someone in need in the hospital or pray with someone at church after the service, I may not know much about the person. During such times, I begin speaking and trust I will say the words the person needs to hear. Bernstein (2016) believes, "we change the world when we shift spiritually – when our attitudes become more loving, when we forgive, when we heal our wounds from the past, and when we embrace the present moment" (p. 172). Just like it helps people heal emotionally and physically, writing can help people heal spiritually. The journal can be a place to explore thoughts and feelings for self-forgiveness, or a place to work through a difficult conversation if it would help to forgive someone else. If the person who needs forgiveness is not willing to have a conversation or longer alive, forgiving can still take place for the writer in journal pages. Bernstein (2018) explains, "putting pen to paper is a prayer. It's an offering. You humbly look at your judgment, choose again, and then pray for that judgment to be replaced with love" (p. 186). By writing, we acknowledge our pasts, remind ourselves to remain mindful in the present, and share hope for the future.

My research and writing became part of my life's purpose. By writing about my experiences, I saw the connections between the moments that happened to me. It's a magical feeling when ideas weave together like threads of a tapestry. If my mom hadn't died, would I still feel that research and writing exist in my life as part of a larger purpose? I do know that helping other people makes me feel that I can use the pain of my life experiences to make a meaningful contribution to the world. I understand that some people may see everything as coincidences, but my spirituality leads me to believe in what Rushnell and DuArt (2017) call Godwinks, which they define as, "Godwinks are those little events that defy human understanding. In the beginning you were tempted to call them coincidences, but inwardly you sensed there was something more going on – and that God had something to do with it" (p. ix). Whatever you believe, I hope writing helps you discover your personal gifts. I then encourage you to share your gifts with others who may benefit from the knowledge.

THE PROCESS

If you are a church leader or anyone who wants to use writing as a spiritual resource:

- If you are contemplating a question or need to make a decision, start writing and see what answers your intuition discovers.
- If you find yourself being your own worst critic, practice self-compassion and write about your strengths in your journal.
- Create a gratitude journal and make a list of things for which you are grateful. Use daily, weekly, or as often as you need.
- If you feel discouraged by acts of hate in the world, shift the focus to love and create an observation journal of random acts of kindness that you practice or witness others practicing throughout the day.
- Write a prayer for yourself or someone else.

THE ART OF WRITING

Throughout this narrative, I cite research studies illustrating the healing benefits that can happen with writing. Even with the technical dimensions of research, creativity drives the artistic writing process. I view writing as an art form, where self-expression becomes essential for the writer. Writing provides a safe space for expression, since the page will not judge the author. Even sharing the story with oneself in the pages of a journal can provide healing benefits. Sharing writing with a supportive reader can build trust and provide additional support for the writer. Romano (2015) describes of sharing stories, "it's been good to write about it and give it to readers" (p. 21). The writer decides who to trust; finding the right reader leads to a source of encouragement and helps the writer build resilience. Writing serves as a coping mechanism for life's fragile moments and can transform negative thoughts into positive ones by reframing the stories.

Multigenre writing provides one method of writing as art. Romano (2000) describes multigenre papers as, "genres of narrative thinking require writers to be concrete and precise." (p. 26). A multigenre format enables me to explore different dimensions of my story. I follow the artistic genres with a technical end notes section which references research, but does not disrupt the momentum of the narrative. Romano (1995) believes, "because of the magnitude and atypical nature of the multigenre project, I also wanted students to experiment with various genres in their learning journals, not simply wait until the research was completed to write their papers" (p.114). This writing symbolizes my learning journal and my experimentation as I apply the theories discussed previously in this chapter to my experiences. Romano (2013) explains, "when I read students' multigenre papers, I know I'm going to learn, but I want to know more. I want to know what will remain invisible unless students tell me" (pp. 169-170). Multigenre writing gives me the opportunity to simultaneously think critically and creatively about a narrative. Romano (2004) writes, "one of the hardest things I do as a teacher is listen to students, listen to their voices in the classroom, listen to their voices on paper" (p. 98). As a teacher, I agree with his statement of the value of listening to student voices, and for this writing I wanted to capture my voice while illuminating my narrative.

Write, and then share. Participate in your own story. Dovetail creativity, imagination, and facts, as well as research and experience to tell the intellectual and emotional truth. Defy expectations, but be responsible. Tell your story and find your voice.

Is multigenre research a documentation of academic theory or the practice of creative writing? Both. Picture a figure skating routine. The technical score focuses on the required elements, such as the number of jumps and spins. Without the technical dimension of figure skating, skaters circle the ice with no direction or purpose. The artistic score focuses on the creativity of the routine. Without the artistic dimension of figure skating, a routine is a series of jumps and spins with no coherence or unity to pull the routine together. Just like skating routines, multigenre research dovetails technical research, where writers share facts learned from research, with artistic interpretation, where writers can choose a creative method such as poetry or artwork to share their knowledge.

Planning a successful multigenre paper is a lot like a teacher planning a lesson or a city planner planning a city. Harper (1996) writes, "monitoring implementation is the only way to know if a plan is becoming effective" (p. 196). She's writing about city planning, but multigenre writers also need to monitor if the implementation of ideas is effective. Throughout my life, I have heard my dad use the terms survey, analysis, plan, implementation, and feedback to describe the city planning process. Whether working with a city or a multigenre paper, careful planning is required. So I became a planner, just like my dad; I just plan lessons and writing pieces instead of cities.

Just as a painter glides across a blank canvas with a paintbrush, the writer glides across a blank page with a pen. Heard (1995) writes, "when I return to writing, the lessons from art guide me. Painting and writing are both about relationships. In painting, paint thickness, brush strokes, image, canvas texture, color, and outline all work together. In writing, the words, images, rhythm, voice, and meaning must work together as well. (p. 119). In the stories captured in the pages of a journal, the writer may search for meaning instead of starting with a specific destination in mind. Journal writing focuses on the journey. During the process, the writer's voice, as unique as a speaking voice, shines through on the page. Trusting first impressions gets the writer closest to the truth of what is on the mind and in the heart. Cameron (1998) explains, "yes, writing is an art, but 'art' is part of the verb 'to be' – as in 'Thou art truly human.' To be truly human, we all have the right to make art. We all have the right to write" (pp. 232-233). Writing means connecting with the self. Take my words and paint a picture with your own words. I provide you with points to ponder as you begin your writing journey.

THE PROCESS

If you want to begin your own writing story:

- Use writing to illuminate your narrative. Trust the words that appear on the page to capture the truth of your thoughts and feelings.
- Show yourself some compassion. No one is perfect. It's okay to feel what you feel.
- Take turtle steps. Whatever your personal journey may be, change takes time.

- Be authentic. No one else is you. Don't feel you need to pretend to be someone else on the page. It won't comment on your writing.
- Show grit. Passion and perseverance will help you achieve goals you set for yourself.
- Track progress. You do not have to reread previous writing, but it can help you see patterns and appreciate accomplishments.
- Share your story. You do not have to share your story, but a supportive reader can offer support and encouragement on your journey.

MY STORY

In my high school English classroom, I encourage my students to write in journals. Almost every weekday, we begin class with journal writing time. I stand in front of teenagers who sit in their bright blue chairs as I show my own black and white composition book and give the instruction to just keep writing. Journals provide a place for students to share their thoughts and feelings and traditionally exist as private writing. I ask my students to show me their best writing, meaning there are pages I never read. I feel fine with that; students tell me the practice of writing helps them relieve stress, process their ideas, and become better writers. One of my favorite teaching moments happens when I conference with each student about his or her writing process.

Soon after my mom died, I never could have imagined my experiences of using writing to cope with grief would become something positive. Handler (2013) believes, "distance from the event that caused your grief can shed light that's necessary when you're writing about the tough stuff. What caused your grief is in the past, and your perspective has changed naturally as you've continued to survive" (p. 16). I also wanted to do more than survive; I wanted to use my pain to help others.

I agree with writer Katie Dalebout (2016), who elaborates, "by putting these deep thoughts and fears down on paper, I acknowledged their presence – and was one step closer to releasing them, along with each of my failed attempts at control" (p. 9). Getting thoughts on paper transforms fears from the mind to the page and gives the writer the chance to let them go.

It did not prove as difficult as I thought it would to write about my mom's life. Bernstein (2016) believes, "true healing occurs when you give yourself permission to feel whatever feelings live below the triggers" (p. 44). Time provided comfort and fun nostalgia instead of tears when I wrote about my mom. Pennebaker and Smyth (2016) describe this as, "writing about emotional topics is more than learning how to put a story together. It is a way for us to learn more about our own emotions, relationships, and thought patterns" (p. 162). I linked my mom's story with mine so I could explore my own thoughts and feelings about both our experiences. Like Strauss (2010), "I wrote and wrote and listened close for whatever the past was trying to say to me" (p. 177). Getting to know my mom again through writing about her makes me proud to be her daughter.

I followed the advice of Files (2016) who suggests, "when it's emotional truth you seek, trust memory's details to find it" (p. 79). Brown (2015) concurs, "stay in the story until you touch every part of it" (p. 92). This process of trusting my memories until I touched every part of the story meant reconnecting with my mom and knowing I honor her whenever I write about research or help a student or patient.

As writer Anne Lamott (1994) observes, "you don't even have to know how or in what way, but if you are writing the clearest, truest words you can find and doing the best you can to understand and communicate, this will shine on paper like its own little lighthouse" (p. 235). May my writing become a lighthouse for others to find their way and may I continue to live a life that would make my mom proud of me.

YOUR STORY

Practicing the art of expressive writing can lead to emotional, physical, and spiritual healing. Cameron (2018) shares, "you direct your attention to the page, open your mind, and make the invisible visible by seeing what comes through on the page" (p. 45). She adds, "the greatest discoveries of your life could appear on those paper or on-screen pages" (p. 48). To begin your writing practice, start by writing whatever comes to your mind and see where it takes you.

Sharp (2000) offers anyone wanting to write the encouragement, "someone who takes the time to sit down, perhaps with pen or pencil in hand, and express themselves in their own words – this is a person who has something to say and the commitment to say it". (p. 133). Everyone has a unique writing voice, so let your writing voice shine. Goldberg (1996) provides the reminder, "when you finish a piece, you're refusing to be silenced or ignored. Writing is brave" (p. 201). I encourage you to find the courage to share your story, whether you share it with yourself or a larger audience.

Writing helps students in a classroom, patients in a hospital, and readers of this narrative who want to pick up a pen and write a new chapter. Hale (2015) offers the advice, "I urge you to save some room for the unexpected. Stay open to plot twists, to edits, to rewrites, to uncertainty" (p. 194). The next chapter in your life is yours to write. Each day offers a chance to fill another blank page with hopes and dreams. May you make the most of it.

ACKNOWLEDGMENT

The preceding chapter contains excerpts from the following previous IGI publications:

Bird, J.L. (2019). Narratives of writing as healing. In J. Bopp, A.M. Grebe, & J.H. Denny (Eds.), *Healing through the arts for non-clinical practitioners*. Hershey, PA: Information Science Reference.

Bird, J.L. (2017). Writing healing narratives. In V.C. Bryan & J.L. Bird (Eds.), *Healthcare community synergism between patients, practitioners, and researchers*. Hershey, PA: Information Science Reference.

Bird, J.L. (2015). Preface. In J.L. Bird (Ed.), *Innovative collaborative practice and reflection in patient education* (pp. xiv-xxi). Hershey, PA: Information Science Reference.

REFERENCES

Anderson, C. M., & MacCurdy, M. M. (2000). Introduction. In C. M. Anderson & M. M. MacCurdy (Eds.), *Writing and healing* (pp. 1–22). Urbana, IL: National Council of Teachers of English.

Beck, M. (2001). *Finding your own North Star*. New York, NY: Three Rivers Press.

Beck, M. (2008). *Steering by starlight*. New York, NY: Rodale.

Bernstein, G. (2010). *Add more –ing to your life*. New York, NY: Harmony Books.

Bernstein, G. (2016). *The universe has your back*. Carlsbad, CA: Hay House.

Bernstein, G. (2018). *Judgment detox*. New York, NY: North Star Way.

Brown, B. (2015). *Rising strong*. New York, NY: Spiegel & Grau.

Brown, B. (2017). *Braving the wilderness*. New York, NY: Random House.

Caldwell, K., Gray, J., & Wolever, R. Q. (2013). The process of patient empowerment in integrative health coaching: How does it happen? *Global Advances in Health and Medicine: Improving Healthcare Outcomes Worldwide*, *2*(3), 48–57. doi:10.7453/gahmj.2013.026 PMID:24416672

Cameron, J. (1998). *The right to write*. New York: Tarcher/Putnam.

Cameron, L. (2018). *The mindful day*. Washington, DC: National Geographic.

Carter, C. (2015). *The sweet spot*. New York, NY: Ballantine.

Chulack, C., Crichton, M., Wells, J., & Zabel, D. (1994-2009). *ER* [Television series]. Burbank, CA: Warner Brothers.

Clandinin, D. J., & Connelly, F. M. (2000). *Narrative inquiry*. San Francisco, CA: Jossey-Bass.

Conner, J. (2008). *Writing down your soul*. San Francisco, CA: Conari.

Dalebout, K. (2016). *Let it out*. Carlsbad, CA: Hay House.

Duckworth, A. (2016). *Grit*. New York, NY: Scribner.

Enayati, A. (2015). *Seeking serenity*. New York, NY: New American Library.

Evans, J. F. (2010). Introducing wellness & writing connections conference papers. In J. F. Evans (Ed.), *Wellness & Writing Connections* (pp. 3–10). Enumclaw, WA: Idyll Arbor, Inc.

Files, M. (2016). *Writing what you know*. New York, NY: Allworth.

Fitzgerald, F. S. (1925). *The great Gatsby*. New York, NY: Scribner.

Germer, C. K. (2009). *The Mindful path to self-compassion*. New York, NY: The Guilford Press.

Goldberg, B. (1996). *Room to write*. New York, NY: Tarcher/Putnam.

Goldberg, N. (2013). *The true secret of writing*. New York, NY: Atria.

Gruwell, E. (2007). Teach with your heart. New York, NY: Broadway.

Gruwell, E., & the The Freedom Writers. (1999). The Freedom Writers diary. New York, NY: Broadway.

Hale, M. (2015). *Beautiful uncertainty*. Nashville, TN: Thomas Nelson.

Handler, J. (2013). *Braving the fire*. New York, NY: St. Martin's Griffin.

Harper, A. N. (1996). Tooling up for effective planning. In B. W. McClendon & A. J. Catanese (Eds.), *Planners on planning* (pp. 190–198). San Francisco, CA: Jossey-Bass.

Haugk, K. C. (2000). *When and how to use mental health resources*. St. Louis, MO: Stephen Ministries.

Hawthorne, N. (1955). *The scarlet letter*. New York, NY: Washington Square Press. (Original work published 1850)

Heard, G. (1995). *Writing toward home*. Portsmouth, NH: Heinemann.

Heifetz, R. A. (1994). *Leadership without easy answers*. Cambridge, MA: The Belnap Press of Harvard University Press.

Johnson, L. (1998). *Two parts textbook, one part love*. New York, NY: Hyperion.

Lamott, A. (1994). *Bird by bird*. New York: Anchor Books.

Matousek, M. (2017). *Writing to awaken*. Oakland, CA: Reveal Press.

Neff, K. (2011). *Self compassion: the proven power of being kind to yourself*. New York, NY: HarperCollins.

Niequist, S. (2016). *Present over perfect*. Grand Rapids, MI: Zondervan.

Pennebaker, J. W. (1997). *Opening up: the healing power of expressing emotions*. New York, NY: The Guilford Press.

Pennebaker, J. W., & Smyth, J. M. (2016). *Opening up by writing it down*. New York, NY: The Guilford Press.

Rankin, L. (2013). *Mind over medicine*. Carlsbad, CA: Hay House.

Rankin, L. (2015a). *The fear cure*. Carlsbad, CA: Hay House.

Rankin, L. (2015b). *The anatomy of a calling*. New York, NY: Rodale.

Romano, T. (1995). *Writing with passion*. Portsmouth, NH: Heinemann.

Romano, T. (2000). *Blending genre, altering style*. Portsmouth, NH: Heinemann.

Romano, T. (2004). *Crafting authentic voice*. Portsmouth, NH: Heinemann.

Romano, T. (2013). *Fearless writing*. Portsmouth, NH: Heinemann.

Romano, T. (2015). *Write what matters*. Lexington, KY: Zigzag.

Rushnell, S., & DuArt, L. (2017). *The Godwink effect*. New York, NY: Howard Books.

Rzeznik, J. (1998). Iris [Recorded by Goo Goo Dolls]. On City of angels soundtrack [CD]. Burbank, CA: Warner Brothers.

Sandberg, S., & Grant, A. (2017). *Option B*. New York, NY: Knopf.

Sharp, C. (2000). *A writer's workbook*. New York, NY: St. Martin's Press.

Strauss, D. (2010). *Half a life*. New York, NY: Random House.

Szabo, R., & Hall, M. (2007). *Behind happy faces*. Beverly Hills, CA: Alegra.

Tindle, H. (2013). *Up: How positive outlook can transform our health and aging*. New York, NY: Hudson Street Press.

Whitman, W. (1993). O Me! O Life! In *Leaves of Grass* (p. 341). New York, NY: Random House. (Original work published 1855)

Zimmermann, S. (2002). *Writing to heal the soul*. New York, NY: Three Rivers Press.

KEY TERMS AND DEFINITIONS

Anxiety: Different clinicians have different definitions of anxiety, and a person who lives with anxiety will describe it from a different point of view than a clinical definition in a textbook, but the general definition of anxiety is chronic fear or stress that can result in panic attacks and a person feeling an inability to cope with life's stresses.

Expressive Writing: Writing that is exploratory and focuses on meaning and first impressions.

Journal Writing: The process of responding to prompts and writing about thoughts and feelings. While journal writing is typically associated with writing classrooms, writing teachers including Julia Cameron and Natalie Goldberg advocate that journal writing can be done by anyone, anywhere.

Medical Professionals: People in the medical profession such as primary care doctors, specialists, physical therapists, and emotional therapists. Medical doctors Hilary Tindle and Lissa Rankin discuss that patients experience improved health when they have a positive outlook and a willingness to share their stories with their doctors.

Narrative Inquiry: Described by F. Michael Connelly and D. Jean Clandinin, narrative inquiry is a qualitative interpretative form of research which focuses on the telling, retelling, and sharing of stories.

Pain Journal: A journal describing symptoms designed to be shown to a medical professional.

Self-Compassion: The act of demonstrating the same kindness for oneself that one would demonstrate for other people.

Spirituality: Regardless of religion, spirituality and a belief in a higher power can lead to increased health and provide both hope and strength.

Writing as Healing: Numerous studies have been conducted investigating the influence of writing on physical and emotional health. James Pennebaker is a leader in the field which explores the health benefits of writing.

Writing Prompts: Questions used as starters to encourage writers to develop ideas.

Chapter 10
Narratives of Writing as Healing

Jennifer Lynne Bird
Oxbridge Academy, USA

Eric T. Wanner
Palm Beach Sports Medicine and Orthopaedic Center, USA

ABSTRACT

This narrative provides an introduction to the concept of multigenre writing and explains methods of multigenre writing used in the field of medicine to create the concept of multigenre medicine. The authors use the theory of narrative inquiry and the practice of multigenre writing to explain the implications of using writing to assist in healing from physical pain. The collaborative qualitative research project illustrates how writing can lead teachers to a stronger self-awareness of what patients need both physically and emotionally to heal.

PART I: INTRODUCTION TO WRITING AS HEALING (2012)

My name is Jen, and I live in a multigenre world. My education students at Florida Atlantic University love pointing to page 177 in Tom Romano's *Crafting Authentic Voice* and finding an example of their professor's writing. They love hearing the story that Tom Romano taught my teaching methods class at Miami University, the place where I first learned the amazing multigenre ideas I now share with them in my own teaching methods class.

DOI: 10.4018/978-1-7998-1931-8.ch010

During the past few years, my life settled into a predictable and comfortable pattern. Each semester my students read wonderful works of literature and created poems, scenes from characters' perspectives, mix CDs, artwork and various other innovative projects based on those wonderful works of literature. They wrote detailed rationales explaining their project choices and shared their masterpieces with classmates on presentation day. This was a day where I always skipped meals because several people in the class usually brought food for a genre connected to the text. My life and teaching progressed in a splendid manner until another twist of fate in my life led me to see multigenre writing as more than an academic research project. Multigenre writing became a way for me to help heal my physical pain. This is a story of using writing as healing told from the perspectives of both the patient and the physical therapist; the lessons learned from this experience led to additional research and advice to help others.

Background of Multigenre Writing

This chapter is an example of multigenre writing. Multigenre writing enables writers to see life from different perspectives. Romano (2000) defines the concept and explains, "a multigenre paper is composed of many genres and subgenres, each piece self-contained, making a point of its own, yet connected by theme or topic and sometimes by language, images, and content" (pp. x-xi). In the following pages you will read a first person narrative told from two perspectives and view artifacts such as a neck pain journal and a list of strategies of how you can apply life lessons from the narrative you read to your own life. You will also see everything tied together using the narrative thread of writing as healing. That's multigenre writing.

When asking my students to complete a multigenre research project, I want them to illustrate their knowledge of a topic using a variety of pieces. They design numerous creative projects, such as poems from the perspective of a character and artwork representing a scene, which demonstrate both their creativity and their comprehension of the text. Romano (1995) elaborates, "each genre offers me ways of seeing and understanding that others do not. I perceive the world through multiple genres. They shape my seeing. They define who I am" (p. 109). I love multigenre papers because I can see a text from multiple perspectives.

Multigenre projects provide for innovation typically not seen in traditional research projects while simultaneously retaining the analysis required of research. Romano (2008) continues, "a multigenre paper arises from research, experience, and imagination" (p. 184). I enjoy seeing my students' unique writing voices shine through in their writing. I learn more about each student's perspective and opinions when reading their multigenre projects than if I asked them to write a book report with no sense of voice. I also find it fun to complete my own multigenre research projects because they represent both the artistic and technical of writing. Multigenre papers provide the author with an opportunity for creativity while retaining the academic rigor associated with traditional research papers. In addition to providing multiple perspectives on a text such as a work of literature, I learned multigenre writing can provide additional insight into life experiences.

Background of Narrative Inquiry

Pain and I know each other well. My mom died an unexpected and tragic death during my time as a doctoral student. Refusing to sink under the weight of the emotional pain that gripped me, I used the theory of narrative inquiry as a lifeboat to help me heal. Connelly and Clandinin (2000) describe narrative inquiry as "stories lived and told" (p. 20). I forever remain grateful to my doctoral dissertation committee for giving me the opportunity to use writing as healing and complete a study that enabled me to tell the stories of other teachers as writers while simultaneously and most importantly living and telling my own story.

I used the theory of narrative inquiry and the practice of multigenre writing to analyze my story, as well as the stories of the teachers I interviewed. Romano (2000) argues, "theory about narrative thinking provides scholarly underpinning for multigenre writing" (p, 18). Both multigenre writing and narrative inquiry support the telling of stories as research. They encourage researchers to look not only outward at others but also inward at themselves and hold a mirror to their own lives. Clandinin and Connelly believe, "narrative inquiries are always strongly autobiographical. Our research interests come out of our own narratives of experience and shape our narrative inquiry plotlines" (p. 121). At the time I conducted my original narrative inquiry, I had no idea that a few years later I would need to critique my own life and eliminate patterns that caused me pain.

I felt emotionally drained after writing about issues related to the death of my mom. I also experienced a major life change by accepting a university job that transformed me from a high school English teacher in Ohio to a professor of future teachers in Florida. I felt happy as long as life remained calm and uneventful. Uneventful didn't last long for me. The ongoing stress in my life created pain in my neck, which resulted in the need for physical therapy.

In the qualitative interpretive research field of narrative inquiry, when we tell our life stories to other people, we choose how we frame and share information. We don't just share our stories with other people; for better or worse, the stories we retell ourselves can influence our perception of life. Clandinin and Connelly (2000) explain, "therefore, difficult as it may be to tell a story, the more difficult but important task is the retelling of stories that allow for growth and change" (p. 71). If I keep telling myself the same story, I am never going to change.

During my physical therapy for neck pain, if I told myself the story, "I am in a lot of pain right now," it would force me to dwell on how much I hurt. I needed to rewrite that story as, "I am in a lot of pain right now, but I am getting better." Even though I felt intense physical pain, my goal became to approach each therapy session with a positive attitude and a willingness to complete the lesson plan of exercises designed for me to help me feel better. Connelly and Clandinin (1988) suggest writing down stories and to "keep an open mind and try to see what patterns emerge" (p. 37). When I wrote down the stories of how I felt, it led to the creation of a neck pain journal and a new perspective on healing. Sometimes, however, we can't see the patterns of our own stories and need others to help us view the story from a new perspective.

The Importance of Writing While in Pain

My physical therapist, Dr. Eric Wanner, always took the time to answer my endless questions about why my neck felt a certain way and what exercises I could do to make it feel better. He also would not let me get away with telling him I felt fine when I didn't. It helped him plan my exercises and treatment if I assigned my pain level a number at the beginning of each session and gave some examples of what I did between sessions to make the pain feel better or worse.

One particular week I looked at the yellow flurry of post-it notes on which I wrote all my observations about my pain I wanted to tell Eric so I didn't forget anything. When presented with chaos my reaction becomes to organize everything. Because of the pain, just teaching my classes became a large effort leaving me with no energy to write any interesting articles. I missed writing. Cameron (1998) believes, "there is something very right about simply letting yourself write. And the way to do that is to begin, to begin where you are" (p. 5). So I grabbed a sheet of paper and assigned a high and low numeric value to my pain level for each day. I also wrote down what I was doing to cause the pain. Of course, my writing voice needed to shine through on paper. Instead of being content to write, "I did my exercises today," I wrote, "9:30pm + home from work late + still need to do second set of exercises = Neck Exercise Disco Dance Party!! Turn on Kylie Minogue CD for motivation and actually have to remind myself to slow down the exercises."

My neck pain journal entertained me, but I couldn't make any sense of why my neck hurt at certain times and not others. I didn't know how Eric was going to react to my writing, but Goldberg (2007) states, "trust what you put down, even if the editor or critic inside you says it's wrong or you made a mistake" (p. 2). In the past I placed drafts of my writing in progress on display for an entire class of students without even thinking about it, so an audience of one physical therapist shouldn't have worried me. This writing, however, seemed more personal. I couldn't eliminate things, because each piece of the neck pain puzzle might make more sense when all the pieces were examined as a whole.

I gave Eric a copy of my neck pain journal at my next physical therapy session. I don't remember the exact conversation, but it went something like this:

"This is your copy. I decided to write everything down in a neck pain journal."

"I like it."

"Really?"

"Looks like your neck hurts whenever you look down for a long period of time, and when you are under a lot of stress."

It impressed me that within minutes Eric looked over my writing and found a pattern to my neck pain. He adjusted the treatment plan that session and my neck felt better.

Too often writers censor themselves and prevent themselves from creating. Murray (1996) believes, "there is no censorship in the world as powerful as self-censorship" (p. 9). The narratives we tell ourselves sometimes cause us to not write something for fear of what others might think. A supportive audience can frequently see patterns in your writing and use that information to help you; consequently, you feel comfortable taking writing risks because you know you will have support. I agreed with Lamott (1994) who writes, "take the attitude that what you are thinking and feeling is valuable stuff, and then be naïve enough to get it all down on paper" (p. 113). It felt nice to know that whatever I wrote, Eric would use the information to help me. So I kept writing and Eric kept reading. My projects became more innovative as my sessions continued, and Eric liked them and continued to read every word. The collection of creative artifacts added to my chart included:

- A journal entry
- A collection of stories
- A flyer from the musical I performed in once I started feeling better
- A playlist of the songs I listened to while I did my exercises
- A picture of the beach where I went to relax
- A line graph charting my neck pain.

Without realizing it, throughout my treatment I wrote a multigenre paper. Romano (2004) describes the concept and illustrates "a multigenre paper is about a single topic but is composed of many different genres that hang together" (p. 34). I didn't start out to write a multigenre paper; the project evolved because I think about life in multiple genres in my classroom and that same thought process translated into the perspective I used to view my pain. Romano (2000) elaborates, "each genre is a color slide, complete in itself, possessing its own satisfying composition, but also working in concert with the others to create a single literary experience" (p. 4).

My journey to healing became comprised of an entire collection of projects illustrating how I felt on any given day. I wrote about my neck pain, my mom who died, and things that made me happy. I put together a playlist of the songs I listened to while doing my exercises and used the advertisement for the musical I would sing in once I healed to motivate me. I looked at the pictures I took at the beach to help me relax and designed a unique method of answering the question my physical therapist asked of how I was feeling.

I also noticed Eric wrote notes on all my projects and pulled together a narrative thread to diagnose my neck pain. Unlike traditional multigenre papers, I did not write my own end notes because I did not have the medical knowledge to make connections, which is why I appreciated Eric's expert knowledge. During the process of completing multigenre projects, students follow the example of Romano (1995) who "asked students to write a note page that explained some of the nitty-gritty, the ins and outs of particular pieces" (p. 142). When students write multigenre papers, they provide end notes of why they created a poem, mix CD, or drawing. With a medical issue such as my neck pain, I lacked the expertise to write my own end notes and felt grateful Eric saw the patterns and connections in my projects and used that information in a treatment plan that helped me heal. I often wondered what Eric really thought as I handed him pages of writing and other artifacts, so I decided to ask him.

A Physical Therapist's Perspective

My name is Eric and I am a Physical Therapist. I went to The Ohio State University for my bachelors in Exercise Science and then continued my education at The University of Dayton, where I completed my Doctor of Physical Therapy Degree.

In the DPT program at the University of Dayton they really stressed the importance of research as well as investigating several complex case studies to find the answers on our own. We then took an eclectic approach going over these studies together. In each case study we had to find out what was causing the patient's symptoms, how each medication could cause adverse reactions, whether or not the patient would need to be referred out to a specialist, their prognosis, how to come up with a treatment plan, goals, etc. I never truly understood the importance of this type of style, until getting into the workforce.

As a physical therapist, I like trying to put the pieces together in order to help patients heal the best they can. Sometimes all you have to do is listen. With Dr. Jennifer Bird, this was easy. She was very thorough with her thoughts and most importantly did not leave anything out while writing in her journal. Writing became part of her healing process. With that, it was easy to find contributing factors to what caused her neck pain and helped her stay motivated.

Like most patients, stress and the ergonomic environment were key components that caused her pain. Having stress can tighten key musculature and lead to more pain whether leading to headaches, referred pain, etc. For example, the muscles in the back of your neck can become more taut which may irritate a nerve and cause a headache. Or, one may have neck pain but it refers down from the neck, to their trapezius, and into their shoulder. Stress will only put more tension on these muscles causing them to pull more on the cervical spine, and again, lead to more pain. Also, as stated by Seaward (2012), "Stress has been linked to all the leading causes of death, including heart disease, cancer, lung ailments, accidents, cirrhosis, and suicide. Some health experts now speculate that perhaps as much as 70-85% of all diseases and illnesses are stress-related" (p. 4). Now do you see why it is very important to try to eliminate stress as much as possible? Those are only a few out of possible thousands of examples.

Jen was going through a lot and had to work long days while grading papers and writing. This created a lot of tension on her neck. Having to look down for a prolonged period of time can not only put more stress on the neck but can make the posture worse. Having poor posture can lead to more neck, upper back, and shoulder pain. It slowly turns into a snowball effect. I had Jen prop up her papers on top of two books while she was grading to see how that worked out for her. I asked her, and she said that she was able to grade longer with less neck pain! She then had her desk elevated to make sure that it was at the proper height so that she would not have to look too far down for several hours at a time.

I also stressed the importance of taking breaks and to "think like a turtle." The meaning behind thinking like a turtle is to try to take on one thing at a time. Realize that if you are doing a task while thinking about something else at the same time, it will not only be less productive, but also may experience more stress or tension. Stress is much more common than people realize. Harris's survey performed by the APA's Mind/Body Health Campaign showed that "most Americans are moderately to severely stressed and 44% stated that their stress levels are increasing" (http://www.apa.org/monitor/2011/01/stressed-america.aspx). Having a lot on your mind at one time most likely means that you are stressed. I told Jen to try to surround herself with as many things that make her feel happy as possible and eliminate as many stressors as she could. After doing so, her neck got much better (along with doing everything at Physical Therapy and her home exercises). Getting Jen back to being pain free would not have been possible without her staying motivated and writing down what she was going through each day to help us figure out her everyday stressors.

Keeping a positive outlook not only decreases stress but also increases compliance with exercises that one should be doing leading to elite results. Perhaps next time you are in pain it would be a good idea to write about it, to become more aware of what is causing you to be in more pain.

New Directions for Multigenre Projects

I told Eric he was the first person in my life to tell me to think like a turtle. In my professional education world (and admittedly in my personal life as well) people equate the name Jen with a multitasking whirlwind who probably hasn't taken on one thing at a time since earning teaching credentials. It's not uncommon. As teachers, we make numerous decisions every minute as we prepare lessons while assessing and reflecting on the reactions of the class of students in front of us. Eric discussed the value of listening; I realized I was listening to everyone except myself and what my body was trying to tell me. So "think like a turtle" became my mantra. I bought a turtle necklace at Target and wear it as a reminder to slow down and enjoy life instead of focusing on checking off items on a list.

I've designed more strategies to empower students so I have more time for creativity and less time grading papers. I started recording my comments about student essays as audio files and sending each student an email with the comments. They experience more insights when transcribing my advice and my neck thanks me for it. I'm not perfect at turtle thinking and at moments my former multi-tasking self resurfaces, but I've also experienced more moments of not worrying and overall feel happier.

As I lived my story, my primary focus became to heal. Only in the retelling of the story did I realize the possibility of using collaborative multigenre projects as healing. Multigenre writing gives us the opportunity to see life from different perspectives. Romano (1995) explains, "the multigenre research paper recognizes that there are many ways to see the world, many ways to show others what we see" (p. 130).

When multigenre projects are used as physical or emotional healing, the topic is your life. The genres you choose to tell the story are the ones that bring you both happiness and understanding. When I felt overwhelmed with pain, I needed to surround myself with people, places, and things that brought me joy in order to feel better. How did I know what would make me happy? According to Heard (1995), "with the map you've already made in your heart. That's where the real home is: inside" (p. 2).

For my final genre to show Eric on my last day of physical therapy, I designed a heart map. Picture a large heart drawn on a sheet of paper with a beautiful list written inside the heart of everything from my favorite songs to people I love. Thinking of my heart map and the journey that led to it makes me smile.

In sharing my story, I hope to inspire educators to think of new directions for multigenre projects in their personal lives as well as their professional lives. Writing reminds me of past loves and present dreams that can lead to future change. I knew multigenre projects helped my students transform the way they write. My learning experience occurred when I realized a multigenre project could transform the way I live.

As educators, we spend a significant time helping other people and often not enough time helping ourselves. Using multigenre projects to work through pain and finding an understanding audience can lead to powerful breakthroughs. Goldberg (1990) elaborates, "trusting your own mind is essential for writing" (p. 1). Trusting both myself and Eric was essential for helping me heal. I know not all patients arrive to treatment sessions like I did with various creative forms of expressing how they feel. I want to believe everyone in the medical field is as compassionate and open to new research ideas as Eric was when reading my writing, even though that may not be true. So perhaps my experience with using multigenre projects as a method of healing existed only in one physical therapy clinic during one moment in time. But in sharing stories, existing theories can transform into new practices which can help others and transform lives.

This is my multigenre journey. What's yours?

In narrative inquiries, there are always new chapters to stories. I hoped my writing could help me heal, but at the time I wrote my neck pain journal I didn't know that it would lead to helping other people and future possibilities for research. In the following conversation, Eric and I explain our future goals for using multigenre writing as healing. We also provide ideas of how you can apply advice from this story to your life.

Our narrative inquiry research about my healing led to another research idea. This research, which involves studying the relationships between patients writing down their feelings and their healing process, is ongoing and we hope to write more about it in future publications. It will be interesting and exciting to see how what we learn can contribute to both the fields of education and medicine.

Future Trends and Future Research: Eric's Perspective

While Jen was a patient of mine, she always expressed her interest in research and how she wanted to do something related to her multigenre writing in a medical type of setting. I myself, have a great interest in research, and thought that this idea could really lead to something positive with my patients. We decided to make this happen and designed a survey together to try to see how patients view different aspects of physical therapy during their treatments. This research is currently being done, but would not be possible if it was not for the writing that Jen did herself.

We both hope to do more research in the future to try to enable people to be able to freely express their feelings during a healing process, and see if it affects their recovery in a more positive way. When patients have a positive view during their recovery the thought is that they will be more willing to do their home exercises, try harder while in physical therapy, and thus accelerate their healing process. Hopefully this will open up the minds of clinicians on how to give each patient the best chance toward a full recovery.

Future Trends and Future Research: Jen's Perspective

While Eric was my physical therapist we always discussed research and writing. At the end of my treatment, I knew I would not miss the neck pain, but I realized how much I was going to miss those conversations. I enjoy research and my students and I discuss how writing helps people heal emotionally. Until I lived the experience, I didn't realize that expressing my feelings could also lead to physical healing. I also thought this idea could lead to something positive for other patients and like Eric said, we decided to make this happen.

We used Eric's expert knowledge in medicine and mine in writing to design a survey that provides a unique perspective of how patients view their physical therapy treatments. We both hope our current research project leads to more research and more writing that enables patients to share their feelings and enhance the recovery process for each patient.

Eric's Advice for Finding Time for Yourself

While reading through Jen's writing, I found a trend and gave her advice. She seems to do best in less stressful situations when she does not have ten different things going on at the same time. I gave her advice on how important it was to find time for herself. Is this possible to do when someone has a very hectic schedule, kids to take care of, and has to grade papers on top of this? Yes, and all the more reason to find time for yourself. Start by giving ten minutes to yourself a day. Put yourself in an environment that you enjoy where nothing is stressing you out.

I told Jen to watch comedies or listen to a song she really enjoyed to help her relax. Laughing increases your endorphin levels which help you feel good. After that, it will help you think clearer and allow you to tolerate things around you easier. Try this out yourself and you might just realize that it isn't too hard to find just ten minutes out of your day, and how much better you feel.

Jen's Advice for Finding Time for Yourself

Sometimes it takes someone else to tell you things you can't see for yourself. Eric noticed I always seem to have ten different things going on at once. I do struggle to say yes to myself and no to other things. I love helping people and often have the attitude that if I do one more thing, perhaps one more person's life will be better in my classroom or my community. Most teachers share this belief. In conversations with other teachers, the topic of the guilt we feel and the worry we have that we just aren't doing enough to help our students becomes a frequent topic of discussion. Nevertheless, I learned I cannot sacrifice my health or my happiness for other people. Now I try to do less but live more in the present moment instead of always checking my calendar; this attitude does lead to clearer thinking. So I watched more comedies, listened to songs I enjoyed, and realized Eric's advice should be adopted by teachers.

Find ten minutes a day to relax! You will feel better as you continue your life's journey.

Advice for Educators

Hopefully this story inspires you to take a look at the educator in the mirror and examine your own story. It may also inspire you to complete some writing of your own. Goldberg (2000) elaborates, "writing is an immediate mirror: it reports back to you. You can't fool anyone, especially yourself" (p. 218). Those of us in helping professions frequently give our time and energy to others without leaving anything for ourselves. Writing provides an opportunity for reflection. Some educators complain they have no time during a busy day for reflection, but reflection becomes a method to get in touch with ourselves and think about what went well during a day and also what could be improved. Graves (2001) writes, "teaching is an emotional roller coaster" (p. 1). Anyone who has been in a classroom or any other education profession experiences the highs and lows that result from frequent interactions with others.

Sometimes it becomes easy to worry about everyone except ourselves because we are trained to focus on the problems of others and not our own. Johnson (1998) explains, "teaching can steal your time and sap your physical and emotional energy very quickly, so it's important to conserve your precious resources whenever possible." (p. 259). But how often do we actually do this? We're guessing not enough.

Be honest. Are you reading this right now and thinking of the ten other items on your to do list? Or maybe you are thinking there just aren't enough hours in the day. Or maybe you aren't thinking much of anything because you are too tired. There will always be one more student to help, one more paper to grade, or one more patient that needs attention. The more time we give, the more people we can help. However, who is that really helping by having that mentality? As Gold and Roth (1993) point out, "stress and burnout are so prevalent in teaching that they have an enormous detrimental effect on the teaching-learning process. Stress and burnout may be viewed as disabilities which are manifest in teachers performing far below their maximal potential, regardless of how well prepared and committed they are" (p. vii).

If you aren't helping yourself, it makes it more difficult to help anyone else. Graves (2001) argues, "awareness that grows out of the specifics of your own situation produces energy" (p. 11). To become more aware of the events in your life, it may help to write down everything you do in a day and see where in your schedule you can find a few extra minutes. If you don't think that you can pencil in time after doing this, do it anyway. Sometimes it's not just a matter of finding time, but more so making time. It may also help for you to write down how you are feeling about your daily experiences. Goldberg (1986) describes of writing, "it is an opportunity to write down, without thinking, wishes at the periphery of our perceptions" (p. 59). What do you really want? Writing can help you find the answers.

Everyone has obligations. Even though it is impossible to spend every minute of every day doing things that you want to do, if you are not spending any time with people and things that bring you joy you will not be as happy. Those of you who are teachers can also be a writing role model for your students. If students know their teacher is writing, they will be more likely to complete writing of their own. Romano (1987) argues, "but despite the demands of my job and the impossibility of writing with my students each time they do, I must and can show my students I write" (p. 48). Writing leads to increased self-awareness, whenever a teacher encourages a student to write a multigenre project about a work of literature, a doctor encourages a patient to write down symptoms, or you write your thoughts and feelings to connect with yourself.

With narrative inquiry and multigenre writing, stories lead to other stories. Life stories will always be ongoing. The next chapter in your story is still unwritten, but you can live it with a greater self-awareness of how you are feeling during the journey and offer others more in return. As the authors of this chapter, we also look forward to seeing how the next chapter of our writing and research unfolds with exciting possibilities for the future.

PART II: CONNECTING MULTIGENRE WRITING TO MEDICINE (2014)

Multigenre perspectives present two sides of a story as researchers live their narratives through creative genres and then step back to report on the research, much like a journalist reporting the news. When we write, our words on the page capture who we are. We need to trust our words. Too often, the self-censor wonders what other people will think. Quindlen (2004) advises journalism students, "but still I urge them to write, uncompensated, even if they have no plans to become writers, for one reason only, and that is to know themselves, for now and for later. Their written words are their personal histories, as they have been mine" (p. 233). But it always remains our choice whether or not to share our writing with anyone. All writers have written words that no one ever sees, that are hidden in a storage box or ripped up and destroyed. Because, in those instances, keeping the writing private is what the writer needs. But sharing the writing can also be beneficial. Writing gives others a glimpse into our hopes, dreams, and personalities. It can give medical professionals insights into how we feel so they can design a treatment plan that can help us. It helps friends, acquaintances, or even strangers who are experiencing similar events in their lives to find strength in our stories.

This is the tension Jen experienced when she began experiencing migraine headaches two years after writing the original chapter about her neck pain journal. She had just started her health coach certification program at Duke Integrative Medicine. The irony was that she was training to counsel patients on dealing with their own health issues while experiencing one of her own. She was supposed to be listening to the stories of other people, not adding another one of her stories to the collection. How she viewed her story would influence her healing.

Jen's Journal

I cannot believe I am going to be a physical therapy patient again. The irony is that I have no neck pain, but I can't live with these migraines. My cousin Robin asked if stress was causing them, but I'm relaxed and content with my life. Seriously, in the past few days I've made egg salad, a pizza, a vegetable dish, and an apple crisp. When I create edible meals it means I am not stressed. Since Eric is now working at the hospital he can't be my physical therapist, so he is recommending that I see his colleague Ryan. I'm really hoping this pain doesn't get so bad that I end up in the hospital, although there were a couple nights when my head hurt bad enough to consider it. Ryan was Eric's student awhile ago and Eric has complete confidence in Ryan's ability to relieve my symptoms. Robin's going to physical therapy with Ryan too so we will have fun (and provide Ryan with hours of entertainment) scheduling our physical therapy sessions together and cheering each other on when doing exercises. It's exciting knowing that I will be going to a very good physical therapist in a clinic right across the street from where I live. There are too many other patients Eric and I need to save with our research and writing for me to be in the hospital! Although Eric and Ryan are constantly reminding me I need to take care of myself before I take care of other people. The weird thing is that my original neck pain journal led to this research and writing journey, but now I can't even keep a pain journal. The pain is ALL THE TIME! AHHHHHH!!!!

Now if only I could sleep……

Back to Sleep

Lucy the cat knows

Whenever Jen can't sleep, Lucy is there

She curls up next to her person and starts purring

Lucy's brother Andy runs around in a circle chasing his tail

He stops his game and joins Lucy to start a chorus of purrs

Jen's breathing slows and for a moment forgets her pain

Thanks to pet therapy

Animals Provide Comfort

Dr. David Dosa, a geriatrician, witnessed the story of Oscar the cat when checking on patients at a nursing home. Oscar, a cat who lived in the nursing home, sensed which elderly patients were the sickest and about to die, so he would visit their rooms, curl up next to them on their beds, and provide comfort. Dosa (2010) reports that "I'd like to think Oscar embodies empathy and companionship. He is a critical cog in a well-oiled and dedicated health care team" (p. 218). Animals may not have medical training, but they know when they are needed.

Eric's Perspective

The beauty of this situation by having Jen go through these symptoms, she will have more of an understanding what my patients may be going through when coaching them. Having an understanding of what patients feel versus memorizing from a textbook what they should be feeling makes a significant difference. If patients understand that you went through a similar situation that they are going through, they will be much more willing to listen what you have to say and actually be compliant for what you recommend. Jen will also be able to explain things more accurately from a firsthand perspective. Will writing about headaches always cure it? No. It depends on the situation for what's causing it, but it could lead to physicians and physical therapists making more accurate diagnoses for the patient. On top of that, when patients write about their symptoms including their outlook it has been shown to decrease their stress levels, increase self-awareness, and increase goal setting which in turn can speed up their recovery process. This eclectic approach is where healthcare should be going.

Jen's Perspective

Healthcare does need an eclectic approach. The Wheel of Health from Duke Integrative Medicine (2010) encourages patients to reflect on multiple dimensions of health including movement, exercise and rest; nutrition; personal and professional development, physical environment; relationships and communication; spirituality; mind-body connection; and mindful awareness

(p. 5). This makes health become a comprehensive plan that focuses on the person, not just the disease. I didn't want to be a patient and experience pain again, but it is amazing seeing both sides of the story from perspective of patient and health coach. It is going to make me a better clinician. Eric and I have learned about the power of writing to influence healing from our research. I love that I am going to be able to use my writing training to help patients in a clinic as well as students in a classroom. However, I've learned that writing is not the only answer. My cousin Robin loves writing, but music motivates her more. So a "PT CD mix" of music to motivate her to do her at home exercises inspired her more than a journal. Other patients may want to use painting, watching sitcoms, or reading an inspirational book as resources to help them heal. I also had to adjust my own expectations. With my original neck pain journal, I wrote information that helped Eric find patterns to my pain. With my migraines, creating that style of journal didn't work because the headaches were constant, so my notes to Ryan about how I felt after each physical therapy session helped him the most. Clinicians achieve success with treatment plans by individualizing them for each patient.

Acrostic Poem About Migraines

Maddening

Intolerable

Gigantic

Relentless

Agitating

Inflexible

Nonstop

Endless

Text Message Conversation Recalled from Memory

Eric: I just sent you a few different sites about headaches. Let me know which one sounds more like your symptoms. Seems like it could be cervicogenic.

Jen: So my neck could be causing my headaches? Headache sounds like cervicogenic.

Eric: If cervicogenic, you may still have some facet restrictions or over-facilitated musculature without pain due to the posture teachers naturally tend to be in while grading papers.

Jen: I'm still taking your advice and propping papers on a pile of books when grading them. It helps me not look down as much and makes writing comments on essays easier too.

Eric: There are many more things that can cause this type of headache, but those would be most likely for you since the imaging and tests came back unremarkable.

Jen: It was a relief that the MRI and all the other diagnostics came back normal, and given my history of neck pain it makes sense that there is a connection.

Eric: Facet restrictions can also lead to over-facilitated muscles which in turn can put pressure on upper cervical nerve roots or peripheral nerves causing a headache.

Jen: Thanks so much! Stupid facet joints! The weird thing is I have no neck pain.

Eric: Headaches don't always make sense. They can be very tricky to diagnose. With your past history of neck pain though, I wouldn't be surprised if this was the case. Might want to ask your physician what they think about doing physical therapy to help your symptoms.

And Now a Word from the Medical Dictionary

According to the North American Spine Society (2014), "headache caused by neck problems is called cervicogenic or neck-related headache. It may be caused by injury to an upper cervical disc, facet joint or higher joints called the atlanto-occipital or atlanto-axial joints. Cervicogenic headache can also make migraines worse" (http://www.knowyourback.org/Pages/SpinalConditions/Injuries/Whiplash.aspx).

Jen's Journal

Ryan thinks my atlantoaxial joint is out of alignment, which could be causing the migraines. He suggested I look it up if I wanted more information, and he's probably not surprised I'm writing about it. Thanks to Ryan's physical therapy treatment plan, I had my first headache free day in three months. I've been on five different medications that didn't help much, and it makes sense. Medicine wouldn't put this joint back where it belongs. Finally, I have hope.

Conversations in Physical Therapy Clinics (Theory)

In order for physical therapists to effectively treat patients, it helps them to know their patients' stories. This helps the physical therapist properly diagnose patients, determine their prognosis, and development an appropriate intervention. By learning patients' stories, physical therapists can also help patients set goals. Randall and McEwen (2000) discuss the value of physical therapists collaborating with patients to write patient-centered functional goals and elaborate, "physical therapists who incorporate a patient-centered approach to writing functional goals may see a change in how they interact with their patients and the decisions they make regarding patient care. Therapists may spend more time getting to know their patients and the self-care, work, or leisure activities that are important to them" (p. 1202). Clinicians need to believe in the value of goal setting and take time to discover a patient's story. When the patient sets out goals it brings them more onboard to achieving them and increases accountability for the patient.

Most patients want to know that their clinician understands them and cares about them as individuals, not just names on charts. As Croft (1980) explains, "the therapist does not need to accept each patient's beliefs and values as his own in order to be empathetic toward that patient. What is important is that the patient has something to say that is important to him at that time. The therapist, then, needs to convey to the patient that nothing at the moment is more important to him than listening to and helping the patient as much as possible" (p. 1034). Because when a patient is in pain, having an empathetic clinician who listens becomes essential. This can also increase the patient's outlook for their recovery process, allow the patient to become more optimistic, work harder at reaching their goals, and increase their compliance. All of those combined leads to a quicker recovery!

Conversations in Physical Therapy Clinics (Practice)

While it is not possible every day due to their busy schedules, at least once a week Jen and Robin schedule their physical therapy sessions at the same time. Of course neither one of them wanted to be in pain, but since the situation is what it is, it helps to have a family member who cares about you and cheers you on during your recovery from pain. We seem to be entertaining our physical therapist Ryan too with our different personalities. Ryan and Robin are enjoying talking about concerts they've attended while he gives her instructions for exercises, while Jen needs the occasional reminder from both of them to relax while she does her exercises (she remembers Eric's advice to "think like a turtle" and make slow and steady progress). Ryan shares this sentiment. While Jen and Robin relax with moist heat packs on physical therapy tables next to each other, Ryan reminds both of them that it took time for the pain to occur, so it is going to take time to heal too.

Definition of Thinking like a Turtle

Turtle Thinking (n): Slowing down and realizing the healing process is a journey. Can also be used as a slang phrase. Example: If someone says, "think like a turtle," to you, it probably means you are moving too fast or multitasking too much. Slow down.

Eric's advice to Jen during physical therapy: "Think like a turtle."

Ryan's advice to Jen during physical therapy: "Relax."

Robin's advice to Jen as her cousin: "Laugh."

Headache Journal

For any patient in pain, it can help clinicians make a diagnosis if the patient keeps a journal of symptoms. Dr. Hagen and the Mayo Clinic Staff (2001) recommend that for recurrent headaches, keep a headache diary and include the following factors: severity, frequency and duration, related symptoms, location, family history, and triggers (p. 83). But don't feel you need to follow a specific format if a different writing style works for you.

Jen's Journal

Pain free for four days after Wednesday's PT session!!! Yay!!! Dull headache started Sunday after church when I looked down while praying (oh, the irony.....) I know the fast neck movement triggered it, but it is still only a dull ache instead of a sharp pain. Have not needed pain medicine indomethacin in a week and this morning neurologist said that if the cortisone shot and PT is working I can stop taking pain medicine unless needed. I forgot what it is like to be pain free!!!

Beach Picture Break

In the book, this photo will appear in black and white, but try to imagine the beautiful colors of sunrise at the beach. Jen took this photo at Carlin Park in Jupiter, Florida on a Saturday morning as the sun was rising over the Atlantic Ocean. The stairs leading through the trees to the sand symbolize the journey patients often feel when the pain fades away and healing leads to new possibilities. Eric once said the beach can be healing, but even if you live nowhere near a beach you can search for places of tranquility and serenity to bring you peace.

Using The Wanner Bird Healing Survey for Pain Recovery for Health Coaching

Physical pain hurts, but the way patients share their pain narratives can lead to either more or less emotional pain. As Beck (2003) explains, "therapists from a branch of psychology called ACT (short for Acceptance and Commitment Theory) coined the terms 'clean pain' and 'dirty pain' to refer to suffering that comes from real events, as opposed to suffering that comes from the stories we tell ourselves about those events" (p. 37). Beck describes clean pain as a person's actual pain and dirty pain as a reflection of what the person thinks about the actual pain. She concludes, "in other words, most of your pain comes not from reality, but from your stories about reality" (p. 38). Health coaching and conversations about the responses to both written and numerical subjective questions can help patients illuminate the health stories they tell themselves. Health coaching can also build a bridge between helping patients decode complex medical terms and comprehending their treatment plan.

Figure 1. Photograph by Jennifer Bird of the beach of Carlin Park in Jupiter, Florida

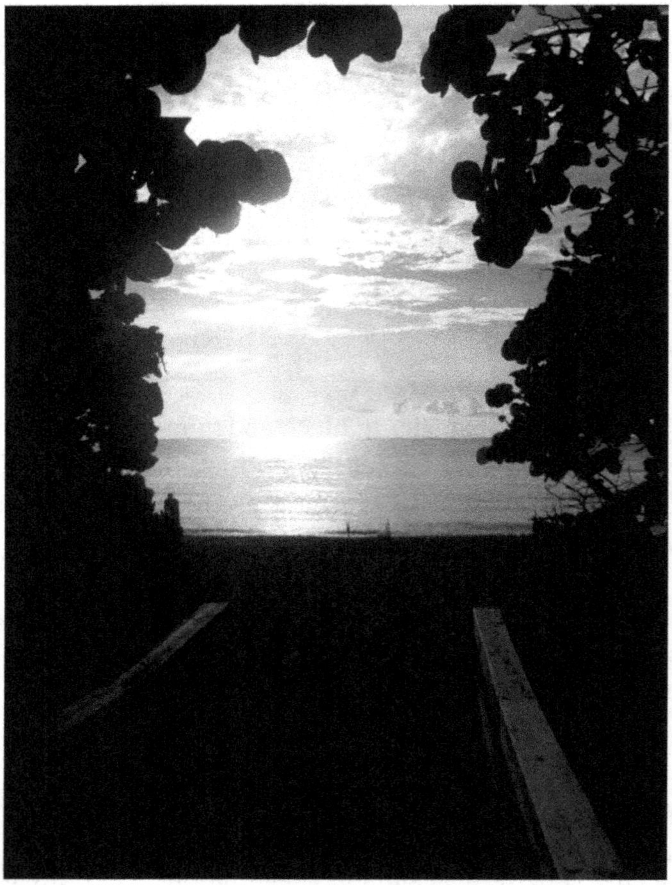

Brown (2010) argues, "our stories are not meant for everyone. Hearing them is a privilege, and we should always ask ourselves this before we share: 'Who has earned the right to hear my story?' (p. 47). When patients feel that their medical practitioners and health coaches earn the right to hear their stories, the sharing of narratives can become healing conversations.

Eric and Jen combined their expertise in the fields of medicine and writing to design *The Wanner Bird Healing Survey for Pain Recovery*. They completed a successful research project with Dr. Claudia Jayne Brahler at the University of Dayton that they hope to publish in a physical therapy journal discussing the numerical subjective and written subjective questions they asked physical therapy patients to complete. The study illustrated that patients with a strong positive outlook and a clear articulation of goals scored higher on existing objective physical therapy measures.

However, due to the busy pace of the physical therapy clinic environment, patients wrote their answers to the written subjective and numeric subjective questions but did not have the opportunity to discuss their answers with anyone. After she began her training to become a health coach, Jen wondered if talking to patients about their answers to survey questions would add another dimension to *The Wanner Bird Survey for Pain Recovery*. Robin began physical therapy for reversal of increased cervical lordosis. The cervical spine naturally has a lordotic curvature to it. This cannot be reversed; however, if it has an increased lordotic curvature, the muscles can stabilize it better and put the spine in a more efficient postural position. Jen's original plan was to practice asking Robin the survey questions before she needed to coach strangers about their health goals as part of her clinical internship. This was not a research project, although Robin's answers would provide answers into future research possibilities. Because of her migraines, Jen ended up also completing the survey questions she and Eric wrote during her own physical therapy treatment.

Remember to Laugh

For the survey question of what helped her most in physical therapy, here is part of Jen's answer: "I love being encouraged to laugh and have fun with my exercises. I can be a very serious person so the reminder to lighten up will help me and my patients as a health coach." Ryan believes in the value of humor, because laughter makes a difference if patients aren't excited about being in physical therapy. It's true that most adults don't find time in their lives to laugh. As Beck (2003) writes, "consider that a typical small child laughs over four hundred times a day. For the average adult, the number is a paltry fifteen" (p. 152). Whenever patients are getting too serious at the clinic, Ryan will lighten the mood by telling jokes. He once set several timers to go off at once (and admitted that a similar joke was Eric's introduction to his sense of humor on the first day they ever worked together).

Robin has renamed the chin tuck exercises that are part of her home exercise plan, "the double chin exercises" so she smiles when she does them. Jen was also forced to laugh at herself when she said "I love you" to her cousin Robin on the way out of the clinic one day. The other patients and physical therapists joked if she knew Robin or was just going around telling random strangers at the clinic that she loved them! Beck discusses the healing value of laughter and explains, "laughter – even the anticipation of laughter – shifts our internal chemistry measurably, reducing stress hormones and increasing the number of natural virus-killer cells available to fight disease from colds to cancer. It also triggers the release of endorphins, hormones that lessen the perception of distress and make us feel fabulous. The cliché is true; laughter really is good medicine – so much so that some hospitals have 'laugh mobiles' that hand out videotaped comedy routines and squirt guns to their patients" (p. 154). So consider that watching your favorite comedy on television may not be a waste of time; the laughter may just help you heal.

And in the End

Jen and Robin both healed from their pain with Ryan's help. Jen and Eric worked at the same hospital and researched the benefits of health coaching for physical therapy patients. Concluding a narrative inquiry feels similar to leaving the theater before the end of a play, but then the researcher must have faith there will be other stories to tell and other chapters to write.

By writing those chapters in a multigenre format, like this chapter, writers see and share such stories from multiple perspectives. As Gruwell (1999) writes of her students, the Freedom Writers, "I realized that in order for them to grow, they had to branch out and explore new ground" (p. 273). This statement applies not only to students in a writing classroom, but also patients in a clinic. While it certainly helps to have a health coach guiding you through the process, all patients can benefit from a reminder they have the power to write the next chapter in their lives and achieve their optimal health visions.

PART III: JEN'S REPRISE OF PAIN IN A HAIKU (2019)

Wake up with headache

Occipital neuralgia

Pain journal again

And Now a Word from the Medical Dictionary

According to the National Institute of Neurological Disorders and Stroke (2019), "occipital neuralgia is a distinct type of headache characterized by piercing, throbbing, or electric-shock-like chronic pain in the upper neck, back of the head, and behind the ears, usually on one side of the head. Typically, the pain of occipital neuralgia begins in the neck and then spreads upwards" (https://www.ninds.nih.gov/Disorders/All-Disorders/Occipital-Neuralgia-Information-Page)

And in the Beginning

Occipital Neuralgia. Inflamed nerves which cause headaches. Once again, my headaches and neck pain required medical attention. This time, however, an MRI scan revealed a herniated disc in my neck which also pressed on a nerve. Hence, the headaches and neck pain. Usually I feel positive, but this seemed overwhelming. I followed the advice of Arioto (2019), who believes, "life is short, too short to spend our time dwelling on mistakes or what we don't have. Too short to feel like a shell of a human being, going through the motions but never really living" (p. 175). I needed to stop dwelling on the pain and start focusing on my treatment plan to fix it. But first, I had to find the energy. Graves (2001) feels, "emotional roller coasters demand energy – high energy – and you need to know how to maximize what gives you energy and minimize what takes it away" (p. 2). Graves discusses teaching in this example, but the same words apply to dealing with a complicated medical situation. I knew I had minimum energy when going to various medical specialists; I knew I had maximum energy when writing. So it made sense to balance something that gave me energy with something that took it away.

Because I had a complex case, I needed to become a prepared patient. In her nursing career working with patients, Goldberg (2019) advises, "a provider's license to practice medicine does not mean that they know you or your body best. They will come to better decisions about how to use their expertise if you meet them in making decisions about your health" (p. 7). So I made the decision: *All right, medical professionals. You will see me. You will know me.*

I chose a new journal, one with black and gold sequins, and started taking notes. When discussing writing as healing, Pennebaker (1997) states, "planning to show your writing to someone can affect your mind-set while writing" (p. 41). Throughout my years of teaching, I watch my students write with more confidence if they can practice writing techniques in their journals before showing me the final draft of their essays. Writers do write differently when we know we will share our writing. Pennebaker continues, "from a health perspective, you will be better off making yourself the audience. In that way, you don't have to rationalize or justify yourself to suit the perspective of another person" (p. 41). In the case of my pain journal, however, I needed to share it so the medical providers I saw could help me. I wrote my notes in my black and gold sequined journal, typed up the relevant information, and handed it to the receptionist at each medical office. I also kept a copy for myself and I took notes during each appointment. I felt like Niequist (2016), who writes, "brave is articulating my feelings, especially when the feelings are sad or scared or fragile instead of confident or happy or light" (p. 126). Sharing writing made an emotionally and physically painful process easier. I felt scared, but I also refused to let my health issues define me.

Reflections on Research

At the commencement of my writing as healing odyssey, I could not predict the amount I would learn on my journey to become pain free. I also could not predict the new insights I would have about the research when becoming a patient again: People feel vulnerable when sharing stories with others, pain can change patient perception, bullet points can provide reflection for people who prefer not to write journal entries, it becomes essential to find your motivation, and practicing self-care becomes necessary when feeling pain.

VIBES

I could control the vibe I gave during treatment. In theory, I should act calm whenever I walked into an exam room. In practice, I would sometimes act stressed and anxious. To remember the lessons I learned when confronting chronic pain, I used the acronym VIBES.

Vulnerability helps you.
Identify your emotions.
Bullet journals share information.
Embrace your why.
Self-care matters.

Patient Lesson #1: Vulnerability Helps You

As a patient, I needed to be my own best advocate. Yes, this specialist is recommending that treatment, but is it the best thing for me? Agreeing to have an occipital nerve block injection in both sides of my neck caused fear with the procedure, and more fear when I still felt pain. Goldberg (2019) explains to patients, "vulnerability and distress intensify when we don't know the source of the pain, the symptom, or the side effect" (p. 159). Each time I needed to share my story, I needed to find the courage to share my story. Seeking medical help means being vulnerable. Sitting on an examination table while having my reflexes tested and often having to wear a medical gown does not instill the same confidence I feel when sitting behind my classroom desk, looking professional while wearing my sassy high heels and ready to conquer the world (or at least whatever student dramas unfold that day).

Writing teacher Romano (2015) believes, "in writing we seek to capture some of this experience of living" (p. 4). While those of us who are English teachers see the value of narratives in our lives and our classrooms, most people who seek medical help do not share an English teacher's perspective on writing. It takes vulnerability to share writing with others, whether the person reading the writing is an English teacher looking through a student's journal in a classroom or a physical therapist looking over a patient's insights about pain in a clinic.

Vulnerability often prevents people from speaking, even if they know that sharing information can help them. In her research as a social worker, Brown (2007) describes times when people have told her they share too much with someone and later regret "what I call the vulnerability hangover. The vulnerability hangover directly relates to our fear of vulnerability, and unfortunately, most of us have experienced it" (p. 206). If someone showed vulnerability in the past and experienced rejection, the person will feel even more vulnerable when sharing again. I experienced a moment of vulnerability hangover when I shared my original neck pain journal with Eric. My thoughts at the time: I have just shared with this physical therapist more about my life than he probably ever wanted to know. Fortunately, Eric responded as a compassionate clinician and actually encouraged me to share more. Anyone on the receiving end of writing needs to demonstrate compassion or the writer will no longer want to share. I feel grateful Eric demonstrated compassion with me as a patient, and I remind myself to demonstrate compassion with my students as a teacher.

Patient Lesson #2: Identify Your Emotions

As a patient, I didn't always feel positive. I knew a positive attitude would help me heal, although sometimes pain makes positivity difficult. Physical and emotional pain can eclipse other feelings. Dooley (2019) writes, "I want to live my story, even the hard and long and messy days" (p. 211). I needed to accept the difficult days in addition to the happy ones and give myself permission to feel what I felt.

Making sure to monitor that my mood did not cross into depression, I accepted the occasional sad days and knew some days I would feel happier than others. A medical explanation exists for this as Rankin (2013) explains, "the stress response also reduces serotonin, the most important neurotransmitter responsible for a positive mood" (p. 134). When I feel pain, my internal narrative resembles the following: I'm in pain. Why won't the pain go away? This is so annoying! Therefore, pain clouds my judgement even when I know to maintain a positive attitude, seek medical attention, and write my symptoms so I can help my doctor help me. According to Tindle (2013), one change makes a difference because, "regardless of how dark our own health situation has been and regardless of for how long, even the spark of one idea to do things differently can light our path to better health" (p. 134). So once again, vulnerability becomes necessary because if I can't find the optimism and courage to make that change, I need to ask for help and lean on others to serve as the light in the dark as I progress through my healing journey.

Feeling gratitude keeps me grounded and can improve my mood. As Brown (2012) shares from one of her studies, "research participants consistently described both joyfulness and gratitude as spiritual practices that were bound to a belief in human connectedness and a power greater than us" (p. 123). Stopping in the moment of pain to appreciate the red Poinciana flowers on the tree outside my window or the two purring cats, Lucy and Andy, who sit next to me and play with their toy mice as I write these words can be enough to interrupt my negative pain thoughts and redirect them into more positive ones. Anything that provides even a little bit of light or joy, whatever that may be for you, can be enough to get you through until you feel better.

Patient Lesson #3: Bullet Journals Share Information

As a patient, I learned I did not have much of a doctor's time. Therefore, as much as I liked narratives and sharing my story, I needed to quickly get to the point. My new pain journals contained bold headings and bullet points describing my medical history and symptoms. The specialists I with whom I shared them found the notes helpful because of the details and context.

When rereading the original notes that Eric and I completed, I noticed we used the process of bulleted, organized lists now known as dot journals. According to Wilkerson Miller (2017), "dot journaling helps you record all of the things that are going on in your life, and makes it easy to keep track of everything you want to do in the future" (p. 8). Our note system helped keep track of current patient symptoms and future goals. Since the original research, dot journals, also known as bullet journals, experienced growth in popularity. Carroll (2018) describes a bullet journal as, "it will help you get organized by providing simple tools and techniques that can inject clarity, direction, and focus into your days" (p. 11). Bullet journals provide another resource for patients, since the writer can complete a bulleted list instead of a longer narrative in a journal. Patients might find completing a bullet journal easier because it does not take as much time and looks more like a list than a written narrative. Some patients may feel more comfortable sharing observations in a list format.

Patient Lesson #4: Embrace Your Why

As a patient, I needed to find reasons to stay motivated. Knowing why you want something, not just what you want, leads to achieving a goal. Hollis (2019) explains, "you have to have the leverage – you have to know your why – or you will never make change. You have to know what to focus on, or you will never make progress" (p. 107). I knew my why: I want to kick this pain into oblivion and be healthy so I can do the things I love to do with my family and friends. I needed to keep that goal in front of me on the days when I felt frustrated or the pain felt worse. Soukup (2019) believes, "it's not enough to set big goals; we have to know why they're important to us. Because truthfully? If you don't know your why, your reason may not justify the sacrifices you need to make to get there" (p. 148). The why of this writing and research journey started as a way to help me cope with the emotional pain of losing my mom and later the physical pain in my neck joints. It would have been enough that my writing helped me. But what if my writing could help other people through difficult experiences?

My sense of purpose transformed into using my passion for writing to help others. Leonard (2018) describes her writing experience as, "I picked up my journal to write down thoughts that had come to me while I was walking. My journaling started as random words, disconnected thoughts, and sometimes even sketches. But after a couple days, my thoughts were beginning to take shape" (p. 224). The description of my journal would sound similar, but what if I found the courage to share and find a narrative thread to my random thoughts? I find the courage every day I teach to discuss writing with students; maybe other people would listen too. Hollis (2018) advises people going through pain, "you are a warrior because of the trials you are going through, but don't you dare squander the strength you have earned just because the acquisition of it was painful. Those are the most important stories to share" (pp. 68-69). If my story inspires someone else, the pain I lived through will have purpose and the power to provide comfort for others as they write their narratives.

Patient Lesson #5: Self-Care Matters

As a patient, I needed to let myself feel a range of emotions. I would feel confident when sharing my story in a medical office, but break down and cry when I returned home. I would feel energetic when swimming in the pool to loosen my muscles, but exhausted and needing to rest an hour later because of a headache and neck pain. Soukup (2016) provides the reminder, "we discovered that while we often think balance is something we can do, balance actually happens when we stop doing and just rest" (p. 180-181). I gave myself permission to remove items from my calendar. I became determined to create positive moments during the time I felt well. I invited my dad, stepmom, aunts, uncles, and cousins over for an indoor picnic. I laughed, I cried, and I prayed.

While I respond to others with compassion and appreciate when I receive compassion, I am my own worst critic and don't always show myself compassion. Neff and Germer (2018) elaborate, "although a simple way to think about self-compassion is treating yourself as you would treat a good friend, the more complete definition involves three core elements that we bring to bear when we are in pain: self-kindness, common humanity, and mindfulness" (p. 10). When I am in pain, it can feel difficult to remain present, know that other people experience pain too, and show myself kindness. On some days, I feel I still need to learn the value of being kind to myself and practicing self-care. Pink (2018) explains, "imagine what someone who cares about you might say. He would likely be more forgiving than you" (pp. 143-144). He adds, "but mix understanding with action. Add a few sentences on what changes you can make to your life and how you can improve in the future" (p. 144). Whether setting a goal for a physical therapy treatment plan or another part of life, it becomes important to combine reflection with action.

Eric once told me to "think like a turtle." Similarly, writing often takes time to work. Grant (2016) elaborates, "James Pennebaker has demonstrated that expressing our thoughts and feelings about a stressful or traumatic event is most salutary after we've had some time to process the event, when we're not blinded by anger or consumed by distress" (p. 240). Trying to write in a journal after an injury, life changing event, or other emotional experience may not be effective because processing an event takes time. I couldn't write anything immediately after my mom's death, and I did not arrive with a pain journal during my first physical therapy session with Eric. Writing became part of my emotional and physical healing only after I began to process the original trauma. Sandberg and Grant (2017) explain, "immediately after a tragedy or crisis, journaling can backfire: the event is too raw for some to process" (p. 63). Pain often prevents a person from writing. So if writing doesn't initially work, the pain may be too new; put the notebook down for awhile and pick up a pen again when ready.

Jen's Journal

It's exhausting having a low grade headache all the time, in addition to neck pain. When I finished physical therapy the last time, I thought that would be the end of needing physical therapy. I'm learning that life, like healing, is a journey. I love being a high school writing and reading center director and don't feel stressed, but my neck is telling me a different story. I'm grateful to be at the clinic where Eric is a director working with an outstanding physical therapy team of Dak and David. My new neck pain bullet journals are entertaining Dak, and the entire clinic team creates a fun environment for doing exercises.

Haiku of Revelation

Journal advocate

But when a patient in pain

Writing takes effort

Moment of Insight

For fun, I answered the survey questions Eric and I designed and compared it to my responses when I had headaches five years ago. Interestingly, I wrote similar responses.

August 2014: For the question of being close to achieving my short term goals, I circled a 3 (in the middle) for the numerical subjective question and for the written subjective question wrote: "My goals are still to be healthy and free of migraines! I am optimistic I can follow the treatment plan and get there."

August 2019: For the question of being close to achieving my short term goals, I circled a 3 (in the middle) for the numerical subjective question and for the written subjective question wrote: "I still have the goal of being pain free and realized healing takes time."

Later, when asked to identify obstacles, I admitted (both then and now) I needed to relax. I also found it interesting that while by numerical responses stayed the same, my narratives changed slightly. My writing five years ago was more optimistic than my recent writing, but maybe too optimistic? Maybe I'm more realistic now? Since Eric and I designed the survey, more patient education exists about the value of narratives. As a medical practitioner, Goldberg (2019) advises patients, "it's helpful to create a narrative or story around the situation prior to going to the appointment. This will give your symptoms context and provide meaning to the timeline, and you'll naturally equip your provider with key information you may not even realize is relevant" (p. 123). She advises practitioners, "it is vital for medical providers not only to hear but also to help create their patients' narratives" (p. 168). When patients find the courage to share their narratives and when medical practitioners demonstrate the compassion to listen, the collaboration can help the patient's healing process.

Sharing narratives can illuminate contributing factors which may interfere with healing. When I reread my journal, I notice I used words like "exhausting" and "stressed" twice as much as words like "grateful." Evidence exists to illustrate the influence of environmental and social factors on stress. As medical doctor Harding (2019) explains, "the essentials of health start with recognizing the role of the hidden factors on stress and their impact on physical and mental health" (p. 143). Looking over my recent pain journal, I could finally see how the puzzle pieces fit together.

As a daughter of a city planner, I saw the importance of communities to help people.

As a teacher, I saw the impacts of stress on students.

As a patient with an autoimmune disease, I saw the results of reworking my lifestyle.

As a health coach, I saw the benefits of a positive attitude for patients.

As a Stephen Minister, I saw the value of faith in the unseen.

As a writer, I saw the evidence of capturing narratives on paper.

And I realized the value of narratives because stories provide a snapshot of life.

Harding (2019) elaborates, "here is what I wish I had known when I was starting in medical school and life: our social conditions (hidden factors) profoundly shape our physical and mental health. Kind and loving choices that support emotional well-being and reduce stress may help prevent or delay the onset of many diseases" (p. 193). My pain journal discussed my symptoms, but what if I looked closer at contributing factors?

Snapshots of Healing

During the physical therapy session where I felt the strongest, I was too busy laughing to overthink my exercises. The continual rock/paper/scissors competition with Dak, David, and Eric (that Dak usually won) provided lighthearted moments in the clinic in addition to the serious exercises. Because the physical therapy team likes to have fun while working, the result means that laughter helps their patients.

Being both the director of a Writing and Reading Center as well as teaching five English classes can cause stress, but I notice I feel happier when performing random acts of kindness such as bringing carnations for my colleagues to display on their desks or encouraging students to live their best lives. When I turn my focus inward and worry, I feel stressed. When I turn my focus outward to help others, I feel better. That said, I've learned not to help others at the expense of my own energy. Returning to the home I decorated and inviting friends and family over brings me peace. Even writing this book you now read brings me joy and does not feel stressful because using writing to help people is part of my purpose in life.

Paying attention to contributing factors won't replace my physical therapy exercises in helping me feel better, but if I repeat unhelpful stressful life patterns, I won't receive the maximum benefit from the exercises. As Harding (2019) believes, "when new mental or physical symptoms arise, we can check in with ourselves as a first step" (p. 163). And it also helps to share my thoughts about my check in with my medical team.

Jen's Journal

Finally, I can see some hope. Each day, I now have a few headache free hours. I do my exercises at my school's clinic on the days I don't have physical therapy. I'm experimenting with different ways to carry books and papers through the school hallways. My goals are to be pain free and avoid surgery, so I need to commit to lifestyle changes.

Jen's Journal (A Few Weeks Later)

Tuesday was first headache free day in five months!!!

I'm getting my life back – honestly forgot what it felt like to be pain free!!

Jen's Journal (A Few Weeks Later)

Overall the best week yet as far as pain levels. No pattern to anything, so I have to stop overanalyzing what might be causing the pain.

Pain level is tolerable if I had to live with it but my goal is still to be pain free!

Writing Epiphany

One day in class, I discussed pain journals with my students and the importance of setting goals. I brought my black and gold sequined journal with me. When looking over my notes, I realized I wrote my symptoms, pain levels, and how I felt. However, I had not written my goals. Bernstein (2019) advises, "affirm in your journal how you want to feel" (p. 29). While I learned from research how setting specific goals can help the healing process, I forgot this step when I became a patient. Following Bernstein's advice to "write your affirmation in your journal" (p. 29), I wrote:

I am in pain.

I want to get back to 100% pain free.

I believe I can get better with the help of my physical therapy team.

After I wrote my intention in my journal, was I suddenly pain free? No.

After I wrote my intention in my journal, did I still need to do my exercises? Yes.

After I wrote my intention in my journal, I articulated my goal, which helped me.

After I wrote my intention in my journal, I finally believed I would heal from pain.

Full Circle

My name is Jen, and I live in a multigenre world. Seven years ago, when I wrote the sentence which opens this chapter, I never imagined the impact researching the connections between the fields of research and writing would have on my life.

Seeing my words in front of me reminded me to stay optimistic about my healing journey and stress less about the process. Dalebout (2016) reports the existing foundation of research as, "though we've witnessed the power of the mind in healing the body again and again in numerous studies on the placebo effect, we still often forget the supremacy of our beliefs" (p. 154). Granted, I couldn't just meditate and write my way to being one hundred percent pain free without the help of my physical therapy team because positive thoughts and a notebook wouldn't change the herniated disc in my neck and my occipital neuralgia. But I can, however, use methods that help me relieve stress in addition to my home exercise plan. Bernstein (2014) believes, "as we release stress in our lives, we help others do the same" (p. 4). When Eric and I gave presentations encouraging the audience to "take initiative and manage stress" (Bird and Wanner, 2013, 2014), I needed to control my stress so I could inspire others to do the same. So I looked back through the notes and reminded myself to take my own advice! Narratives never have a definitive ending; the end of one narrative leads to the beginning of another.

As a researcher, I love the theory of using writing as healing. Life as a patient taught me that while the practice of journal writing is excellent, different styles of journals need to exist. Whether used with patients in a clinic or students in a classroom, writing can illuminate a person's thoughts and coalesce the swirl of ideas in the mind. Medical doctor Tindle (2013) recommends to patients, "we need to come face-to face with our own internal dialogue so that we can learn whether we truly believe the things we are telling ourselves" (p. 95). How to capture a patient's inner dialogue? Write about it. Writing teacher Cameron (1998) shares with writers, "things do come to us through writing, and they are not always so intangible as insights. Moving our hands across the page, we make a handmade life" (p. 28). The survey Eric and I designed built on the existing foundation of research while adding a unique interdisciplinary collaboration and interpretation. We connected our own insights and perspectives with existing research in the field. Medical doctor Harding (2019) describes the lasting impact of Pennebaker's initial research showing the health benefits of writing as, "subsequent follow-up studies show benefits across age, gender, social class, culture, and even personality type in as little as fifteen minutes a day of writing for three days" (p. 137). I discovered the success of the research I did with Eric, Jayne, and others we added to our team exists in the lives of the people who we help by the information we learned and decided to share.

It feels vulnerable to share a story. Even after writing about my experiences in book chapters, I still feel vulnerable sharing my pain narrative, but experts like my physical therapists Eric, Ryan, and Dak always showed willingness to help. I feel vulnerable sharing narratives of my life with you, the reader of this story, but I share my story with the wish it will inspire you to write your own narrative and make it a good one. Lamott (1994) writes, "against all odds, you have put it down on paper, so that it won't be lost. And who knows? Maybe what you've written will help others, will be a small part of the solution" (p. 235). I want my research and writing to continue to help others. I hope to live my life in a way similar to the words of Hale (2018) when she says, "so I urge you to put yourself out there. Be vulnerable. Take a chance. Step outside your comfort zone. Try something new and daring and audacious" (p. 23). I'm grateful that years ago I took a chance and shared my pain narrative with Eric because he helped me and we then used our research and writing to help others.

My purpose in sharing my narrative reflects my life's larger purpose of using my passion for writing, especially narrative writing, to help others. Hollis (2019) explains, "this goal, this mission of yours, this dream, this place that you're headed – this is not a temporary thing" (p. 185). I want to continue to write narratives which educate and inspire because I agree with Hollis (2018) who shares, "writing – for me –is its own kind of worship" (p. 150). As an English teacher, I believe in the value of writing. I agree with Heard (1995) who writes, "writing is an act of faith: faith that what I have to say, how I see the world, are important" (p. 27). I want my students to have faith that writing can lead the way to heal from the past, honor the present, and articulate goals for the future.

ACKNOWLEDGMENT

The preceding chapter contains excerpts from the following previous IGI publications:

Bird, J.L., Wanner, E.T., Urenda, R., & Perry, R. (2015). Multigenre medicine. In J.L. Bird (Ed.), *Innovative collaborative practice and reflection in patient education* (pp. 1-19). Hershey, PA: Information Science Reference.

Bird, J.L., & Wanner, E.T. (2013). Multigenre narratives as a healing process. In V.C.X. Wang (Ed.), *Handbook of research on teaching and learning in K-20 education* (pp. 416-428). Hershey, PA: Information Science Reference.

REFERENCES

Arioto, M. (2019). *Have more fun*. Grand Rapids, MI: Zondervan.

Beck, M. (2003). *The joy diet*. New York, NY: Crown.

Bernstein, G. (2014). *Miracles now*. Carlsbad, CA: Hay House.

Bernstein, G. (2019). *Super attractor*. Carlsbad, CA: Hay House.

Bird, J. L., & Wanner, E. T. (2013). Take initiative and manage stress. *Learn Green Conference*.

Bird, J. L., & Wanner, E. T. (2014). Take initiative and manage stress. *Learn Green Conference*.

Brown, B. (2007). *I thought it was just me*. New York, NY: Gotham Books.

Brown, B. (2010). *The gifts of imperfection*. Center City, MN: Hazelden.

Brown, B. (2012). *Daring greatly*. New York, NY: Gotham Books.

Cameron, J. (1998). *The right to write*. New York: Tarcher/Putnam.

Carroll, R. (2018). *The bullet journal method*. New York, NY: Portfolio/Penguin.

Clandinin, D. J., & Connelly, F. M. (2000). *Narrative inquiry*. San Francisco: Jossey-Bass.

Clay, R. A. (2011). *Stressed in America*. Retrieved from http://www.apa.org/monitor/2011/01/stressed-america.aspx

Connelly, F. M., & Clandinin, D. J. (1988). *Teachers as curriculum planners*. New York: Teachers College press.

Croft, J. (1980). Interviewing in physical therapy. *Physical Therapy*, *60*(8), 1033–1036. doi:10.1093/ptj/60.8.1033 PMID:7403279

Dalebout, K. (2016). *Let it out*. Carlsbad, CA: Hay House.

Dooley, J. L. (2019). *Own your everyday*. New York, NY: Waterbrook.

Dosa, D. (2010). *Making rounds with Oscar*. New York, NY: Hyperion.

Duke Integrative Medicine Staff. (2010). *Personalized health plan manual*. Durham, NC: Duke Integrative Medicine.

Gold, Y., & Roth, R. A. (1993). *Teachers managing stress*. London: The Falmer Press.

Goldberg, N. (1986). *Writing down the bones*. New York: Bantam.

Goldberg, N. (1990). *Wild mind*. New York: Bantam.

Goldberg, N. (2000). *Thunder and lightning*. New York: Bantam.

Goldberg, N. (2007). *Old friend from far away*. New York: Free Press.

Goldberg, S. (2019). *How to be a patient*. New York, NY: Harper Wave.

Grant, A. (2016). *Originals*. New York, NY: Viking.

Graves, D. (2001). *The energy to teach*. Portsmouth, NH: Heinemann.

Gruwell, E., & the The Freedom Writers. (1999). The Freedom Writers diary. New York, NY: Broadway.

Hagen, P. T. (Ed.). (2001). *Mayo clinic guide to self-care*. Rochester, MN: Mayo Clinic.

Hale, M. (2018). *You are enough*. New York, NY: FaithWords.

Harding, K. (2019). *The rabbit effect*. New York, NY: Atria.

Heard, G. (1995). *Writing toward home*. Portsmouth, NH: Heinemann.

Hollis, R. (2018). *Girl, wash your face*. Nashville, TN: Nelson Books.

Hollis, R. (2019). *Girl, stop apologizing*. Nashville, TN: HarperCollins Leadership.

Johnson, L. (1998). *Two parts textbook, one part love*. New York: Hyperion.

Lamott, A. (1994). *Bird by bird*. New York: Anchor Books.

Leonard, L. (2018). *Brave love*. Grand Rapids, MI: Zondervan.

Miller, R. W. (2017). *Dot journaling*. New York, NY: The Experiment.

Murray, D. (1996). *Crafting a life*. Portsmouth, NH: Heinemann.

National Institute of Neurological Disorders and Stroke. (2019). *Occipital neuralgia information page*. Retrieved from https://www.ninds.nih.gov/Disorders/All-Disorders/Occipital-Neuralgia-Information-Page

Neff, K., & Germer, C. (2018). *The mindful self-compassion workbook*. New York, NY: Guilford.

Niequist, S. (2016). *Present over perfect*. Grand Rapids, MI: Zondervan.

North American Spine Society. (2014). Whiplash and whiplash associated disorder. *Knowyourback.org*. Retrieved from http://www.knowyourback.org/Pages/SpinalConditions/Injuries/Whiplash.aspx

Pennebaker, J. W. (1997). *Opening up: the healing power of expressing emotions*. New York, NY: The Guilford Press.

Pink, D. (2018). *When*. New York, NY: Riverhead.

Quindlen, A. (2004). *Loud and clear*. New York, NY: Ballantine.

Randall, K. E., & McEwen, I. R. (2000). Writing patient-centered functional goals. *Physical Therapy*, *80*(12), 1197–1203. PMID:11087306

Rankin, L. (2013). *Mind over medicine*. Carlsbad, CA: Hay House.

Romano, T. (1987). *Clearing the way*. Portsmouth, NH: Heinemann.

Romano, T. (1995). *Writing with passion: life stories, multiple genres.* Portsmouth, NH: Heinemann.

Romano, T. (2000). *Blending genre, altering style*. Portsmouth, NH: Heinemann.

Romano, T. (2004). *Crafting authentic voice*. Portsmouth, NH: Heinemann.

Romano, T. (2008). *Zigzag*. Portsmouth, NH: Heinemann.

Romano, T. (2015). *Write what matters*. Lexington, KY: Zigzag.

Sandberg, S., & Grant, A. (2017). *Option B*. New York, NY: Knopf.

Seaward, B. L. (2012). *Managing Stress* (7th ed.). Burlington, MA: Jones and Bartlett.

Soukup, R. (2016). *Unstuffed.* Grand Rapids, MI: Zondervan.

Soukup, R. (2019). *Do it scared.* Grand Rapids, MI: Zondervan.

Tindle, H. (2013). *Up: How positive outlook can transform our health and aging*. New York, NY: Hudson Street Press.

Wanner, E.T., & Bird, J.L. (2013). *The Wanner Bird healing survey for pain recovery*. Academic Press.

KEY TERMS AND DEFINITIONS

Integrative Health Coach: Health coaches have a variety of educational backgrounds but participate in specialized training to help patients design personalized health plans. Health coaches help patients clarify their vision and values. They also work with medical professionals to assist patients in comprehending the treatment plan while setting goals to achieve optimal health.

Integrative Medicine: A holistic approach to medicine that treats the person, not the disease. Patients and doctors form a partnership to treat the patient's mind, body, and spirit.

Migraines: A type of painful headache. Migraines have a variety of symptoms and causes. Patients suffering from migraines should consult a medical professional to help with a treatment plan.

Multigenre Healing Project: Jen and Eric designed a multigenre project where Jen wrote about her neck pain and Eric provided the end notes analysis.

This is a different perspective on multigenre projects that connects the field of education and medicine and can lead to greater patient awareness about health.

Multigenre Medicine: Connecting multigenre writing to the field of medicine.

Multigenre Writing: Originally made popular in the field of education by Tom Romano, a multigenre paper consists of two parts: creative writing in multiple genres and the writer's analysis of the genres. The original version of multigenre papers can also be used in classrooms for students of all ages.

Narrative Inquiry: Originally made popular in the field of research by F. Michael Connelly and D. Jean Clandinin, narrative inquiry is a qualitative interpretative form of research that focuses on the telling, retelling, and sharing of stories. Researchers who complete narrative inquiries interpret stories and search for common threads to find patterns. Some narrative inquires begin with a research question, while others, such as Jen's stories of her neck pain and Eric's interpretation of those stories, evolve over time. Narrative inquires adapt to emerging circumstances and frequently change based on new information.

Neck Pain Journal: Jen created a journal of how her neck was feeling and what she was doing when her neck felt pain. Eric read the journal and diagnosed what Jen needed to do to make her neck feel better.

Physical Therapy Interview: The initial intake session where a physical therapist asks patients questions and learns about the patient's story.

Thinking Like a Turtle: This philosophy means taking on one task at a time, which can lead to less stress.

Wanner-Bird Healing Survey for Pain Recovery: An original survey designed by Dr. Eric Wanner and Dr. Jennifer Bird. This survey features a combination of numerical subjective questions, where patients are asked to respond to statements by circling a number from 1-5, and written subjective questions that evaluates patients on a rubric with a score of 1, 3, or 5 to incorporate the technical and artistic dimensions of writing. The survey questions can also be used for health coaching.

Writing Voice: Voice in writing describes how a writer uses word choice and tone when writing a journal entry or other composition that reflects the personality of the writer. Just like each person has a unique speaking voice, each writer has a unique writing voice.

APPENDIX: CREATING YOUR MULTIGENRE HEALING PROJECT

You can use the following ideas as inspiration to create your own multigenre healing project.

1. How do you best express what you are feeling, both physically and emotionally? It may be building a model of a boat, comparing your experiences to your favorite actor or athlete, writing a poem, playing a song you wrote on the piano, or drawing a picture. It may be different on different days. Just remember that multigenre projects are a form of creative expression that do not hurt yourself or anyone else. You may want to share your feelings by throwing rocks at your neighbor's window, but that creates more problems than it solves.
2. If you need help getting started, writers Julia Cameron, Georgia Heard, and Natalie Goldberg suggest thinking of a word as a prompt and reacting to it. Start with something neutral or humorous. For example, I'm looking out a window right now. I could write about the beautiful red flowers that bloom every year in May around my birthday. I could take a picture of the flowers. I could listen to music while I look at the flowers. The word window led me to my next word, flowers. You can continue to use words like these as inspiration or you can try more serious words, such as pain. Stop the activity if you feel physical or emotional pain.
3. If you complete more than one multigenre project, look for patterns. Do these patterns tell you anything? For example, if I spend a lot of time looking out windows to describe what I see, does it mean I am avoiding something by spending too much time looking out windows and not enough time working? Other people can also help you find patterns.
4. Make a list of things you love, including people, pets, activities, television shows, music, movies, sports, and other things that bring you joy and make you smile. Spend ten minutes a day with the people and things on that list.
5. Create a pain journal and share it with your doctor or physical therapist. Refer to Jen's as an example.

Table 1. Jen's Sample Neck Pain Journal

Date	Pain Level 1=Low, 10=High	Observations
Wed 3/28 morning	Left Side = 2, Right Side =2	Feeling great after physical therapy and want to continue trend. Ask tech guy at work if I can prop computer monitor on books so I am looking up, not down. He loves idea and it makes my neck feel better.
afternoon	Left Side =4, Right Side = 4, also dizzy	Pick up podium in classroom and move it. Pick up large box of books in classroom and move it. Have done both dozens of times in my life before neck pain. Apparently my neck isn't ready for furniture moving. Students happily move furniture.
afternoon	Left Side = 3, Right Side =3	Students present text modernizations that are purposefully funny. Romeo and Juliet's families have a dance battle instead of a sword fight. Dorothy and her friends get lost at the mall instead of in Oz. I laugh so much I almost cry and somehow that helps neck.
evening	Left Side = 4, Right Side = 3, also dizzy	Not sure how I feel about the guy I am going out with this weekend, but my neck doesn't like him. It's tightening up while I'm making plans for a date. Maybe my neck is trying to tell me something.
night	Left Side = 3, Right Side = 3	9:30pm + home from work late + still need to do second set of exercises = Neck Exercise Disco Dance Party!! Turn on Kylie Minogue CD for motivation and actually have to remind myself to slow down the exercises.
Thurs 3/29/12 morning	Left Side = 1, Right Side = 3	Second set of exercises in less than 12 hours. Left side is tight but not in much pain. Think I'm still dreaming. Glad I'm not.
afternoon	Left Side = 1, Right Side = 2	Take lunch break to play on the swings by the campus residence halls. Heaven.
afternoon	Left Side = 2, Right Side =4, also dizzy	Playing baseball game in class for semester review and throwing ball around. I'm not getting enough sleep and all I had to eat before teaching was an energy bar. And I wonder why I'm feeling dizzy?!
night	Left Side =0 (gone), Right Side =3	Another late night on campus. Time to turn on the Kylie CD for Neck Exercise Disco Dance Party Part II! The left side of my neck is tight, but there is no pain. Amazing. Forgot what that feels like. The right side still hurts but not as bad.
Summary	Left side is tight with occasional pain but mostly gone. Need to get over final hurdle with right side pain.	I needed to laugh more! Writing this has been entertaining, insightful, and enlightening. Hope you enjoyed it!

Compilation of References

Adams, K. (1990). *Journal to the Self*. New York, NY: Warner Books.

Alexander, E. (2012). *Proof of Heaven*. New York, NY: Simon and Schuster.

Alexander, E. (2014). *The map of Heaven*. New York, NY: Simon and Schuster.

Allen, C. A. (2001). *The multigenre research paper*. Portsmouth, NH: Heinemann.

American Institute of Stress. (2013). Stress statistics. *American Psychological Association*. Retrieved from http://www.statisticbrain.com/stress-statistics/

Anderson, C. M., & MacCurdy, M. M. (2000). Introduction. In C. M. Anderson & M. M. MacCurdy (Eds.), *Writing and healing* (pp. 1–22). Urbana, IL: National Council of Teachers of English.

Arioto, M. (2019). *Have more fun*. Grand Rapids, MI: Zondervan.

Arterburn, S. (2011). *Healing is a choice*. Nashville, TN: Thomas Nelson.

ASCM Staff. (2011). ACSM issues new recommendations on quantity and quality of exercise. *American College of Sports Medicine*. Retrieved from http://www.acsm.org/about-acsm/media-room/news-releases/2011/08/01/acsm-issues-new-recommendations-on-quantity-and-quality-of-exercise

Atwell, N. (1987). *In the middle*. Portsmouth, NH: Heinemann.

Austen, J. (2005). *Pride and prejudice*. New York, NY: Penguin. (Original work published 1813) doi:10.5117/9781904633013

Baldwin, C. (1998). *Calling the circle*. New York, NY: Bantam.

Baldwin, C. (2006). *One to one*. Lanham, MD: Rowman and Littlefield.

Barbieri, M. (1995). *Sounds from the heart*. Portsmouth, NH: Heinemann.

Barrett, D. (2013). What is paintracking? *Pain Pathways*, *6*(1), 36–41.

Baty, K. (2003). *A girl's gotta do what a girl's gotta do*. New York, NY: Rodale.

Beane, J. A. (1997). *Curriculum integration*. New York, NY: Teachers College Press.

Beck, M. (2001). *Finding your own North Star*. New York, NY: Three Rivers Press.

Beck, M. (2003). *The joy diet*. New York, NY: Crown.

Beck, M. (2008). *Steering by starlight*. New York, NY: Rodale.

Beck, M. (2012). *Finding your way in a wild new world*. New York, NY: Free Press.

Berkow, R. (Ed.). (1997). *The Merck manual of medical information*. Whitehouse Station, NJ: Merck & Co.

Bernstein, G. (2010). *Add more –ing to your life*. New York, NY: Harmony Books.

Bernstein, G. (2014). *Miracles now*. Carlsbad, CA: Hay House.

Bernstein, G. (2016). *The universe has your back*. Carlsbad, CA: Hay House.

Bernstein, G. (2018). *Judgment detox*. New York, NY: North Star Way.

Bernstein, G. (2019). *Super attractor*. Carlsbad, CA: Hay House.

Bezner, J. R. (2015). Promoting health and wellness: Implications for physical therapist practice. *Physical Therapy*, *95*(10), 1433–1444. doi:10.2522/ptj.20140271 PMID:25908523

Bird, J. L., & Wanner, E. T. (2013). Take initiative and manage stress. *Learn Green Conference*.

Blaylock, R. (2013). Exercise repairs the brain. *Newsmax Health*. Retrieved from http://www.newsmaxhealth.com/

BMR Calculator. (2013). *BMI Calculator*. Retrieved from http://www.bmi-calculator.net/bmr-calculator/bmr-formula.php

Bradley, E. H., Bogardus, S. T. Jr, Tinetti, M. E., & Inouye, S. K. (1999). Goal setting in clinical medicine. *Social Science & Medicine*, *49*(2), 267–278. doi:10.1016/S0277-9536(99)00107-0 PMID:10414834

Brady, L., & Vega, P. (2009). 5 keys to structural success. In Orthopedics and spine (pp. 107-132). Danvers, MA: HCPro.

Brickman, J. (2015). *Soothe*. New York, NY: Rodale.

Brown, B. (2007). *I thought it was just me*. New York, NY: Gotham Books.

Brown, B. (2010). *The gifts of imperfection*. Center City, MN: Hazelden.

Brown, B. (2012). *Daring greatly*. New York, NY: Gotham Books.

Brown, B. (2015). *Rising strong*. New York, NY: Spiegel & Grau.

Brown, B. (2017). *Braving the wilderness*. New York, NY: Random House.

Brown, B. (2018). *Dare to lead*. New York, NY: Random House.

Caldwell, K., Gray, J., & Wolever, R. Q. (2013). The process of patient empowerment in integrative health coaching: How does it happen? *Global Advances in Health and Medicine: Improving Healthcare Outcomes Worldwide*, *2*(3), 48–57. doi:10.7453/gahmj.2013.026 PMID:24416672

Cameron, J. (1998). *The right to write*. New York, NY: Tarcher/Putnam.

Cameron, J. (2002). *The artist's way* (2nd ed.). New York, NY: Tarcher/Putnam.

Cameron, L. (2018). *The mindful day*. Washington, DC: National Geographic.

Caregiver.com Inc. (2015). Today's caregiver. *Caregiver.com*. Retrieved from http://caregiver.com/index.htm

Carroll, R. (2018). *The bullet journal method*. New York, NY: Portfolio/Penguin.

Carter, C. (2015). *The sweet spot*. New York, NY: Ballantine.

Catanese, A. J. (1996). Lessons learned. In B. W. McClendon & A. J. Catanese (Eds.), *Planners on planning* (pp. 287–295). San Francisco, CA: Jossey-Bass.

Centers for Disease Control and Prevention. (2011). Health Related Quality of Life. *Health Related Quality of Life Surveillance Program*. Retrieved from http://www.cdc.gov/hrqol/hrqol14_measure.htm

Charon, R. (2006). *Narrative medicine: honoring the stories of illness*. New York, NY: Oxford University Press.

Cheo, K. (2012). Goal setting: why 90% of us don't do it effectively. *Boston Business Journal*. Retrieved from http://www.bizjournals.com/boston/blog/mass-high-tech/2012/09/goal-setting-why-90-of-us-dont-do.html?page=all

Chua, C. (2009). *6 important reasons why you should set goals*. Retrieved from http://personalexcellence.co/blog/6-important-reasons-why-you-should-set-goals

Chulack, C., Crichton, M., Wells, J., & Zabel, D. (1994-2009). *ER* [Television series]. Burbank, CA: Warner Brothers.

Clandinin, D. J., & Connelly, F. M. (2000). *Narrative inquiry*. San Francisco, CA: Jossey-Bass.

Clark, A. H. (2018). *Hack your anxiety*. Naperville, IL: Sourcebooks, Inc.

Clark, C. C. (2006). *Living well with anxiety*. New York, NY: HarperCollins.

Clay, R. A. (2011). *Stressed in America*. Retrieved from http://www.apa.org/monitor/2011/01/stressed-america.aspx

Cleary, L. M. (1991). *From the other side of the desk*. Portsmouth, NH: Heinemann.

Cleaver, J. (2002). *Immediate fiction*. New York, NY: St. Martin's Press.

Coates, V. E. (1999). *Education for patients and clients*. New York, NY: Routledge.

Codell, E. R. (1999). *Educating Esme*. Chapel Hill, NC: Algonquin Books.

Cohen-Sandler, R. (2005). *Stressed-out girls*. New York, NY: Viking.

Connelly, F. M., & Clandinin, D. J. (1988). *Teachers as curriculum planners*. New York, NY: Teachers College press.

Conner, J. (2008). *Writing down your soul*. San Francisco, CA: Conari.

Covey, S. R., Merrill, A. R., & Merrill, R. R. (1994). *First things first*. New York, NY: Free Press.

Creative Health Care Management Staff. (2003). *Re-igniting the Spirit of Caring*. Minneapolis, MN: Creative Health Care Management.

Croft, J. (1980). Interviewing in physical therapy. *Physical Therapy*, *60*(8), 1033–1036. doi:10.1093/ptj/60.8.1033 PMID:7403279

Dalebout, K. (2016). *Let it out*. Carlsbad, CA: Hay House.

Daniels, H., & Zemelman, S. (2004). *Subject matters*. Portsmouth, NH: Heinemann.

DeBecker, G. (1997). *The gift of fear*. Boston, MA: Little, Brown and Company.

DeSalvo, L. (1999). *Writing as a way of healing*. Boston, MA: Beacon Press.

Dimitrius, J. (1998). *Reading people*. New York, NY: Ballantine.

Dooley, J. L. (2019). *Own your everyday*. New York, NY: Waterbrook.

Dosa, D. (2010). *Making rounds with Oscar*. New York, NY: Hyperion.

Driscoll, M. (2012). *Edith Wharton: 10 best quotes on her 150th birthday*. Retrieved from http://www.csmonitor.com/Books/2012/0123/Edith-Wharton-10-best-quotes-on-her-150th-birthday/Giving-happiness-to-others

Duckworth, A. (2016). *Grit*. New York, NY: Scribner.

Duke Integrative Medicine Staff. (2010). *Personalized health plan manual*. Durham, NC: Duke Integrative Medicine.

Duke Integrative Medicine Staff. (2010). *Personalized Health Plan Manual*. Durham, NC: Duke Integrative Medicine.

Dweck, C. (2006). *Mindset*. New York, NY: Ballantine.

Enayati, A. (2015). *Seeking serenity*. New York, NY: New American Library.

Evans, J. F. (2010). Introducing wellness & writing connections conference papers. In J. F. Evans (Ed.), *Wellness & Writing Connections* (pp. 3–10). Enumclaw, WA: Idyll Arbor, Inc.

Files, M. (2016). *Writing what you know*. New York, NY: Allworth.

Fitzgerald, F. S. (1925). *The great Gatsby*. New York, NY: Scribner.

Fletcher, R. (2013). *What a writer needs* (2nd ed.). Portsmouth, NH: Heinemann.

Garber, C. E., Blissmer, B., Deschenes, M. R., Franklin, B. A., Lamonte, M. J., Lee, I. M., ... Swain, D. P. (2011). Quantity and quality of exercise for developing and maintaining cardiorespiratory, musculoskeletal, and neuromotor fitness in apparently healthy adults: Guidance for prescribing exercise. *Medicine and Science in Sports and Exercise*, *43*(7), 1334–1359. doi:10.1249/MSS.0b013e318213fefb PMID:21694556

Gaughan, J. (1997). *Cultural reflections*. Portsmouth, NH: Heinemann.

Gaughan, J. (2001). *Reinventing English*. Portsmouth, NH: Heinemann.

Germer, C. K. (2009). *The Mindful path to self-compassion*. New York, NY: The Guilford Press.

Gillespie, P., & Learner, N. (2008). *The Longman guide to peer tutoring* (2nd ed.). New York, NY: Pearson.

Go, A. S., Mozaffarian, D., Roger, V. L., Benjamin, E. J., Berry, J. D., Borden, W. B., ... Turner, M. B.American Heart Association Statistics Committee and Stroke Statistics Subcommittee. (2013). Heart disease and stroke statistics—2013 update: A report from the American Heart Association. *Circulation*, *127*, e6–e245. Retrieved from http://www.heart.org/idc/groups/heart-public/@wcm/@sop/@smd/documents/downloadable/ucm_319588.pdf PMID:23239837

Goldberg, B. (1996). *Room to write*. New York, NY: Tarcher/Putnam.

Goldberg, N. (1986). *Writing down the bones*. Boston, MA: Shambhala.

Goldberg, N. (1990). *Wild mind*. New York, NY: Bantam.

Goldberg, N. (2000). *Thunder and lightning*. New York, NY: Bantam.

Goldberg, N. (2007). *Old friend from far away*. New York, NY: Free Press.

Goldberg, N. (2013). *The true secret of writing*. New York, NY: Atria.

Goldberg, N. (2016). *The great spring*. Boulder, CO: Shambhala.

Goldberg, S. (2019). *How to be a patient*. New York, NY: Harper Wave.

Gold, Y., & Roth, R. A. (1993). *Teachers managing stress*. London: The Falmer Press.

Grant, A. (2016). *Originals*. New York, NY: Viking.

Graves, D. (2001). *The energy to teach*. Portsmouth, NH: Heinemann.

Graves, D. H. (1994). *A fresh look at writing*. Portsmouth, NH: Heinemann.

Greenberg, M. A., Wortman, C. B., & Stone, A. A. (1996). Emotional expression and physical health: Revising traumatic memories or fostering self-regulation. *Journal of Personality and Social Psychology*, *71*(3), 588–602. doi:10.1037/0022-3514.71.3.588 PMID:8831163

Greene, M. (1995). *Releasing the imagination*. San Francisco, CA: Jossey-Bass.

Greenfield, B. H., & Jensen, G. M. (2010). Understanding the lived experiences of patients: Application of a phenomenological approach to ethics. *Physical Therapy*, *90*(8), 1185–1201. doi:10.2522/ptj.20090348 PMID:20539020

Greenfield, B. H., Jensen, G. M., Delany, C. M., Mostrom, E., Knab, M., & Jampel, A. (2015). Power and promise of narrative for advancing physical therapist education and practice. *Physical Therapy*, *95*(6), 924–933. doi:10.2522/ptj.20140085 PMID:25524869

Groopman, J. (2007). *How doctors think*. New York, NY: Mariner Books.

Gruwell, E. (2007). Teach with your heart. New York, NY: Broadway.

Gruwell, E. (2009). Teaching hope. New York, NY: Broadway.

Gruwell, E., & the The Freedom Writers. (1999). The Freedom Writers diary. New York, NY: Broadway.

Gruwell, E., & the The Freedom Writers. (2009). The Freedom Writers diary (2nd ed.). New York, NY: Broadway.

Guh, D. P., Zhang, W., Bansback, N., Amarsi, Z., Birmingham, C. L., & Anis, A. H. (2009). The incidence of co-morbidities related to obesity and overweight: a systematic review and meta-analysis. *BMC Public Health*. Retrieved from http://www.biomedcentral.com/1471-2458/9/88

Hagen, P. T. (Ed.). (2001). *Mayo clinic guide to self-care*. Rochester, MN: Mayo Clinic.

Hale, M. (2013). *The single woman*. Nashville, TN: Thomas Nelson.

Hale, M. (2014). *I've never been to Vegas but my luggage has*. Nashville, TN: Thomas Nelson.

Hale, M. (2015). *Beautiful uncertainty*. Nashville, TN: Thomas Nelson.

Hale, M. (2018). *You are enough*. New York, NY: FaithWords.

Handler, J. (2013). *Braving the fire*. New York, NY: St. Martin's Griffin.

Harding, K. (2019). *The rabbit effect*. New York, NY: Atria.

Harper, A. N. (1996). Tooling up for effective planning. In B. W. McClendon & A. J. Catanese (Eds.), *Planners on planning* (pp. 190–198). San Francisco, CA: Jossey-Bass.

Harvard Medical School Family Health Guide. (2006). *Good nutrition: should guidelines differ for men and women?* Harvard Health Publications. Retrieved from http://www.health.harvard.edu/fhg/updates/update0906b.shtml

Haugk, K. C. (2000). *When and how to use mental health resources*. St. Louis, MO: Stephen Ministries.

Haugk, K. C. (2012). *Christian caregiving*. St. Louis, MO: Stephen Ministries.

Havrilesky, H. (2018). *What if this were enough?* New York: Doubleday.

Hawthorne, N. (1955). *The scarlet letter*. New York, NY: Washington Square Press. (Original work published 1850)

Heard, G. (1995). *Writing toward home*. Portsmouth, NH: Heinemann.

Heard, G. (1999). *Awakening the heart*. Portsmouth, NH: Heinemann.

Heard, G. (2002). *The revision toolbox*. Portsmouth, NH: Heinemann.

Heard, G. (2016). *Heart maps*. Portsmouth, NH: Heinemann.

Heifetz, R. A. (1994). *Leadership without easy answers*. Cambridge, MA: The Belnap Press of Harvard University Press.

Helgoe, L. A., Wilhelm, L. R., & Kommor, M. J. (2005). *The anxiety answer book*. Naperville, IL: Sourcebooks, Inc.

Helldorfer, M., & Moss, T. (2007). *Healing with heart*. Orinda, CA: Moss Communications.

Helpguide. (2013). Stress symptoms, signs, causes. *Helpguide.org*. Retrieved from http://www.helpguide.org/mental/stress_signs.htm

Hoch, C. (1995). Teaching ethics and planning theory. In S. Hendler (Ed.), Planning ethics (pp. 281-300). New Brunswick, NJ: Rutgers.

Holden Leadership Center. (2009). *Great leadership quotes*. Retrieved from http://leadership.uoregon.edu/resources/quotes

Hollis, R. (2018). *Girl, wash your face*. Nashville, TN: Nelson Books.

Hollis, R. (2019). *Girl, stop apologizing*. Nashville, TN: HarperCollins Leadership.

Hubbard, R. S. (1996). *A workshop of the possible*. York, ME: Stenhouse.

Johnson, B. (2009). *But now! Awakening faith in an age of anxiety*. Belleville, Canada: Essence Publishing.

Johnson, L. (1998). *Two parts textbook, one part love*. New York, NY: Hyperion.

Johnson, L. (2005). *Teaching outside the box*. San Francisco, CA: Jossey-Bass.

Johnson, W. C. (1997). *Urban planning and politics*. Chicago, IL: American Planning Association.

Jones, J., Brady, L., & Gaunt, R. (2009). The philosophy of patient-centric care. In Orthopedics and spine (pp. 81-105). Danvers, MA: HCPro.

Jones, J., Steele, D., & McClennan, C. (2009). Defining and pursuing excellence. In Orthopedics and spine (pp. 11-50). Danvers, MA: HCPro.

Juhan, D. (1998). *Job's body* (2nd ed.). Barrytown, NY: Station Hill.

Kabat-Zinn, J. (2013). *Full catastrophe living* (2nd ed.). New York, NY: Bantam.

Kamenetz, A. (2013). Power of the pen. *Oprah*, *14*(12), 140–141.

Kearns, J. (1997). *Where to begin: a guide to teaching secondary English*. Portsmouth, NH: Heinemann.

Kepler, H. B. (1973). *Basic graphical kinematics* (2nd ed.). New York, NY: McGraw Hill.

Kinsella, W. P. (1982). *Shoeless Joe*. New York, NY: Ballantine.

Koloroutis, M. (2004). *Relationship-based care*. Minneapolis, MN: Creative Health Care Management.

Kolt, G. S. (2003). Psychology of injury and rehabilitation. In G. S. Kolt (Ed.), *Physical therapies in sport and exercise* (pp. 165–183). London, UK: Churchill Livingstone.

Lamott, A. (1994). *Bird by bird*. New York: Anchor Books.

Lamott, A. (2005). *Plan B: further thoughts on faith*. New York, NY: Riverhead.

Larson, J. (2005). Seasons of love [Recorded by the cast of Rent]. On Rent: Original motion picture soundtrack [CD]. Burbank, CA: Warner Brothers Records.

Lee, I. F. (2018). *Joyful*. New York, NY: Little, Brown Spark.

Leonard, L. (2018). *Brave love*. Grand Rapids, MI: Zondervan.

Lepore, S. J., Greenberg, M. A., Bruno, M., & Smyth, J. M. (2002). Expressive writing and health: self-regulation of emotion-related experience, physiology, and behavior. In S. J. Lepore & J. M. Smyth (Eds.), *The writing cure* (pp. 99–117). Washington, DC: American Psychological Association. doi:10.1037/10451-005

Linton, S. J., & Shaw, W. S. (2011). Impact of psychological factors in the experience of pain. *Physical Therapy*, *91*(5), 700–711. doi:10.2522/ptj.20100330 PMID:21451097

Madigan, S. (2011). *Narrative therapy*. Washington, DC: American Psychological Association.

Marshall, J. D., Sears, J. T., & Schubert, W. H. (2000). *Turning points in curriculum*. Upper Saddle River, NJ: Merrill/Prentice Hall.

Matousek, M. (2017). *Writing to awaken*. Oakland, CA: Reveal Press.

Mayo Clinic Staff. (2010). Weight loss: 6 strategies for success. *Mayo Clinic*. Retrieved from http://www.mayoclinic.com/health/weight-loss/HQ01625

Mayo Clinic Staff. (2011). 7 benefits of regular physical activity. *Mayo Clinic*. Retrieved from http://www.mayoclinic.com/health/exercise/HQ01676

McCall, C. (2011). *Writing and healing*. Retrieved from http://www.psychologytoday.com/blog/overcoming-child-abuse/201103/writing-and-healing

Michele, L. (2015). *You first: journal your way to your best life*. New York, NY: Crown Archetype.

Miller, R. W. (2017). *Dot journaling*. New York, NY: The Experiment.

Miller, W. R., & Rollnick, S. (2002). *Motivational interviewing* (2nd ed.). New York, NY: The Guilford Press.

Murray, D. (1996). *Crafting a life*. Portsmouth, NH: Heinemann.

Murray, D. M. (1985). *A writer teaches writing* (2nd ed.). Boston, MA: Houghton Mifflin.

National Institute of Neurological Disorders and Stroke. (2019). *Occipital neuralgia information page*. Retrieved from https://www.ninds.nih.gov/Disorders/All-Disorders/Occipital-Neuralgia-Information-Page

Neal, M. C. (2012). *To Heaven and back*. Colorado Springs, CO: WaterBrook Press.

Neff, K. (2011). *Self compassion: the proven power of being kind to yourself*. New York, NY: HarperCollins.

Neff, K., & Germer, C. (2018). *The mindful self-compassion workbook*. New York, NY: Guilford.

Neporent, L. (2011). Does exercise really boost your metabolism? *That's Fit*. Retrieved from http://www.thatsfit.com/2011/03/23/does-exercise-really-boost-your-metabolism/

Niequist, S. (2016). *Present over perfect*. Grand Rapids, MI: Zondervan.

Noppe-Brandon, G. (2004). *Find your voice*. Portsmouth, NH: Heinemann.

North American Spine Society. (2014). Whiplash and whiplash associated disorder. *Knowyourback.org*. Retrieved from http://www.knowyourback.org/Pages/SpinalConditions/Injuries/Whiplash.aspx

Nutrition Policy Staff. (2013). Why good nutrition is important. *Center for Science in the Public Interest*. Retrieved from http://www.cspinet.org/nutritionpolicy/nutrition_policy.html

Nutrition Source. (2008). Healthy eating plate and healthy eating pyramid. *Harvard School of Public Health*. Retrieved from http://www.hsph.harvard.edu/nutritionsource/what-should-you-eat/pyramid/

O'Brien, T. (1990). *The things they carried*. New York, NY: Broadway Books.

Pennebaker, J. W. (1997). *Opening up: the healing power of expressing emotions*. New York, NY: The Guilford Press.

Pennebaker, J. W. (1997). *Opening up: The healing power of expressing emotions*. New York, NY: The Guilford press.

Pennebaker, J. W., & Evans, J. F. (2014). *Expressive writing: words that heal*. Enumclaw, WA: Idyll Arbor.

Pennebaker, J. W., & Evans, J. F. (2014). *Expressive writing: Words that heal*. Enumclaw, WA: Idyll Arbor.

Pennebaker, J. W., & Smyth, J. M. (2016). *Opening up by writing it down*. New York, NY: The Guilford Press.

Pennebaker, J., & Chung, C. K. (2010). Expressive writing, emotional upheavals, and health. In J. Evans (Ed.), *Wellness and writing connections* (pp. 11–52). Enumclaw, WA: Idyll Arbor.

Pink, D. (2009). *Drive*. New York, NY: Riverhead Books.

Pink, D. (2018). *When*. New York, NY: Riverhead.

Pipher, M. (1994). *Reviving Ophelia*. New York, NY: Grosset/Putnam.

Pipher, M. (2006). *Writing to change the world*. New York, NY: Riverhead.

Poetter, T. S. (2013). Stemming the tide. *Kappa Delta Pi Record*, *49*(3), 100–104. doi:10.1080/00228958.2013.819195

Putz, M. (2006). *A teacher's guide to the multigenre research project*. Portsmouth, NH: Heinemann.

Quindlen, A. (2004). *Loud and clear*. New York, NY: Ballantine.

Randall, K. E., & McEwen, I. R. (2000). Writing patient-centered functional goals. *Physical Therapy*, *80*(12), 1197–103. PMID:11087306

Rankin, L. (2013). *Mind over medicine*. Carlsbad, CA: Hay House.

Rankin, L. (2015a). *The fear cure*. Carlsbad, CA: Hay House.

Rankin, L. (2015b). *The anatomy of a calling*. New York, NY: Rodale.

Rasminsky, A. (2012). The story doc. *Oprah*, *13*(7), 88.

Rasminsky, A. (2012). The Story Doc. *Oprah*, *13*(7), 88.

Richardson, L. (1997). *Fields of play*. New Brunswick, NJ: Rutgers University Press.

Rief, L. (1992). *Seeking diversity*. Portsmouth, NH: Heinemann.

Rief, L. (1999). *Vision and voice*. Portsmouth, NH: Heinemann.

Roberts, L., & Bucksey, S. J. (2007). Communicating with patients: What happens in practice? *Physical Therapy*, *87*(5), 586–594. doi:10.2522/ptj.20060077 PMID:17405807

Rodriguez, N. R., DiMarco, N. M., & Langley, S. (2009). American College of Sports Medicine position stand. Nutrition and athletic performance. *Medicine and Science in Sports and Exercise*, *41*(3), 709–731. PMID:19225360

Rollnick, S., Miller, W. R., & Butler, C. C. (2008). *Motivational interviewing in health care: helping patients change behavior*. New York, NY: The Guilford Press.

Romano, T. (1987). *Clearing the way*. Portsmouth, NH: Heinemann.

Romano, T. (1995). *Writing with passion*. Portsmouth, NH: Heinemann.

Romano, T. (1995). *Writing with passion: life stories, multiple genres*. Portsmouth, NH: Heinemann.

Romano, T. (2000). *Blending genre, altering style*. Portsmouth, NH: Heinemann.

Romano, T. (2004). *Crafting authentic voice*. Portsmouth, NH: Heinemann.

Romano, T. (2008). *Zigzag*. Portsmouth, NH: Heinemann.

Romano, T. (2013). *Fearless writing*. Portsmouth, NH: Heinemann.

Romano, T. (2015). *Write what matters*. Lexington, KY: Zigzag.

Routman, R. (2003). *Reading essentials*. Portsmouth, NH: Heinemann.

Rushnell, S. (2012). *Divine alignment*. New York, NY: Howard Books.

Rushnell, S., & DuArt, L. (2017). *The Godwink effect*. New York, NY: Howard Books.

Ryan, N. P., Wade, J. C., Nice, A., Shenefelt, H., & Shepard, K. (1996). Physical therapists' perceptions of family involvement in the rehabilitation process. *Physiotherapy Research International*, *1*(3), 159–179. doi:10.1002/pri.56 PMID:9238732

Rzeznik, J. (1998). Iris [Recorded by Goo Goo Dolls]. On City of angels soundtrack [CD]. Burbank, CA: Warner Brothers.

Sadker, M., & Sadker, D. (1994). *Failing at fairness*. New York, NY: Charles Scribner's Sons.

Sandberg, S. (2013). *Lean in*. New York, NY: Alfred A. Knopf.

Sandberg, S. (2014). *Lean in for graduates*. New York, NY: Alfred A. Knopf.

Sandberg, S., & Grant, A. (2017). *Option B*. New York, NY: Knopf.

Schmidt, S. (2012). Obesity and exercise. *American College of Sports Medicine*. Retrieved from http://www.acsm.org/access-public-information/articles/2012/01/19/obesity-and-exercise

Schunk, D. H. (1990). Goal setting and self-efficacy during self-regulated learning. *Educational Psychologist*, *25*(1), 71–86. doi:10.120715326985ep2501_6

Seaward, B. L. (2012). *Managing Stress* (7th ed.). Burlington, MA: Jones and Bartlett.

Shandler, S. (1999). *Ophelia speaks*. New York, NY: HarperCollins.

Sharp, C. (2000). *A writer's workbook*. New York, NY: St. Martin's Press.

Sharp, C. (2000). *A writer's workshop*. New York, NY: St. Martin's Press.

Simmons, L. A., & Wolever, R. Q. (2011). *Health coaching: Research summary (report)*. Durham, NC: Duke Integrative Medicine / Duke University Health System.

Smith, D. (2012). *Monkey mind: A memoir of anxiety*. New York, NY: Simon & Schuster.

Smith, L. L., Lake, N. H., Simmons, L. A., Perlman, A., Wroth, S., & Wolever, R. Q. (2013). Integrative health coach training: A model for shifting the paradigm toward patient-centricity and meeting new national prevention goals. *Global Advances in Health and Medicine: Improving Healthcare Outcomes Worldwide*, *2*(3), 66–74. doi:10.7453/gahmj.2013.034 PMID:24416674

Smith, L., & Wroth, S. (2011). *Duke integrative health coach professional training manual.* Durham, NC: Duke Integrative Medicine.

Soukup, R. (2016). *Unstuffed.* Grand Rapids, MI: Zondervan.

Soukup, R. (2019). *Do it scared.* Grand Rapids, MI: Zondervan.

Starratt, R. J. (1993). *The drama of leadership*. London, England: The Falmer Press.

Steele, M. K. (2009). Orthopedics and spine. Danvers, MA: HCPro.

Stephen Ministries Staff. (2000). *Stephen Ministry Training Manual.* St. Louis, MO: Stephen Ministries.

Stossel, S. (2013). *My age of anxiety.* New York, NY: Alfred A. Knopf.

Strauss, D. (2010). *Half a life.* New York, NY: Random House.

Szabo, R., & Hall, M. (2007). *Behind happy faces.* Beverly Hills, CA: Alegra.

Tindle, H. (2013). *Up: how positive outlook can transform our health and aging*. New York, NY: Hudson Street Press.

Tindle, H. (2013). *Up: How positive outlook can transform our health and aging*. New York, NY: Hudson Street Press.

Tindle, H. (2013). *UP: How positive outlook can transform our health and aging*. New York, NY: Hudson Street Press.

Tolstoy, L. (2000). *Anna Karenina*. New York, NY: Penguin. (Original work published 1873)

Tompkins, G. E. (2011). *Literacy in the early grades* (3rd ed.). Boston, MA: Pearson.

U.S. Department of Agriculture. (2005). The new food pyramid. *The Washington Post*. Retrieved from http://www.washingtonpost.com/wp-srv/nation/daily/graphics/diet_042005.html

U.S. Department of Health and Human Services. (2011). Dietary guidelines for Americans, 2010. *Office of Disease Prevention and Health Promotion*. Retrieved from http://www.health.gov/dietaryguidelines/2010.asp#overview

University of Maryland Medical Center Staff. (2013). Stress. *University of Maryland Medical Center*. Retrieved from http://umm.edu/health/medical/reports/articles/stress

University of Maryland Medical Center. (2014). *Stress*. Retrieved from http://umm.edu/health/medical/reports/articles/stress

University of Scranton. (2012). New Year's resolution statistics. *Journal of Clinical Psychology*. Retrieved from http://www.statisticbrain.com/new-years-resolution-statistics/

Vacca, R. T., Vacca, J. L., & Mraz, M. (2014). *Content area reading* (11th ed.). Boston, MA: Pearson.

Vinz, R. (1996). *Composing a teaching life*. Portsmouth, NH: Heinemann.

Wanner, E.T., & Bird, J.L. (2013). *The Wanner Bird healing survey for pain recovery*. Academic Press.

Wanner, S. Y. (1994). *On with the story*. Portsmouth, NH: Heinemann.

Warren, R. (2012). *The purpose driven life: What on Earth am I here for?* Grand Rapids, MI: Zondervan.

Weiner-Davis, M. (1995). *Fire your shrink*. New York, NY: Simon & Schuster.

Welch, S. (2009). 10-10-10. New York, NY: Scribner.

Wharton, E. (1920). *The age of innocence*. New York, NY: Collier.

Wheelan, C. (2013). *Naked statistics*. New York, NY: W.W. Norton.

Whitman, W. (1993). O Me! O Life! In *Leaves of grass* (p. 341). New York, NY: Random House. (Original work published 1855)

Whitman, W. (1993). O Me! O Life! In *Leaves of Grass* (p. 341). New York, NY: Random House. (Original work published 1855)

Wilder, T. (1938). *Our town*. New York, NY: HarperPerennial.

Willamette University. (2011). *Research program brings together scholars from different disciplines*. Retrieved from http://www.willamette.edu/people/archives/2011/08/larc.html

Winfrey, O. (2014). *What I know for sure*. New York, NY: Hearst Communications.

Winner, J. (2008). *Take the stress out of your life*. Philadelphia, PA: Da Capo.

Younger, J., Gandhi, V., Hubbard, E., & Mackey, S. (2012). Development of the Stanford expectations of treatment scale (SETS): A tool for measuring patient outcome expectancy in clinical trials. *Clinical Trials*, *9*(6), 767–776. doi:10.1177/1740774512465064 PMID:23169874

Zimmermann, S. (2002). *Writing to heal the soul*. New York, NY: Three Rivers Press.

About the Contributors

Jennifer Bird, PhD, is the Director of the Writing and Reading Center (WRC) and teaches literature and writing classes at Oxbridge Academy in West Palm Beach, Florida. She previously taught current and future teachers at Florida Atlantic University. She received her Bachelor of Science in Education in Secondary English Education, Master of Education in Secondary English Education, and Doctor of Philosophy degrees from Miami University in Oxford, Ohio and her health coach certification from Duke University Integrative Medicine in Durham, North Carolina. She is a National Board Certified Health and Wellness Coach. Her research in writing and healing led to the publication of her book *Innovative Collaborative Practice and Reflection in Patient Education* (2015).

* * *

Eric Wanner, DPT, OCS, is the Director of the Physical Therapy Department at Palm Beach Sports Medicine and Orthopaedic Center in West Palm Beach, Florida. He received his Bachelor of Science in Exercise Science degree from The Ohio State University in Columbus, Ohio and his Doctor of Physical Therapy degree from The University of Dayton in Dayton, Ohio. He is a Board Certified Clinical Specialist in Orthopaedic Physical Therapy through the American Board of Physical Therapy.

Index

J

L

M

N

P

S

T

U

W

www.ingramcontent.com/pod-product-compliance
Lightning Source LLC
LaVergne TN
LVHW080600300926
849162LV00005B/1005